WORKING WITH HIGH-RISK ADOLESCENTS

Also by Matthew D. Selekman

Collaborative Brief Therapy with Children

Working with High-Risk Adolescents

A Collaborative Strengths-Based Approach

Matthew D. Selekman

Foreword by Harlene Anderson

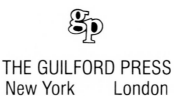

THE GUILFORD PRESS
New York   London

The author has checked with sources believed to be reliable in his efforts to provide
information that is complete and generally in accord with the standards of practice that
are accepted at the time of publication. However, in view of the possibility of human error
or changes in behavioral, mental health, or medical sciences, neither the author, nor
the editor and publisher, nor any other party who has been involved in the preparation
or publication of this work warrants that the information contained herein is in every
respect accurate or complete, and they are not responsible for any errors or omissions
or the results obtained from the use of such information. Readers are encouraged to
confirm the information contained in this book with other sources.

Library of Congress Cataloging-in-Publication Data

Names: Selekman, Matthew D., 1957– author.
Title: Working with high-risk adolescents : a collaborative strengths-based
   approach / Matthew D. Selekman ; foreword by Harlene Anderson.
Description: New York : The Guilford Press, [2017] | Includes bibliographical
   references and index.
Identifiers: LCCN 2016057578 | ISBN 9781462529735 (hardback) |
   ISBN 9781462539215 (paperback)
Subjects: LCSH: Adolescent psychotherapy. | Family therapy. | BISAC:
   PSYCHOLOGY / Psychotherapy / Child & Adolescent. | MEDICAL / Psychiatry /
   Child & Adolescent. | SOCIAL SCIENCE / Social Work. | PSYCHOLOGY /
   Psychotherapy / Couples & Family.
Classification: LCC RJ503 .S446 2017 | DDC 616.89/140835—dc23
LC record available at https://lccn.loc.gov/2016057578

The hardcover edition of *Working with High-Risk Adolescents* has the subtitle "An
Individualized Family Therapy Approach."

To the late Carolyn S. Selekman,
mother and teacher extraordinaire!

About the Author

Matthew D. Selekman, MSW, LCSW, is a family therapist and addictions counselor in private practice and Director of Partners for Collaborative Solutions, an international family therapy training and consulting firm in Evanston, Illinois. He is an Approved Supervisor with the American Association for Marriage and Family Therapy. Mr. Selekman served as the invited Henry Maier Practitioner-in-Residence at the School of Social Work of the University of Washington and is a three-time recipient of the Walter S. Rosenberry Award from Children's Hospital Colorado for his significant contributions to the fields of psychiatry and behavioral sciences. The author of numerous professional articles and seven books, Mr. Selekman consults worldwide to schools and treatment programs serving adolescents and their families. Since 1985, he has given workshops extensively throughout the United States, Canada, Mexico, South America, Europe, Southeast Asia, South Africa, Australia, and New Zealand. His website is *www.partners4change.net*.

Foreword

We live in a fast-changing world, characterized by people on all continents and in all walks of life who demand to have a voice in decisions that affect their lives. They are tired of institutional oppressions: expert, top-down silo structures that declare what people need. People want to have a say in what services they need and how these services are delivered. In the context of therapy, clients are asking to be collaborative partners in their treatment. To meet this need and be coactive partners with clients, it is incumbent upon therapists to challenge the traditions and ethics of family therapy. Collaborative therapies in general, and certainly Selekman's "solution-determined" and "collaborative strengths-based" family therapy model, have taken up this challenge. Collaborative therapies center on the clients and their local knowledge rather than the therapist and his or her knowledge. This is the political and social justice orientation of collaborative therapies.

The political and business institutions that fund psychotherapeutic services want brief, economical, efficient, and evidence-based treatment. This agenda trickles down to local therapeutic institutions and to the therapists in the room. Therapists become constrained as they try to wedge clients into institutional quota demands and one-size-fits-all, predetermined problem designations and solution methods. Therapists consequently risk not only losing their creativity and adaptability, but also interfering with clients' natural strengths and resources.

My colleagues and I have long questioned the traditions of psychotherapy in general and family therapy specifically (Anderson, 1997; Anderson & Goolishian, 1988) as well as therapy with adolescents (Anderson,

1993; Goolishian & Anderson, 1987). Early in my career, when working in the pediatric and child and adolescent psychiatry departments of a state medical school, I wondered why the "revolving-door" families described as multiproblem and unmotivated treatment failures were stereotypically viewed as immune and resistant to help. My curiosity motivated me to ask the families about their experiences with prior "helpers" (e.g., physicians, therapists, teachers, judges). I wanted to learn what was and was not so helpful and what advice they had for these "helpers" (Anderson, 1997). In other words, I wanted to access *the clients'* clinical wisdom. What I learned strongly influenced the development of what I call collaborative–dialogic therapy (Anderson, 1997, 2012; Anderson & Gehart, 2007; Goolishian & Anderson, 1987).

Adolescence is a major discourse in psychology and psychiatry today, such that it is hard to imagine that only the categories *childhood* and *adulthood* were recognized prior to the late 19th century. The concept and category of *adolescence* as the physical, emotional, psychological, social, and cognitive transition from childhood to adulthood acquired visibility in the literature around 1900 (Demos & Demos, 1969). The psychologist G. Stanley Hall is credited with introducing the term *adolescence* (Arnett, 2006). In 1959, the sociologist James Coleman coined the term *adolescent society* and called attention to the role of educational systems in the segmentation of adolescents from adult society and reinforcement of a distinct peer subculture (Coleman, 1959, 1961). Since the 1960s, psychiatrists, psychologists, anthropologists, and sociologists have continued to add to the discourse on adolescence. Most theories highlight the importance of institutions (e.g., education, health, legal, familial) and rapidly changing cultural and societal influences (e.g., economical, environmental, ideological, political, and technological) on this subculture. Collaborative therapies remind us that the provision of therapy and other services for adolescents and their families must keep these influences in mind. Collaborative therapies caution that adolescence is not a category of people branded by fixed characteristics and predictable problems. Rather, each person and their familial and social networks is unique and must be met as such. Selekman's "solution-determined" and "collaborative strengths-based" family therapy model exemplifies the importance of this caution and consideration.

Selekman suggests that our conception of adolescence is critical to delivering successful or unsuccessful services. Adolescence, I suggest, is not a developmental stage, nor does it represent a homogeneous subculture. It is, simply put, the *process* of a child developing into a young adult. Similarly, a family is always in *process*—uniquely developing and adjusting to meet shifting circumstances, regardless of its composition and context or how long the current members have been a family. Although there are similarities across these processes from one adolescent and family to another, Selekman's clinical examples call attention to the importance of bearing in mind that not all adolescents or families are alike, and of the differences in the professional and social systems in which their lives are embedded.

This book's gifts of "clinical practice wisdom" will be of value to readers whether they are therapists, community agency workers, child and adolescent social services staff, or advocates. Selekman endorses empirically supported family therapy and common factors suggested by outcome research as critical to therapeutic success, but I suggest his clinical practice wisdom trumps it. This comes through most clearly in two invaluable lessons the book offers for its readers.

One lesson is the importance of being a "reflective practitioner." The concept of "reflective practitioner," developed by the social scientist Donald Schön, refers to the value of a professional's unarticulated or tacit knowledge gained in everyday work, that which cannot be learned in formal education (Schön, 1983). Schön suggests that for professionals to best learn from their experience, and to put learning into action and build on it, they must take time to pause, step back, and reflect *in* and *on* their work. This theme runs throughout the book, and I believe it has significantly enabled Selekman to learn from his clinical experience.

Schön's "reflective practitioner" is important in today's fast-changing world. For Schön, learning is critical to understanding, adapting to, and managing transformations in our societies and their institutions—and in ourselves. Learning, therefore, is critical to both stability and fluidity. This idea shines through in the importance Selekman accords to honoring and using the resources of therapy traditions while at the same time challenging and supplementing them through reflective learning.

Selekman provides ample examples of his practice of reflection. He offers a session-by-session description of treatment with adolescents, and their family and professional helping system, and includes his reflections for each step. Selekman also emphasizes the importance of session-by-session client feedback—which I think of as "research as part of everyday practice"—about what was helpful or not. This stands in contrast to research conducted after the conclusion of treatment that, although perhaps transferrable to future clients, is not helpful for the "research subjects." Through research as part of everyday practice, the therapist can use what he or she learns from the client to adjust the therapy along the way, thereby increasing the likelihood of therapeutic success.

The other lesson Selekman offers is what can be learned by carefully paying attention to one's "ways of being," which he shows through examples of how he performs as a therapist. Selekman's examples demonstrate his respect, compassion, and trust for what the adolescent and family express they need at the moment. With seemingly contradictory powers of confidence and uncertainty, Selekman creates a sense of client ownership for the therapy and the expectation of hope for his clients' desired futures.

Selekman recognizes that by the time an adolescent and his or her family reach his office, the situation often has a long and complex history and is accompanied by an accumulation of well-meaning—though obviously unsuccessful—helpers. Why wouldn't family members appear suspicious, desperate, insistent, resistant, or hopeless amid such situations? Through it all, Selekman maintains modest expectations of himself, the adolescent, and the family members while also holding firm to the importance of not giving up.

Most, though not all, practices designated as collaborative derive from a movement on the margins of psychotherapy influenced by postmodern, social construction, and related philosophies. Collaborative practice is an epistemological shift in the way we think about the people we work with, ourselves, and what and how we perform together. It strongly emphasizes the role of language and dialogue in the construction of meaning and knowledge. Collaborative practice has relevance beyond the family and the therapy room. As such, Selekman reminds us to never forget that adolescents and their families are embedded in multiple systems and that therapists' collaborative stance *must* extend to those systems as well.

HARLENE ANDERSON, PhD

References

Anderson, H. (1993). On a roller coaster: A collaborative language systems approach to therapy. In S. Friedman (Ed.), *The new language of change: Constructive collaboration in psychotherapy* (pp. 323–344). New York: Guilford Press.

Anderson, H. (1997). *Conversations, language and possibilities: A postmodern approach to therapy*. New York: Basic Books.

Anderson, H. (2012). Collaborative relationships and dialogic conversations: Ideas for a relationally responsive therapy. *Family Process, 52*(1), 8–24.

Anderson, H. & Gehart, D. (Eds.). (2007). *Collaborative therapy: Relationships and conversations that make a difference*. New York: Routledge.

Anderson, H., & Goolishian, H. (1988). Human systems as linguistic systems: Evolving ideas about the implications for theory and practice. *Family Process, 27*, 371–393.

Arnett, J. J. (2006). G. Stanley Hall's *Adolescence*: Brilliance and nonsense. *History of Psychology, 9*(3), 186–197.

Coleman, J. (1959). Academic achievement and the structure of competition. *Harvard Education Review, 29*(4), 330–351.

Coleman, J. (1961). *The adolescent society: The social life of the teenager and its impact on education.* Oxford, UK: Free Press of Glencoe.

Demos, J., & Demos, V. (1969). Adolescence in historical perspective. *Journal of Marriage and Family, 31*(4), 632–638.

Goolishian, H., & Anderson, H. (1987). De la thérapie familiale à la thérapie systémique et au-delà. In F. Ladame, P. Gutton, & M. Kalogerakis (Eds.), *Psychoses et adolescence: Annales internationales de psychiatrie de l'adolescence* (pp. 168–180). Paris: Masson.

Schön, D. (1983). *The reflective practitioner: How professionals think in action.* New York: Basic Books.

Preface

Since the publication of *Pathways to Change: Brief Therapy with Difficult Adolescents,* I have allowed my collaborative strengths-based therapeutic approach for working with adolescents and their families to evolve, logically integrating empirically supported ideas from psychotherapy and family therapy outcome research and clinical evidence-based practice wisdom regarding what may have the best chance of working with specific types of adolescent and family difficulties. One of the biggest challenges for today's clinicians is being referred complex adolescent cases, including adolescents who have experienced multiple treatment failures and come to us quite demoralized. What I have come to discover in working with these clients is that therapeutic flexibility, having an open mindset, learning how to thrive in chaos, and building therapeutic alliances with each family member are essential. Based on the "common-factors" research finding that "client extratherapeutic factors" count the most for treatment success, this is all the more reason we should carefully tailor-fit our therapeutic approach to the unique needs and characteristics of each adolescent and family we work with. When it comes to complex high-risk adolescent cases with extensive treatment histories, using rigid formulaic treatment protocols can do these families a terrible disservice and perpetuate their hopelessness and despair. I contend that these families are the real experts on their stories, knowing what is best for themselves, and that they need to be in the driver's seat in determining the goals for treatment: who participates in family sessions, the frequency of meetings, and when to terminate therapy.

One major theme reverberating throughout the book is that clinicians don't have to be alone in working with these challenging adolescent cases. There are often key resource people who can be tapped for the solution construction process and for helping clients stay on track outside of our offices. With clients' help, mobilizing all of the key resource people from their social ecologies, including actively involved larger systems professionals to serve as members of what I call the "solution-determined collaborative team," we can rapidly co-generate high-quality solutions that can be implemented in every context in which the adolescents are experiencing difficulties. This kind of meaningful and powerful teamwork can help produce deeper and more long-lasting changes with high-risk adolescents and their family systems.

Another important area discussed in this book, which is often neglected in the family therapy literature, is being more mindful about how our innate cognitive biases and mental traps can misguide therapeutic decision making and lead clinicians to make mistakes and inadvertently create therapeutic climates ripe for inevitable treatment failure. In addition to critically reflecting on therapeutic decision making, we need to solicit feedback from clients, session by session, about their perceptions of our relationships with them and how they experience the change process. This valuable client feedback guides us on how to better interact with each family member and what to do more of or abandon therapeutically.

Overview of the Book

Chapter 1 presents key systemic aggravating factors that contribute to both the development and maintenance of adolescent risky behaviors. A comprehensive overview of the collaborative strengths-based family therapy approach is provided.

In Chapter 2, I present several effective empirically supported strategies for engaging challenging adolescents, parents, and families. I discuss special engagement dilemmas, such as engaging reluctant powerful adolescents and absent fathers and other nuclear and extended family members who play major roles in maintaining the adolescent's and family's difficulties.

In Chapter 3, I discuss effective ways to build successful collaborative partnerships with concerned members from the family's social network and pessimistic helping professionals from larger systems. Collaborative tools and strategies are presented for facilitating solution-generating and transformative dialogues and constructively managing inevitable conflicts.

Chapter 4 addresses how to co-construct well-conceived, solution-determined collaborative treatment plans and establish realistic and achievable goals with families, involved helping professionals, and concerned members of clients' social networks. I cover harm-reduction goals as a viable therapeutic option for adolescents with serious self-destructive behaviors, who are either in the precontemplation or contemplation stages of readiness for change or do not wish to pursue total abstinence goals early in treatment.

Chapter 5 covers how to co-develop and select therapeutic experiments that are designed to resolve specific types of adolescent, parental, and family presenting difficulties. For more entrenched and intractable high-risk adolescent case situations, I present some "out-of-the-box," playful, idea-generating strategies that tap the inventiveness of families to spark high-quality solutions worth experimenting with. I also include a transtheoretical compendium of therapeutic experiments and rituals for the adolescent, parents, and the whole family.

Chapter 6 addresses state-of-the-art family social network goal-maintenance and relapse prevention tools and strategies. I cover constructive strategies for managing inevitable slips, addressing client concerns or budding crises outside of targeted goal areas, and preventing prolonged relapse. The use of adolescents' adult "inspirational others," peers, and close relatives as valuable resources for helping adolescents stay on track is also discussed.

Chapters 7 and 8 present full-length case examples with postsession and posttreatment reflections. The serious and potentially life-threatening presenting problems of the family cases in these chapters are the bane of most therapists: an explosive, violent, and gang-involved male adolescent, and a female adolescent with a long career of self-injury, substance abuse, and multiple suicide attempts.

In Chapter 9, I cover therapeutic mistakes, failures, and wisdom gained from these experiences. I offer practical guidelines to help minimize the likelihood of poor clinical decision making, premature dropout, and treatment failures.

Chapter 10 focuses on the creative use of self and how therapists can become more daring, playful, inventive, and improvisational in their sessions with families. It addresses strategic use of self-framework and provides practical guidelines for finding sources of inspiration and utilizing creative ideas from theater, popular TV shows and movies, literature, jazz, art, and science and technology. I discuss how to offer clients alternative ways to view their problem situations, spark epiphanies, and help liberate them from rigid family role behaviors, belief systems, and problem-maintaining interactions. Case examples are provided throughout the chapter.

Finally, my hope is that the plethora of therapeutic ideas, tools, and strategies presented in this book will empower you to have better outcomes with your most challenging high-risk adolescent cases. Ultimately, it is all about the clients. So be sure to listen generously, be patient, and carefully observe for how best to establish cooperative partnerships with them in order to best navigate them in the direction of change.

Acknowledgments

There are several people I wish to acknowledge who greatly contributed to my professional development and the ideas discussed in this book. Early in my family therapy career, my live supervision intensive trainings with Salvador Minuchin, Jay Haley, Harry Goolishian, and Harlene Anderson were some of the most memorable and influential training experiences I have ever had. Later, I had the good fortune to work with a master solution-focused trainer, my friend Michele Weiner-Davis. She showed me the short road to family change by capitalizing on clients' pretreatment changes and the natural gifts, resources, and competencies that all clients bring to us, which are a treasure trove of possibilities. Once I caught the solution-focused fever, which fits nicely with my pathological optimism, I participated in numerous incredible short- and longer-term trainings with Steve de Shazer and Insoo Kim Berg. The narrative therapy approach of Michael White and David Epston had caught my interest, particularly externalization of the problem, their major contribution to the family therapy field. I participated in some excellent workshops with them to learn more about their cutting-edge work. By this time in my career, my collaborative strengths-based family therapy approach was taking shape and was a culmination of all of these previous training experiences. This flexible, collaborative, and ecosystemic approach incorporates the best elements of the aforementioned models with key findings from psychotherapy and family therapy outcome research. Finally, I am grateful to all of the high-risk adolescents and families I have worked with over the past 34 years; when it comes down to it, they were my best teachers.

I would like to thank Harlene Anderson for writing the foreword. In her trademark fashion, she did a beautiful job of describing the evolution of family therapy work with adolescents and their families and situating my approach in the collaborative practice school.

Last, but not least, I want to acknowledge Jim Nageotte, Senior Editor at The Guilford Press, for giving me the green light to write this book and for his helpful editorial recommendations. A special thanks goes to Adam Ornstein for his technical assistance with the figures and forms.

Contents

CHAPTER 1

Navigating through Complex
High-Risk Adolescent Mazes

We are continually faced with great opportunities
which are brilliantly disguised as unsolvable problems.
—MARGARET MEAD

Across the country, economic hardship and state and federal funding cuts for services to high-risk youth and families have forced social
service and child protection agencies, mental health clinics, addictions
programs, residential treatment programs, and even specialized hospital-
based programs to reduce their staff sizes, or even to close down. As a
result, clinicians still working in such settings are being inundated with
many challenging and complex adolescent cases. These kids arrive at
their programs with extensive treatment histories and past traumas, and
come from multiproblem families, which for even the most seasoned family therapist can be very difficult to work with. Furthermore, because of
administrative productivity requirements, health insurance limitations,
and time constraints, clinicians working in the trenches are expected to
see more of these difficult cases for much shorter durations of treatment.

To help combat these clinical challenges, those fortunate surviving
agencies, clinics, and specialized treatment programs that have well-
endowed training budgets are purchasing expensive empirically supported family therapy treatment packages. These include staff family
therapy training, supervision, case consultation with stuck cases, and a
program evaluation component. Unfortunately, the vast majority of these
agencies, clinics, and treatment programs can't afford them. Even if they

could, they lack the staff to implement them and the capacity to provide 24/7 home-based treatment and crisis management.

These empirically supported family models have produced solid therapy outcome data that indicate they work well with high-risk treatment populations such as adolescents who are violent, delinquent, disruptive in school, substance-abusing, eating distressed, self-injuring, severely depressed, and suicidal (Alexander, Waldron, Robbins, & Neeb, 2013; Diamond et al., 2006; Diamond, Diamond, & Levy, 2014; Diamond & Stern, 2003; Henggeler & Schaeffer, 2010; Henggeler, Schoenwald, Borduin, Rowland, & Cunningham, 2009; Henggeler & Sheidow, 2011; Le Grange, 2011; Liddle, 2010; Liddle & Diamond, 1991; MST Services, 2014; Robin & Le Grange, 2010; Robbins, Horigian, Szapocznik, & Ucha, 2010; Rowe, 2012; Schwartz, Muir, & Brown, 2012; Smith & Chamberlain, 2010; Szapocznik, Hervis, & Schwartz, 2003; Szapocznik, Waldron & Brody, 2010). Yet they are not panaceas, and the leading proponents of these models seldom write about or present in-depth data on why some families prematurely drop out or experience treatment failures. Most of these models are heavily problem focused, therapist or/team expert driven. From my perspective, they are not client directed or collaborative enough, and do not incorporate enough important psychotherapy outcome research findings on the *common factors*. Studies in psychotherapy research suggest that 40% of what counts for treatment success is client extratherapeutic factors, a subset of the "common factors" described in the literature, such as utilizing client strengths to the maximum degree, resources, resiliency protective factors, past successes, theories of change, and stages of readiness for change to empower clients to resolve their difficulties (Duncan, Miller, Wampold, & Hubble, 2010; Norcross, 2011; Selekman & Beyebach, 2013; Sprenkle, Davis, & Lebow, 2009). In view of the client extratherapeutic common factor research findings, clinical evidence-based practitioners recognize the dangers in adopting the "one-size-fits-all" treatment philosophy. They view the clients as the experts on their lives and recognize the importance of establishing collaborative partnerships with them so clients have the lead voices with goal setting and all clinical decision making. In addition, clinical evidence-based practitioners recognize that it is best to view these challenging cases through multiple theoretical lenses. These practitioners know they need to include themselves as part of the observations they are making in the clinical encounter; to ask bold and well-thought-out questions from a position of not-knowing and curiosity; and never to lose sight of how the complex interactions among the families they treat involve larger systems professionals, key resource people from their social networks, and the community at large. These other people hold tremendous potential for the co-generation of multiple high-quality solutions.

All family therapy models need to be flexible, and more integrative to better meet the contemporary needs of today's high-risk adolescents and their families. The empirically supported family therapy models will have even better outcome results by adopting a stronger client strengths-based, outcome-informed emphasis, and by integrating some of the ideas from newer therapeutic approaches that are showing clinical promise. In this spirit, this highly practical book presents a *collaborative strengths-based family therapy* (CSBFT) model that combines the best elements of the major empirically supported family therapy approaches with clinical practice wisdom regarding *what works* with high-risk adolescents presenting with both externalizing and internalizing disorders. What is unique about the CSBFT approach is that it *individualizes the treatment for high-risk adolescents and their families*. Under this model, therapists carefully tailor what they do therapeutically with the clients' preferences, theories of change, expectations, goals, and input regarding therapeutic intervention design and selection, throughout the clinical decision-making process.

In this chapter, I first discuss four key dimensions of adolescent risky behaviors including how they are maintained individually, by peers, families, concerned professionals, and members from their social networks. Next, I provide a comparative critical analysis of the strengths and weaknesses of the major empirically supported family therapy approaches and recommendations for ways to further improve treatment outcome results. Two clinically promising family therapy approaches for self-injuring and suicidal adolescents are also discussed. I follow this with a discussion on the importance of evidence-based clinical wisdom and the benefits of combining therapeutic art with family therapy science. I then offer a brief overview of the CSBFT approach, followed by a discussion on *individualizing* what we do therapeutically to the unique needs and characteristics of high-risk adolescents and their families. Finally, I present 16 CSBFT practice guidelines for working with more challenging high-risk adolescents and their families.

Let's start with a perspective on four important dimensions of adolescent high-risk behaviors: (1) adolescent risky behaviors as resources for coping; (2) key findings from recent neuroscience research on the adolescent brain; (3) the need for positive risk taking and collaborative risk management with high-risk adolescents; and (4) how "high-risk" adolescent problem-determined systems are created and maintained.

Adolescent Risky Behaviors as Gifts and Resources for Coping

Having worked for decades with adolescents who were deemed "high risk" by mental health, healthcare, and school professionals, I have observed that there is a logical dimension to their provocative, intimidating, troubling self-destructive and destructive behaviors. For many adolescents, their high-risk behaviors have served as gifts, resources, and attempted solutions to help them to cope with individual, family, and social stressors in their lives. It is no surprise that they gravitate toward particular behaviors that work for them. You probably see these kinds of things in your practices routinely:

- Using anger and aggression to gain power and control over others when one feels disempowered and devalued in one's family, among one's peers, and in life in general.
- Cutting oneself to get quick relief from emotional distress, to soothe oneself, or for numbing out bad thoughts and feelings.
- Engaging in extreme daredevil behaviors as a way to escape from feeling emotionally dead inside.
- Using cocaine, methamphetamine, and other stimulants to elevate one's moods.

That's not to say these behaviors are benign or to be encouraged. The longer adolescents engage in high-risk behaviors, the more uses they find for them and the more fearless they become (Selekman, 2009; Selekman & Beyebach, 2013). Often, these youth will associate with peers who engage in similar behaviors, share the same struggles in their lives, and with whom they feel a strong sense of connection (Hardy & Laszloffy, 2006; Taffel, & Blau, 2001). It is important to note that, developmentally, adolescents must figure out a way to fit in with their peers; failure to do so is equivalent to social death (Selekman, 2009)!

Bear in mind as well that adolescents who turn to high-risk behaviors may do so with distress they feel in the wake of a traumatic experience. According to van der Kolk and his colleagues (van der Kolk, 2014; van der Kolk, MacFarlane, & Weisaeth, 2007), we need to respect the clients' use of self-injury, eating-distressed behaviors, and substance abuse as coping strategies or defensive shields to ward off flashbacks, painful feelings and memories, and suicidal thoughts. Premature removal of these coping strategies can contribute to a youth's being so emotionally vulnerable that he or she becomes suicidal and needs to be hospitalized.

The Adolescent Brain and High-Risk Behaviors

The past decade's neuroscience research on adolescent brain development helps explain why adolescents are risk- and sensation-seeking beings (Siegel, 2014; Steinberg, 2014). The findings from this research help us to understand why adolescents continue to engage in risky behaviors even when they repeatedly lead to quite severe consequences. This research also helps adolescents and their parents or legal guardians understand what is driving these behaviors. Knowing this important information can help prevent unproductive parental and professional social control responses like yelling, lecturing, dishing out severe and lengthy consequences, being medicated, psychiatrically hospitalized, or sent to residential treatment as a response to their risky behaviors. Research indicates that the frontal lobe areas of adolescents' prefrontal cortexes are not fully developed until ages 23–24. The prefrontal cortex area of the brain has to do with impulse control, planning, and judgment. So it makes sense that adolescents with their still-developing prefrontal cortexes would be impulsive, make poor choices, and repeatedly choose ultimately unhelpful means for managing stress and life difficulties they are faced with (Siegel, 2014; Steinberg, 2014).

The adolescent's hypothalamus and amygdale are also immature. These components of the brain have to do with mood regulation and management and serve as our brains' alarm systems (houses our fight-or-flight response) in response to emotional and external threats. This is why even small disappointments or frustrations can evoke intense and extreme emotional reactions in adolescents. In addition, some high-risk adolescents' amygdalae are so hypersensitive that when they are exposed to emotional distress they cope by lashing out at others or engaging in self-destructive behaviors for quick emotional escape. Adolescents' primitive survivalist brains drive them to pursue shortcuts to pleasure by engaging in risky behaviors for quick relief from emotional and physical distress. They are more likely to repeat high-risk behaviors that are attached to positive emotional memories and experiences that are stored in their brains' limbic system region. Finally, adolescents are more likely to engage in more extreme risky behaviors when observed and sanctioned by their peers (Schoen, 2013; Siegel, 2014; Steinberg, 2014).

The good news is that due to our brains' *plasticity* (our ability to create new neuronal pathways in our brains), we can develop a repertoire of positive behaviors and habits, such as mindfulness meditation, yoga, dancing, exercising, making art, or writing poetry (Selekman & Beyebach, 2013). These positive habits can become the go-to activities for coping with emotional and physical distress the more consistently they are practiced. Neuroscientists Schwartz and Gladding (2011) teach clients to counter their brains' self-defeating and/or self-destructive behaviors by telling themselves, "I AM NOT MY BRAIN!" Instead, clients are encouraged to pursue a wide range of healthy coping strategies and meaningful activities that they come up with and have been exposed to by their therapists, such as mindfulness meditation.

Positive Risk-Taking Opportunities
and Collaborative Risk Management

Since we know that adolescents, by nature, are risk and thrill seekers, why not provide them with ample opportunities to be challenged by positive risk-taking activities and tasks? Positive school and community activities can take the form of psychological, physical, and social challenges, such as: rock climbing; fund-raising strategies for community or social causes that they are interested in; offering a wide range of service work opportunities; forming new clubs or groups to counter student difficulties like bullying and eating disorders; inviting a gang member to co-facilitate a violence prevention group; or serving on a student advisory council to help school administrative staff make the school experience more inviting, intellectually stimulating, and opportunity rich.

Adolescents who have been deemed "high risk" often possess many strengths and talents that can be accentuated and utilized to empower them and to help turn around their lives and the lives of others. When empowered, they can become positive leaders and peer counselors in their schools and communities. They enjoy and find meaning and purpose in life when helping the less fortunate and doing prevention and outreach work with both their peers and younger children (Selekman, 2009; Selekman & Beyebach, 2013).

Another way we can aid adolescents engaging in risky behaviors is to encourage them to take the lead in making good choices, through looking at their options and reflecting (Steiner, 2014; Welch, 2009). We can ask the following types of questions:

"With your crew (friends), how much and how often do you have to party (drink/do drugs) with them in order to be accepted by them?"

"Do you think it is possible to cut back a little if you chose to and still be accepted by your friends?"

If the answer is "Yes" ask, "How will you decide to cut back and how specifically will you pull that off successfully?"

If the answer is "No" ask, "What will you choose to do, especially if your heavy partying is continuing to cost you big time in most areas of your life?"

"High-Risk" Adolescent and Problem-Determinied Systems

There are two major ways adolescents can be labeled as "high risk" and they and their families can become ensnared in problem-determined systems. The first pathway is by being red-flagged for engaging in risky or intimidating behaviors, like cutting, substance abuse, eating-distressed habits (bulimia, binge eating, obesity, self-starvation), aggressive behavior, and delinquent behaviors, such as bullying or gang involvement. The second pathway is by just coming out of or having a history of incarceration, psychiatric hospitalizations, and residential treatment. This latter group is often placed in specialized support groups at school or in therapeutic day school settings with the belief that they will have grave difficulty surviving emotionally, behaviorally, and academically in regular public or private school settings and need a lot of individual attention. There also may be a strong push from the juvenile court system, the school, or their psychiatrists for them to receive intensive multimodal outpatient treatment, which often includes being on psychiatric medications.

According to Anderson (1997) and Anderson, Goolishian, and Winderman (1986), once a "problem" is identified or defined, a system of helping professionals and, in some cases, concerned members from the adolescent's social network coalesce around trying to solve the problem or control identified "high-risk" behaviors. For example, if a female adolescent student is identified as a "self-injurer" at school, often there is a wide range of pressing questions, beliefs, and emotional reactions (fear and anxiety to take immediate action to protect the student from herself) that are triggered in the minds of the school professionals involved, such as: "Is she suicidal?"; "Has she been sexually or physically abused?"; "Does she have 'borderline personality disorder'?" Due to school liability issues, there may be a strong administrative push with her parents for her to be psychiatrically evaluated or worse, hospitalized. This may lead to her being placed on antidepressant medication and either referred to a specialized adolescent outpatient program for self-injurers or a short stint in a psychiatric hospital, with the thinking that she might be at high risk for a suicide attempt. Once she gets involved in the specialized intensive outpatient program or gets out of the hospital, she will be tightly monitored and seen quite regularly at school by her school social worker or counselor and may be placed in a special group for students just coming out of hospital and residential treatment programs. Within the context of the problem-determined system, a negative self-fulfilling prophecy and an oppressive dominant story can inadvertently get set in motion. This can lead to the adolescent's questioning her own abilities to cope and to her return to self-injuring and possibly concurrent self-destructive habits. Even if the adolescent refrains from cutting herself, appears happier, and is avoiding associating with former toxic peers, these positive *sparkling moments* often go unnoticed because they do not fit with the dominant story of her having "poor coping skills," or that "self-injurers are sneaky and I bet she is still doing this behind the scenes," and so on. If caught at school cutting again, the parents will be notified their daughter may need to be placed in a therapeutic day school setting and they need to closely monitor her at home, which means loss of her privileges and freedom. These interactions can go on endlessly between the professionals, parents, concerned members of their social networks, and the identified "high-risk" adolescents. Often, the adolescent and the parents lose their decision-making voices in the problem-determined system. Interactions with the professionals in power positions can enforce response and action as long as they are concerned. Problem-determined systems and their concomitant oppressive dominant stories and problem life-support systems are not just limited to school systems. They can get set in motion by the complex interactions between multiple larger systems professionals, the family, concerned members from the family's social network, and the lightning-fast spread of concern and rumors among adolescents' peers' communications via social media.

When collaborating with members of the "high-risk" adolescent problem-determined system, the therapist needs to be sensitive to how his or her thinking and ways of responding to participants either opens up space for meaningful dialogue or inhibits conversational flow. We can never attain a God's-eye view from which to observe and study the problem-determined system members' interactions because we are part of the same system once we enter the conversation about an identified "problem" (Anderson, 1997; Hoffman, 1988). In addition, we need to adopt a curious stance and come to know the various participants' stories of involvement, attempted solutions, concerns, problem explanations, best hopes, and expectations. Finally, as therapists we need to be sensitive to the role context plays in determining what the participants will be able to see, hear, and understand (Anderson et al., 1986). For example, if we work in a mental health or psychiatric setting, the first order of business will be conducting a psychosocial assessment and coming up with a DSM-5 diagnosis based on an adolescent client's symptomatology and behavior (American Psychiatric Association, 2013). If the diagnosis is depression, more than likely a combination of cognitive-behavioral therapy and antidepressants will be strongly recommended and pursued. This treatment regimen will be pursued because there is a body of empirical research that supports this therapeutic course of action for depression, as the root of the patient's psychopathology is his problematic thinking patterns and unbalanced biochemistry. For the therapist who enforces this in-house clinic treatment protocol with every depressed adolescent who comes through the office door, he or she may experience grave difficulty opening the adolescent up to alternative problem formulations and courses of treatment by other members of the problem-determined system.

The Major Empirically Supported Family Therapy Models: A Comparative Analysis

The major empirically supported family therapy models being used both in this country and abroad with high-risk adolescents exhibiting externalizing and internalizing disorders are *multisystemic therapy* (MST; Henggeler & Schaeffer, 2010; Henggeler & Sheidow, 2011;MST Services, 2014; Weiss et al., 2013); *functional family therapy* (FFT; Alexander et al., 2013; Waldron & Brody, 2010); *multidimensional family therapy* (MDFT; Diamond et al., 2006; Liddle, 2010; Liddle & Diamond, 1991; Rowe, 2012); *brief strategic family therapy* (BSFT; Muir, Schwartz, & Szapocznik, 2004; Robbins et al., 2010; Szapocznik et al., 2012; Szapocznik et al., 2003; Szapocznik & Kurtines, 1989); *attachment-based family therapy* (ABFT; Diamond et al., 2014; Diamond & Stern, 2003); *Maudsley family-based treatment* (MFBT; Le Grange, 2011; Lock & LeGrange, 2005; Perkins, Murphy, Schmidt, & Williams, 2006; Robin & Le Grange, 2010); and *multidimensional treatment foster care* (MTFC; Smith & Chamberlain, 2010). I have critically reviewed the strengths and weaknesses of the models based on what the developers and research teams of these approaches have indicated after a decade or more of pilot projects and larger-scale outcome studies.

It is possible to offer guidelines regarding which of these models appear to work best for both adolescent *externalizing disorders* and *internalizing disorders*. By externalizing disorders, the researchers are referring to adolescents exhibiting the following behavioral difficulties: antisocial and delinquent behaviors, substance abuse, school disruptive behavior, sexually risky behaviors, and aggressive and violent behaviors. Adolescents with internalizing disorders exhibit problems with depression, eating disorders, self-injury, and suicidal behaviors. Many high-risk adolescents exhibit a combination of both externalizing and internalizing symptoms, but often exhibit more symptoms and behaviors from one of these categories of disorders. Below, by disorder category I discuss which empirically supported family therapy approaches are best suited for particular types of adolescent behavioral difficulties.

Externalizing Disorders

Out of all of the empirically supported family therapy models, MST has the best short- and long-term outcome results with antisocial, delinquent, aggressive, and violent adolescents. MTFC also has highly positive outcome results with delinquent adolescents, particularly with female adolescent juvenile offenders. Both MST and MTFC have successfully reduced adolescents' involvement with negative peer groups. In addition, MTFC has shown great outcome results at reducing sexually risky behaviors among juvenile offending females. Both models provide a team approach, 24/7 in-home coverage for sessions and for managing crises, and target all of the systems levels in the adolescents' social ecologies for intervention. One can argue that this gives these family treatment models the advantage over FFT, MDFT, and BSFT. Adolescents in foster care are often deemed "high risk" due to having experienced multiple placements out of their homes and/or having experienced emotional neglect and/or past traumas. MTFC's strong emphasis on parental and adolescent skill development and tightly monitored behavioral management systems tailored to the unique needs of the adolescents and their biological parents or caretakers make it a most ideal model for foster care programs.

Although one can argue that a lot of high-risk adolescents abuse substances to self-medicate, regulate their moods, or escape from their problems, this behavior has been considered as an externalizing behavior by the leading proponents of the empirically supported family therapy models. This is because substance abuse often co-occurs with juvenile offending behaviors in their studies. FFT has had good outcome results with adolescent marijuana and alcohol abusers after integrating cognitive-behavioral tools and strategies into the treatment regimen. MDFT and BSFT have had the best outcome results with decreasing and stabilizing substance-abusing behavior, particularly with culturally diverse adolescents and their families. The researchers behind these models have found that they also decrease juvenile offending and improve school functioning behaviors. BSFT in particular has produced excellent outcome results with Latino adolescents and their families. Finally, the central research team behind BSFT developed an innovative one-person family therapy approach for adolescent substance abusers that has been proven to be just as effective as BSFT with whole-family groups. The implications of the one-person family therapy approach are far reaching in that it can potentially be used in clinical situations where conjoint family therapy may be contraindicated due to the parents' intense marital discord or post-divorce battles that overshadow the adolescent's needs; the parents refusal to participate in conjoint family therapy, in spite of the therapist's efforts to engage them; intense conflicts and verbal exchanges between the adolescent and the parents that are too disruptive and prove conjoint family work to be counter-productive; one or both parents suffering from severe mental health or substance abuse difficulties; and an older adolescent who is struggling to launch from the family and can benefit from independent living skills and support. The one-person family therapy approach also demonstrates that it is possible to both stabilize the identified adolescent clients' behaviors and produce significant family changes through one family member.

Internalizing Disorders

A newer and highly effective empirically supported family treatment approach for depressed and suicidal adolescents is ABFT. Histories of self-injury are often seen in the backgrounds of severely depressed and suicidal adolescents. For these adolescents, self-injury is designed to help ward off or "numb" painful thoughts and feelings. Some of these adolescents also use self-injury as a form of self-punishment. Adolescents with long careers of self-injury have conquered their fears of death and may perceive death as a "beautiful thing," which puts these youth at high risk for suicide attempts (Joiner, 2005; Selekman, 2009; Selekman & Beyebach, 2013). The researchers and therapists behind the ABFT model have observed and demonstrated that what works best with depressed and suicidal adolescents is achieving the following outcomes: disrupting emotionally invalidating family interactions, repairing parent–adolescent relationship ruptures, strengthening the parent–adolescent relationship, and supporting the adolescent's needs for more autonomy.

MFBT has demonstrated good outcome results for adolescents with anorexia and their families who have shorter-term histories with this disorder (Le Grange, 2011; Robin & Le Grange, 2010). Further research is needed to help determine whether this model or a modified version of it is equally effective with adolescents presenting with bulimia and binge-eating difficulties. Furthermore, the central research teams behind MFBT need thorough model expansion to look for additional methods to better meet the needs of long-term anorexic adolescents and their families.

Clinically Promising New Family Therapy Approaches in Need of Further Research

Two clinically promising family therapy approaches that require a great deal more research on their efficacy are the *DBT multifamily group* (Miller, Rathus, & Linehan, 2007; Rathus & Miller, 2015) and *collaborative strengths-based family therapy* (Selekman, 2009; Selekman & Beyebach, 2013; Selekman & Schulem, 2007). Miller, Rathus, et al. (2007) are the first to apply dialectical behavior therapy (DBT) methods to families of self-injuring and suicidal adolescents. They have had success varying the treatment format by concurrently running parenting and adolescent skills groups or seeing individual families using DBT techniques and strategies. Randomized controlled studies in the United States and Norway have indicated that the DBT multifamily group and its variations can improve management of emotional distress and greatly reduce depressive symptoms and self-harming behaviors well into outcome follow-up (Goldstein et al.,

2012; Rathus & Miller, 2015). The major problems with the existing studies were the small sample sizes, which compromises generalizability.

In a qualitative study of CSBFT, 20 culturally diverse high school-age self-harming adolescents and their families were randomly interviewed by an independent researcher (parents and adolescents separately) across the course of their treatment experiences and up to 2 years of follow-up. The adolescents were self-injuring with concurrent eating-distressed, substance-abusing, and sexually risky behaviors. In the research interviews, the families shared important feedback regarding therapist relationship and structuring skills, specific techniques and change strategies they found useful, and things the therapists said and tried with them that were not helpful. One consistent and quite surprising research finding was the adolescents' strong desire to grow into their relationships with their parents, no matter how much conflict was in their relationships. They wanted to know that their parents loved and appreciated them and wanted them to provide emotional support when they needed it. With all families in the research project, the adolescents' self-harming behaviors had greatly decreased and remained stabilized for up to 2 years at follow-up. The parent–adolescent bonds were stronger, and family and school functioning had greatly improved. Across the course of therapy, the researcher spoke with the families and interviewed the therapists and related back to them what the families felt about what was working and what they needed to do differently. This greatly helped the therapists better meet the clients' needs of and increase their satisfaction with their treatment experiences. We found the client interviews to be quite rich, particularly what specific interventions they found most beneficial. We also learned what was off the mark and where therapists needed to shift gears to find better fit with certain family members. The major problems with our study were the small sample size and the absence of control groups.

Evidence-Based Clinical Wisdom:
Therapeutic Art, Improvisation, and Intuition

Although the leading proponents behind their respective empirically supported family therapy models encourage therapists to use their relationship skills to build strong alliances with their clients and be active in sessions, they must stay true to the model in order to demonstrate treatment efficacy. They must not lose focus by introducing therapeutic techniques and strategies from other therapy approaches that could contaminate the research results. In fact, most of these empirically supported family therapy models provide specific sets of procedures and activities that therapists are supposed to employ in designated sessions with families.

This indicates fidelity to the model. Yet if therapists are too preoccupied with "doing the model right," this can stifle their ability to stay truly present with their clients. If therapists think a particular technique or strategy from another therapeutic approach might work better, they are discouraged from trying it out. Over several years in different countries, I have heard these complaints and frustrations from therapists and supervisors alike who are tasked to implement and maintain stringent fidelity to the major empirically supported family therapy models in their practice settings. They have reported feeling clinically stifled, like prisoners in the boxes of the models.

It is my contention that family therapists should be free to be daring, to inject an element of surprise into their sessions, be playful, view uncertainty and constraints as opportunities, use large doses of humor, and stretch their imagination and inventiveness as far as they can go without being limited by a particular family therapy approach, as long as what they choose to do has purpose. This is why empirically supported family therapy models need to be allowed to evolve, be flexible, integrate new and older effective therapeutic ideas from other individual and family therapy approaches outside of their base models. The therapist can be free to take more risks and tap into a wider range of therapeutic techniques and strategies. Once liberated from the box of a particular family therapy model, the therapist becomes an improvisational artist. He or she is free to bring in ideas from the arts, literature, science, and philosophy as rich sources of inspiration for offering clients new ways of viewing their presenting problem situations and for co-designing with them high-quality strategies.

For evidence-based practitioners, *intuition* plays an important role in clinical decision making in both in session and between sessions. Like chess players, they rely on *pattern recognition* and a vast reservoir of past *action maps* in their heads about what has the best shot at working based on their past therapeutic experiences with particular types of adolescent difficulties, family problem-maintaining patterns of interactions, and therapist–family member interactions in sessions, such as engaging reluctant members to talk, how best to respond to "yes . . . but" client responses, and so forth. Back in 1986, I remember hearing Salvador Minuchin saying in a weeklong family therapy training, "I have seen this before" while sitting with a couple in a live consultation session (Minuchin, 1986). In his illustrious and remarkable career as a family therapy pioneer, Minuchin has probably seen just about every couple and family presenting problem and their corresponding problem-maintaining patterns and has perfected sets of interventions that are quite effective at resolving these difficulties, including his incredible use of self as a powerful and highly creative change agent.

Klein (1998, 2002, 2013) studied experienced professionals in crisis management occupations like firefighters, hospital emergency room staff, and air-traffic controllers who have to decide and act quickly. He found that across the board they all relied on their intuition and past action maps to guide their present action plans and problem resolution strategies. They also were quite skilled at future visioning (projecting themselves into the future to see the results of a selected and implemented solution strategy). They used this to look for any loopholes in the selected plan of action and would quickly identify backup plans B, C, or D that might have a better shot with successfully managing a crisis situation.

Nobel Prize winner Daniel Kahneman (2011) has done pioneering research in the areas of intuition and how our cognitive biases can greatly influence on our decision making. He has identified two systems of thinking: *system 1* and *system 2*. According to Kahneman, system 1 thinking should be used with problem situations that are clear, acute, and where logical, straightforward solutions are most likely to work. With system 1, he recommends that you go with your gut (intuition) and clinical solutions that have worked in the past with a particular client problem situation. With more complex and chronic client problem situations, system 2 thinking should be used. For this, he recommends that you step back from the problem situation, reflect, think about your options, and incubate any ideas you come up with before trying out one or more change strategies. Many therapists get into trouble with complex and challenging clinical situations because they do not step back and reflect on potential therapeutic options (system 2 thinking). Instead, cognitive biases drive their actions. They dive into the situation with optimism, overconfidence, and bank it all on a particular therapeutic technique, strategy, or therapy model. Rather than remedying the situation, the client's situation gets worse or the clients lose their faith in their therapist's ability to help them and may drop out of treatment. Kahneman's practical and well-researched framework can serve as a helpful guide for family therapists in the midst of therapeutic action, but we should not allow it to constrict us from taking risks as we see fit when our guts tell us something has a great shot of working based on our past success using it with similar family situations.

Schon (1983) has identified two sets of reflective activities used by experienced practitioners representing a wide range of professional disciplines. These can greatly benefit family therapists both in and out of sessions with their clients. The first is *reflection-in-action*. It involves the therapist stepping outside of his- or herself and carefully observing how family members respond both nonverbally and verbally to whatever he or she tries therapeutically in order to determine what appears to be working. The second therapeutic activity is *reflection-on-action*, which involves taking the time immediately after the session to reflect on the following question: "If I could conduct this session all over again, what would I have done differently?" In response, therapists can compile a list of reflections and questions to ponder and guide them in interacting with particular family members to help build better working alliances and spark the change process. Both of these therapeutic activities can help us keep an open mind, be more curious about our clients' presenting dilemmas, be therapeutically flexible, and stay on target with how we use ourselves in the therapeutic process.

By making room for evidence-based clinical wisdom, therapists using the major empirically supported family therapy models can have even better outcomes. They will also find their work much more meaningful and enjoyable. Both the major empirically supported family therapy approaches and evidenced-based clinical wisdom can complement one another and help us to be much more therapeutically knowledgeable, versatile, and competent family therapists producing better treatment outcomes with our client families (Diamond, 2014; Williams, Patterson, & Edwards, 2014).

A Brief Overview of CSBFT

CSBFT is an approach that helps clinicians integrate empirically supported approaches and clinical wisdom. The model has been evolving since 1985 (Beyebach, 2009; Selekman, 1995, 2005, 2006, 2009, 2010; Selekman & Beyebach, 2013). It is a flexible, collaborative, and integrative family therapy approach that incorporates the best elements of *solution-focused brief therapy* (Berg & Miller, 1992; Miller, 1997; de Shazer, 1985, 1988, 1991; de Shazer et al., 2007; Franklin, Trepper, Gingerich, & McCollum, 2012; McKeel, 2012; Ratner, George, & Iveson, 2012), *solution-oriented and Ericksonian* influences (Erickson & Rossi, 1979; Gilligan, 2002; Gordon & Meyers-Anderson, 1981; Haley, 1973, 1983; Havens, 2003; O'Hanlon, 1987; O'Hanlon & Weiner-Davis, 1989; Rosen, 1991; Short, Erickson, & Erickson-Klein, 2005; Zeig, 1980), *positive psychology* (Csikszentmihalyi, 1990, 1997; Fredrickson, 1999; Lopez, 2013; Lopez & Snyder, 2009; Lyubomirsky, 2007; Peterson, 2006; Peterson & Seligman, 2004; Seligman, 2002, 2011; Tugade, Shiota, & Kirby, 2014), the *stages-of-change model* (Norcross, Krebs, & Prochaska, 2011; Prochaska, DiClemente, & Norcross, 2006), *motivational interviewing* (Miller & Rollnick, 2013; Rollnick, Mason, & Butler, 1999), *MRI brief problem-focused therapy* (Fisch & Schlanger, 1999; Fisch, Weakland, & Segal, 1982; Ray & de Shazer, 1999; Watzlawick, Weakland, & Fisch, 1974), *narrative therapy* (Duval & Beres, 2011; Freeman, Epston, & Lobovits, 1997; Maisel, Epston, & Borden, 2004; White, 2007, 2011; White & Epston, 1990), *client-directed, outcome-informed therapy* (Duncan, 2010; Duncan, Hubble, & Miller, 1997; Duncan & Miller, 2000; Duncan et al., 2010; Hubble, Duncan, & Miller, 1999), *collaborative language systems therapy* (Anderson, 1997; Anderson & Gehart, 2007; Anderson et al., 1986; Goolishian & Anderson, 1988), *Milan systemic therapy* (Boscolo & Bertrando, 1993; Boscolo, Cecchin, Hoffman & Penn, 1987), *Ackerman systemic family therapy* (Sheinberg, 1985; Sheinberg & Fraenkel, 2001), other *postmodern systemic therapy* influences (Andersen, 1991; Friedman, 1995; Hoffman, 1988, 2002; Tomm, 1987; Tomm, St. George, Wulff, & Strong, 2014), and *harm-reduction therapy* (Marlatt, 1998; Tatarsky, 2007).

With many high-risk adolescents, it is simply not enough to utilize their strengths, resources, and past successes at coping to resolve challenging life situations, alter outmoded rigid parental beliefs, and disrupt problem-maintaining family patterns of interaction. These can fail to stabilize their presenting emotional distress and behavioral difficulties. These young people may be experiencing grave difficulty regulating and coping with their powerful emotions; identifying and verbalizing their painful thoughts, feelings, and conflicts; challenging their oppressive thinking patterns; and maintaining self-control. To help remedy adolescents' difficulties in these areas, CSBFT therapists employ the following therapeutic tools and strategies: *mindfulness meditation and self-compassion practices* (Bowen, Chawla, & Marlatt, 2011; Chodron, 2010; Dodson-Lavelle, Ozawa-de Silva, Negi, & Raison, 2015; Germer, Siegel, & Fulton, 2013; Hanh, 1998, 2001; Neff, 2010; Peltz, 2013; Pollak, Pedulla, & Siegel, 2014; Rathus & Miller, 2015; Siegel, 2009; Simpkins & Simpkins, 2009; Willard & Saltzman, 2015), *cognitive skills training* (Andreas, 2012, 2014; Pahl & Barrett, 2010; Stark, Streusand, Krumholz, & Patel, 2010; Weersing & Brent, 2010), *self-control management skills* (Brier, 2010, 2014; Donohue & Azrin, 2012), *art therapy* (Malchiodi, 2003, 2008; Selekman & Beyebach, 2013), and *expressive writing* and *drama therapy* tools and strategies (Malchiodi, 2006; Pennebaker, 2004).

Another important dimension to the CSBFT model is the creative use of self both within and outside the boundaries of any single-therapy approach. Three of the most inspiring and brilliant pioneers of the creative use of self are Salvador Minuchin (Fishman & Minuchin, 1981; Minuchin, 1986; Minuchin, Reiter, & Borda, 2014); Carl Whitaker (Connell, Mitten, & Bumberry, 1999; Whitaker, 1989; Whitaker & Keith, 1981), and Virginia Satir (Satir, 1983, 1988). In my early family therapy training, these three pioneers, through their workshops, training videos, and publications, strongly conveyed the importance of being fearless risk takers, being transparent with our thoughts and emotional reactions, using a lot of humor and playfulness, and tapping into the wild and crazy sides of our personalities. Some of their major therapeutic techniques and strategies may be useful once a therapist has exhausted all of the possibilities within the CSBFT model. Since most of the major empirically supported family therapy models are strongly influenced by structural and strategic family therapy ideas (Fisch et al., 1982; Haley, 1973; Minuchin & Fishman, 1981; Minuchin, Rosman, & Baker, 1978; Stanton & Todd, 1982), it may be worthwhile to integrate some of their techniques and strategies to enhance the effectiveness of the CSBFT approach with more challenging adolescents and their families.

From the initial intake call until family therapy is completed, CSBFT therapists actively collaborate with the referring person and all key resource people from a family's social network and involved larger systems professionals. These important individuals are viewed as part of the *solution developing, solution-determined system* (Selekman, 2009, 1995; Selekman & Beyebach, 2013). The goal is to counteract problem-determined systems, discussed earlier, that usually ensnare high-risk adolescents and their families.

Because the CSBFT model integrates a wide range of individual and family therapy approaches, it offers therapists multiple pathways for intervening on multiple systems levels in high-risk adolescents' social ecologies. This allows therapists to zoom in on the adolescents' and family members' unique needs and struggles, and zoom out to observe their complex interactions with concerned members from their social networks, involved larger systems professionals, and with their communities. CSBFT therapists are mindful of the fact that they can never find an outside place from which to look at their clients. CSBFT therapists realize that their thinking can greatly influence what they see and do in their interactions with everyone involved with the presenting problem situation. After decades of work with high-risk adolescents and their families, I have found it to be most advantageous to view concerned members from the family's social networks and larger systems as potential allies that possess a plethora of strengths and resources that can be tapped for co-constructing multiple high-quality solutions in our collaborative meetings with families.

Individualizing the Family Therapy Approach to the Unique Needs and Characteristics of the Family

The idea of tailoring what we do therapeutically to our clients is not a new idea (Beutler et al., 2011; Pinsof, 1995). The developers of MRI brief problem-focused therapy (Fisch & Schlanger, 1999; Fisch et al., 1982) and solution-focused brief therapy (de Shazer, 1988, 1991; de Shazer et al., 2007) have long encouraged therapists to determine how best to cooperate with each family member. Therapists can do this by carefully observing what family members do and listening to what they say in their in-session responses and between-session management of suggested therapeutic experiments. Such interventions should be in line with the family members' goals, which will then dictate the best way to cooperate with them (de Shazer et al., 2007; Fisch & Schlanger, 1999). One important way to tailor treatment is based on decades of scientific research by Prochaska and his colleagues (2006). They have demonstrated with tens of thousands of individuals worldwide the importance of matching what we do therapeutically with the client's readiness for change. Therapists can gradually move clients through the six stages of change. With families, Friedlander and her colleagues (Friedlander, Escudero, Heatherington, & Diamond, 2011) found that family therapists must strive to accomplish the following in order to optimize positive treatment outcomes: build strong relationship bonds with each family member, maintain emotional safety in sessions, and elicit a shared sense of purpose from the family.

More recently, Lebow (2014, pp. 227–237) has provided 23 practical guidelines for individualizing one's integrative family therapy practice model. Nine of his most important guidelines for family therapists are in line with the key assumptions and mechanics of the CSBFT model:

1. One's family therapy approach should build on and work to enhance the common factors of positive outcomes.
2. Family therapists should shape their own unique combinations of concepts, strategies, and techniques from a wide range of approaches.
3. Client problems are manifested simultaneously on a number of systems levels. No one level should be privileged as more important.
4. In choosing intervention strategies, family therapists make vital choices about who is seen as well as what is done.
5. The integrative family therapist should be attuned to the personal values involved and the unique ethical issues in family therapy.
6. An essential therapeutic operation lies in co-constructing collaborative treatment plans and goals with families.
7. With each family, the therapist in close collaboration with them selects a set of strategies that will optimize achieving their identified treatment goals.
8. In choosing a specific intervention strategy, the therapist also must consider such pragmatic factors as acceptability to the clients and the resources available to best meet their unique needs and goals.
9. An integrative approach is not a static entity but an evolving method, a system open to new ideas to logically add to one's core model.

I wish to underscore those above guidelines that place a strong emphasis on building collaborative partnerships with families. This is where families have the lead voices in deciding what their goals are, are the lead authors of their treatment plans, and have major input in selecting therapeutic tools and strategies that they think can benefit them the most. Taking the individualizing process to the next level, clients can be invited to co-design therapeutic experiments sparked by their own creativity and resourcefulness. The case example below with an Armenian family illustrates how the therapist's and the adolescent's ideas can be combined to co-design a creative therapeutic experiment.

Fifteen-year-old Sabina and her parents came for a live family therapy case consultation in the context of a workshop I was giving. In the past, Sabina and her mother would get into intense power struggles that at times would get quite physical. Sabina also used to have problems with self-injury and self-starvation, which she contended were a result of her mother's controlling and micromanagement behaviors. Sabina alluded to the parents being unhappy that their marriage had become too humdrum. Because Sabina was a talented dancer, I offered her the therapeutic experiment of *adolescent as mentor to her parents* for 1 week (Selekman, 2009). When asked what type of dance she would teach her parents over the week, she shouted, "Hip-hop!" The parents, consulting therapist, and I laughed and thought this was a great idea. Sabina shared with me at the end of the session that she would film the dance lessons and send me a copy of the video. The added bonuses with this therapeutic experiment were that it injected playfulness and new life into the parents' dull marital relationship situation and it was a great opportunity for Sabina to shine as a loving and competent daughter.

In addition to co-designing therapeutic experiments with families, as collaborative partners we need to ensure the following: honoring clients' requests for having more subsystem session time such as with the parental couple or the adolescent wanting to learn more about specific coping tools; deciding who participates in sessions, including key resource people from the family's social networks and involved larger systems professionals that comprise the solution-determined system; the frequency of sessions; and deciding when families are confidently ready to complete treatment.

Collaborative Strengths-Based Family Therapy Practice Guidelines

For CSBFT therapists, therapy begins with the initial telephone contact with the parent. We need to make this initial conversation a very positive and memorable experience. It should instill hope and raise the parents' expectation that something special is going to happen in our work together and it is only a matter of *when*. In addition to using relationship skills like listening generously, validating, and conveying warmth and empathy, there is no better way to begin co-creating a therapeutic context ripe for change than offering the concerned parent a pretreatment therapeutic experiment prior to the first family therapy session (McKeel, 2012; Selekman, 2009; Weiner-Davis, de Shazer, & Gingerich, 1987). The pretreatment experiment is as follows:

> "Over the years, my colleagues and I have been so impressed with how creative, resourceful, and resilient clients are, that well before we have seen them for the first time they have already taken important steps to better cope with or resolve their difficulties, even with the most chronic and severe problems. In order for me to learn more about your and your son's/daughter's strengths and resourcefulness, I would like you on a daily basis to pull out your imaginary magnifying glass and carefully observe any encouraging or responsible steps that you see your son/daughter take that you would like to see continue. In addition, I would like you to pay close attention to what you may be doing during those times that may contribute to preventing your son's/daughter's situation from getting much worse and improving his/her behavior even a little bit. Please write down everything you have observed and discovered and bring your list to our session next week. I look forward to hearing what further progress you made!"

Some of the major benefits of beginning family therapy in this strengths-based fashion are that it accomplishes the following: it increases clients' awareness about their strengths, resourcefulness, and resilience; it can raise their expectancy, hope, and optimism about their ability to resolve their difficulties; it triggers positive emotion, which can neutralize negative emotions and thoughts; therapists learn about key family members' solution-building thoughts, feelings, and actions and can encourage them; and the initial family therapy session becomes like the second session, which can greatly shorten clients' lengths of stay in treatment. In the first session after coming to know family members by their personal and occupational strengths, the therapist can explore with the parents and the adolescent what has gotten better with their problem situation as a result of the pretreatment therapeutic experiment. The therapist can amplify and consolidate all of their pretreatment changes, determine with them what they need to increase doing, and find out from them what next steps will propel them closer to successfully completing treatment.

In the spirit of solution-focused brief therapy (de Shazer et al., 2007), CSBFT therapists place a strong emphasis on underscoring and maximizing clients' strengths, resources, talents, life passions, past successes, and future visions of success. This starts in pretreatment and runs throughout the whole course of family therapy. When families report a wealth of pretreatment changes, their initial complaints at intake are absent from the conversation. Minus problems, they are feeling optimistic about their futures. Their lengths of stay in treatment can be greatly reduced to four to six sessions with longer intervals between the sessions as a vote of confidence to them. Over the years, I have worked with a number of adolescents deemed high risk and their families, some of whom had had extensive treatment histories. They had responded quite well to a fairly pure solution-focused approach, which also involved separate subsystem work with parents and adolescents and active collaboration with the concerned helping professionals from larger systems. Often, once adolescents are labeled "high risk," they will remain on the "watch list" for some time, particularly in school settings even after they make quite dramatic changes. This is why CSBFT therapists offer to serve as advocates for their clients and collaborate with the concerned school personnel until they are less concerned, so the adolescent no longer needs to be tightly monitored. It can help quell school staff members' anxieties and concerns to have monthly or bimonthly collaborative meetings at adolescents' schools to hear about their important changes. Family members are present at the meetings throughout the course of family therapy and for a short period after treatment is completed. Failure to cover this important base can lead to adolescents' having slips in progress areas and family derailments.

At this point, readers are probably asking themselves, "Well, what do CSBFT therapists do when working with more difficult and complex adolescent family cases that do not respond well to the pretreatment experiment" or a pure solution-focused brief therapy way of working?" Below, I provide 16 guidelines for what to do when family members cannot identify any pretreatment changes, past successes, or visualize hypothetical future successes, and the treatment becomes more problem-focused. In addition, CSBFT therapists will expand their base model and incorporate the most effective therapeutic strategies and techniques from the major empirically supported family therapy approaches. It is important to note that within the solution-focused brief therapy model there are many therapeutic options to pursue even with the most demoralized and pessimistic clients (de Shazer et al., 2007). Therefore, the guidelines begin with what CSBFT therapists do once they exhaust all of the possibilities within the base solution-focused model component of their therapeutic approach.

1. With families that have had long treatment histories, it is important to provide them with plenty of floor time to share their long problem-saturated stories by using open-ended *conversational* questions, curiosity, and generous listening, being careful not to be a narrative editor by prematurely moving the conversation to finding out about pretreatment

changes, past successes, or beginning the goal-setting process (collaborative language systems therapy; Anderson, 1997; Goolishian & Anderson, 1988, 1991).

2. A critical area of inquiry is to find out from the family all of their attempted solutions, including what former therapists and treatment program staff had tried with them that did not work and was upsetting to them. In addition, revisit with the parents or legal guardians and the adolescent whether they can identify some past successful coping or problem solving strategies (MRI brief problem-focused therapy; Fisch & Schlanger, 1999; Fisch et al., 1982).

3. Next, we need to clarify with family members what they view as the *right* problem to begin working on first and break that down into bite-size pieces. It is okay to work simultaneously on separate pieces of the problem that the parents or legal guardians and adolescent identified to begin with. Solution-focused questions are great for establishing realistic behavioral goals with families (de Shazer et al., 2007).

4. Presenting problems can be reframed to offer family members alternative ways of viewing them and pattern intervention strategies can be used to disrupt the problem-maintaining family patterns using MRI brief problem-focused therapy (Fisch & Schlanger, 1999; Fisch et al., 1982); solution-oriented brief, Ericksonian, and strategic family therapies (Haley, 1973, 1983; O'Hanlon, 1987; O'Hanlon & Weiner-Davis, 1989).

5. If the family describes the problem as chronic, oppressive in nature, and warranting extensive treatment, they are ripe for more of a narrative therapy approach (Duval & Beres, 2011; White 2007, 2011; White & Epston, 1990). Here, the main oppressive problem, DSM-5 disorder, habit, lifestyle, or pattern can be externalized and rituals can be employed to empower the family to pioneer a preferred future reality.

6. With high-conflict and chaotic families with adolescents engaging in serious delinquent and aggressive behaviors, using family approaches with core structural–strategic and social learning strategies and techniques like MST, MDFT, FFT, BSFT with Latino families, or MTFC with foster care youth are the best courses of therapeutic action (Alexander et al., 2013; Henggeler & Schaeffer, 2010; Liddle, 2010; Robbins et al., 2010; Smith & Chamberlain, 2010; Stanton & Todd, 1982).

7. Families presenting with adolescents experiencing eating-distressed difficulties like anorexia are most likely to respond well to the therapeutic strategies and techniques from the MFBT family approach (Le Grange, 2011; Robin & Le Grange, 2010). Important components of this model that have produced good clinical results are the *family lunch*

strategy (Minuchin, Rosman, & Baker, 1978) and narrative therapy strategies (Maisel et al., 2004).

8. With families presenting with self-injuring, suicidal, and depressed adolescents, using a combination of the major therapeutic tools and strategies from the ABFT, DBT multifamily group, and the base CSBFT models are the best courses of therapeutic action (Diamond et al., 2014; Rathus & Miller, 2015; Selekman, 2009; Selekman & Beyebach, 2013).

9. Families presenting with adolescents who have serious substance abuse problems and/or delinquent behaviors will respond well to the major therapeutic tools and strategies of MDFT, FFT, and BSFT (Alexander et al., 2013; Liddle, 2010; Robins et al., 2010).

10. With adolescents who are struggling with serious self-destructive habits like disordered eating, self-injury, and substance abuse, family therapy alone is often not enough to stabilize these difficulties. Therefore, individual session time in the context of family therapy needs to be devoted to offering adolescents a wide range of coping tools and strategies to constructively manage emotional distress and other powerful triggers. These tools include mindfulness meditation, self-compassion techniques, visualization, and self-control and cognitive skills and strategies (Bowen et al., 2011; Brier, 2014; Neff, 2010; Pelz, 2013; Selekman & Beyebach, 2013; Stark et al., 2010; Willard & Saltzman, 2015).

11. With families grappling with unresolved traumas, losses, and secrets, using postmodern systemic therapy approaches can be effective, such as collaborative language systems therapy (Anderson, 1997), reflecting team (Andersen, 1991; Friedman, 1995), Milan systemic and Ackerman systemic therapy approaches (Boscolo & Bertrando, 1993; Boscolo et al., 1987; Sheinberg & Frankael, 2001).

12. When the treatment process gets stuck and/or the family is not responding well to any of the above action steps, certain constraints may be keeping things at a standstill. Therapeutic options that can be pursued are using curiosity and wondering aloud with the family about the *negative consequences of change* (Fisch et al., 1982); the Milan systemic approach (Boscolo & Bertrando, 1993; Boscolo et al., 1987); the Ackerman systemic approach of using colleagues as a consultation team joining the family and the therapist debating about the dilemmas of change (Sheinberg & Frankael, 2001; Sheinberg, 1985); using a reflecting team (Andersen, 1991; Friedman, 1995) or the collaborative language systems therapy approach (Anderson, 1997; Anderson & Gehart, 2007) to open up space for possibilities and the revelation of the unexpressed, which may be family secrets that are contributing to the maintenance of the adolescent's behavioral difficulties, keeping treatment at a standstill.

13. Throughout the course of family therapy, CSBFT therapists are free to use themselves as the catalysts for change, which includes carefully observing and listening for opportunities to seize in sessions and improvise when necessary. Also, therapists must actively collaborate at the beginning of family therapy with all involved larger systems providers and concerned key members from families' social networks to gain their allegiance and to tap their expertise in the change effort.

14. In situations where multiple family members are struggling with severe marital discord, intense postdivorce conflicts, or serious mental health and/or substance abuse difficulties, it makes the most sense to work with individuals or subsystems of the family establishing separate goals and work projects. Using a modified one-person CSBFT approach or the one-person family therapy model developed by the BSFT research team can be the best treatment choice with these complex and challenging clinical situations (Selekman, 2006, 2009; Selekman & Beyebach, 2013; Szapocznik et al., 2003; Szapocznik & Kurtines, 1989).

15. Goal maintenance and relapse prevention are a family–social network affair, and this process should begin early in treatment and continue until the family therapy is completed. Solution-focused and other Ericksonian-oriented questions are ideal for consolidating family gains and empowering families to envision a compelling reality of future success (de Shazer et al., 2007; O'Hanlon & Weiner-Davis, 1989; Selekman & Beyebach, 2013).

16. Session by session, therapists must solicit feedback from their clients about the quality of their therapeutic relationship and their perceptions about the change process. This helps to prevent alliance ruptures, premature dropout, and negative treatment outcomes (Duncan, 2010; Lambert, 2010). In response to this invaluable client feedback, therapists need to shift gears, abandon unproductive therapeutic strategies and interactions, and pursue client-informed ways to better connect with dissatisfied family members and strengthen their alliances with them.

These 16 guidelines are not carved in stone, and they by no means capture all the possible therapeutic pathways for intervening with high-risk adolescents and their families. Furthermore, therapists should feel free to try therapeutic experiments and coping tools and strategies from a wide range of individual and family therapy approaches that they think can benefit their clients in any given session.

The most important considerations to keep in mind are that the therapeutic tools and strategies selected need to be theoretically compatible; they should have a good fit with or have been modified to better fit the needs of clients from different cultural backgrounds; and they are in line with the clients' theories of change, stages of change, and treatment goals. Clients have the ultimate say regarding whether they choose to experiment with a strategy in and out of family sessions; their feedback determines whether to continue using selected therapeutic tools and strategies. Finally, with families entering treatment where the threat of suicide is great or some form of violence has occurred, the top priority is to immediately ensure that family members are safe. Stabilize the volatile situation first before pursuing any of the above treatment guidelines.

CHAPTER 2

Family Engagement

Tailor the Relationships of Choice

We are each angels with only one wing.
We fly only by embracing one another.
—LUCIANO DE CRESCENZO

The therapeutic relationship has been found to be one of the most robust predictors of positive treatment outcomes (Muran & Barber, 2010; Norcross, 2010; Norcross & Lambert, 2013; Norcross & Wampold, 2013; Swift & Greenberg, 2015). When therapists establish strong alliances early in family therapy with adolescents in particular, this predicts positive treatment outcomes (Diamond et al., 2014; Robbins, Turner, Dakof, & Alexander, 2006).

Building Therapeutic Alliances

Two of the pioneers in studying the important role of strong therapeutic alliances, John Norcross and Michael Lambert, have identified seven important therapeutic activities that therapists need to engage in to build strong therapeutic bonds with their clients (Norcross & Lambert, 2013, 24–26):

1. Empathy
2. Goal consensus
3. Collaboration
4. Positive regard/affirmation

5. Congruence/genuineness
6. Collecting client feedback
7. Managing countertransference

Empathy

All of the major psychotherapy studies on *empathy* indicated that this key therapist activity played a major role in predicting positive outcomes across different therapy approaches as rated by the clients (Elliott, Bohart, Watson, & Greenberg, 2011). Therapists should go to great lengths to understand their clients' experiences and to demonstrate this understanding. Empathic therapists carefully convey to their clients that their overall goals and moment-to-moment experiences in the therapeutic process are understood. Empathic responses can take many forms: directly conveying that you understand the meaning of clients' experiences; supporting their perspectives; "being with" clients; bringing clients' experiences to life by using evocative language; and making explicit what is implicit (Norcross & Lambert, 2013). Ideally, when clients convey that they "feel felt" by us, we are empathically attuned to them, and this helps strengthen the therapeutic alliance.

Goal Consensus

Goal consensus consists of empowering clients to determine what problems they wish to solve first, what their goals are, and as partners, to co-develop a plan of action for achieving their goals. Tryon and Winograd (2011) found that high agreement between clients and therapists about treatment goals and how they will be achieved often leads to positive outcomes. Therapists who push their own goals and agendas on clients set the stage for negative outcomes.

Collaboration

When collaborative partnerships are established with clients, they will be more motivated to implement therapeutic change strategies, achieve their goals, and succeed in treatment (Tryon & Winograd, 2011). Throughout the course of family therapy, therapists need to solicit clients' input on choosing among intervention options, designing therapeutic experiments together, soliciting feedback on the quality of the teamwork, and client satisfaction with the change process. Give clients the lead voice in determining what key individuals from their social ecologies to collaborate with. Using words like *we, let us,* and *teamwork* also help convey to our clients, "We are in this together." Using this type of language has been highly rated by clients as indicating alliance with their therapists (Bohart & Tallman, 1999, 2010; Creed & Kendall, 2005).

Positive Regard and Affirmation

Research shows therapists' conveying positive regard and affirmation has a moderate association with therapeutic outcomes (Farber & Doolin, 2011). Communicating to clients our positive feelings and respect and underscoring their creative courage, resilience, and resourcefulness fosters cooperative relationships.

Congruence and Genuineness

Congruence and genuineness have both intrapersonal and interpersonal sides. The first has to do with therapists being transparent about using themselves as emotional barometers and letting clients know what they are thinking and feeling. The interpersonal side concerns matching your words with your actions. This may involve use of self-disclosure to help normalize what clients are going through. According to Norcross and Lambert (2013), effective therapists will tailor their congruence style according to their clients' characteristics. Many adolescents like therapists who "talk straight" with them, calling them on their bluffs and manipulative ploys. The case example below of a therapy savvy, street-smart high-risk youth illustrates the benefits of "talking straight."

Sid, a white 16-year-old, had a long history of substance abuse, dealing drugs, running away from home, and both inpatient and outpatient treatment. Earlier in the session, I had learned that Sid had conned his dad into giving him $10 so he could take his girlfriend out. His father had asked him to mow the lawn for $10; Sid got the money prior to mowing the lawn and left the house without doing the job. The parents' goal for Sid was to be "a man of his word" when agreeing to help out around the house or do his chores. While meeting alone with Sid, I noticed he frequently used the "F" word and put down his parents as we discussed the lawn mowing incident, and described how he was a master "wheeler and dealer" by getting the money and leaving the house without "delivering" on the job. I used his favorite "F" word in my response to him, saying how slick he was at conning his father to get the money. Sid responded laughing with, "Oh, he [his father] is just retarded or something like that. . . ." Following this exchange, Sid dramatically changed his tone of voice, started using my words in the conversation, and sitting like me in his chair when I called him on his manipulative ploy with his father. Since this session was a live family therapy consultation in the context of a workshop and Sid had natural leadership abilities, I had him join me in the room with the participants and field questions from the audience about how best to work with tough kids like him. He confidently got in front of the crowd and asked, "Questions!" Sid confirmed that kids like him like therapists who "talk straight, have a good sense of humor, self-disclose about their struggles as teens, know about what the most popular street drugs are, and about gang culture."

Collecting Client Feedback

Researcher Michael Lambert has done the most extensive research in the area of client feedback (Lambert, 2010; Lambert & Shimokawa, 2011; Norcross & Lambert, 2013). Collecting feedback provides opportunities to repair alliance ruptures, enhance social support, and prevent premature dropout and treatment failures. Standardized questionnaires can collect clients' perceptions of the quality of their relationships with their therapists and satisfaction with the change process. With this information, therapists can adjust their therapeutic stances and decision making to better meet the needs of their clients. Two instruments that are widely used to solicit this important information are: the *SRS* (Session Rating Scale) and the *ORS* (Outcome Rating Scale) (Duncan, 2010; Duncan et al., 2010). Lambert and Shimokawa (2011) found that when client feedback was combined with warning signals of at-risk therapy and decision support tools for such cases, the rates of client deterioration decreased by two-thirds and positive outcomes doubled. Some clients balk at having to fill out questionnaires. If this is the case, therapists solicit client feedback at the end of each session by asking the following questions:

> "What was this meeting like for you today?"
> "What ideas do you plan to put to use over the next week?"
> "Was there anything you were surprised I did not ask you about your situation that you think is important for me to know?"
> "Would you like to address that issue in our next session?"
> "Was there anything I said or did in the session that upset any of you that you would like me to stop doing?"

Managing Countertransference

A final area that plays a major role in building strong alliances is how we manage *countertransference*. In a study on countertransference, Hayes, Gelso, and Hummel (2011) found that when therapists were successful at constructively managing their countertransference reactions to clients, it greatly contributed to better treatment outcomes. Therapists who had stronger alliances with their clients employed self-talk, self-reflection, made good use of supervision, and did not respond behaviorally in sessions to negative feelings or unresolved conflicts triggered by their clients.

In addition to self-monitoring strategies, therapists can use countertransference reactions to increase their clients' awareness of the impact they have on others. Therapists might share analogies, metaphors, quotations, stories with a resilience twist, or scenes from popular movies that remind them of a particular triggering interaction.

Next, I discuss two client characteristics that are important for therapists to assess and use in tailoring their approach to the engagement process. Therapists need to carefully assess for and match their strategies with family members' stages of change and their psychological reactance levels (Beutler et al., 2011; Norcross et al., 2011).

Stages of Readiness for Change

One of the most important bodies of research from the 20th century underpins the transtheoretical model, also known as the stages of change (Norcross et al., 2011; Prochaska et al., 2006). After having studied thousands of clinical and nonclinical individuals, Prochaska and his colleagues identified six distinct stages people go through in the process of changing a behavior: precontemplation, contemplation, preparation, action, maintenance, and termination. Sometimes people need to go through the stages multiple times for behavioral and changes to occur and be maintained. Their research indicates that we can increase the likelihood for treatment success by matching therapeutic strategies with each family member's stage of change. We can help clients advance at their own pace from one stage to the next. According to these researchers, only 20% of clients come to therapy in the action stage ready to change, and yet most therapists assume that new clients are armed with goals and ready to change their problem situations. This is the danger in adopting a "one-size-fits-all" treatment mind-set. The mismatch of therapy approach with stage of change may be why some of families prematurely drop out or experience treatment failure. Often the therapists involved blame clients for being "resistant" and "noncompliant." The bottom line is that clients, even the most challenging therapy veterans, do want to cooperate with us. Our job is to be generous listeners for how best to cooperate with them and patient observers of our interactions with each family member. We have to be careful not to become resistant therapists! This is why it is best to be flexible, integrative family therapists and to carefully tailor what we do to the needs and characteristics of our clients. The stages of change are fluid, and it is possible for a family member to advance from one stage to the next in a given session.

Precontemplative Stage

Most high-risk adolescents come to us under duress. Often, their parents drag them in to be "fixed." Others are being forced to see us by social control agents representing larger systems that have the power to enforce attendance. These adolescents are not even window-shoppers for counseling. They may be on the defensive, and will quickly declare that, "I don't have a problem!" What is important to remember is that they are in the *precontemplative* stage of change for good reasons, not due to being in DENIAL! After many unsuccessful outpatient and inpatient treatment experiences, they may be demoralized or skeptical of any treatment ever working to change their depressing and stressful family situations. They also may be stuck in precontemplation because no one in their family has ever modeled the benefits of changing anything. Their parents may have long-standing substance-abuse difficulties with destructive and unproductive ways of managing conflicts and anger. In such circumstances, why should the adolescent be fired up to change his or her problematic behaviors?

Two effective strategies for engaging adolescent precontemplators are the following.

The Two-Step Tango

The first step of the tango is to empathize with the adolescent's dilemma about being forced to see you and what a drag it is to have to be in counseling again. The second step of the tango is, in a nonchalant manner, to plant seeds in his or her mind about the benefits of changing some of the behaviors that led to being forced to see you. The therapeutic stance is one of a gentle back and forth—restraining them from changing ("Go Slow!" messages) and planting seeds regarding the benefits of changing. This kind of dialogue helps raise the adolescent's consciousness level so that he or she begins to think, "Maybe some of the things I have been doing are costing me big time (such as juvenile detention time, having to wear a leg monitor, or having to be locked up in a psych hospital for cutting)."

Compliments

High-risk adolescents who come to their first sessions deserve big compliments for taking responsibility by showing up and cooperating with their parents and social control agents making them go for therapy. During the initial family session, we may learn other important steps the teen has been taking to avoid getting into further trouble, such as staying away from certain people and places, refraining from cutting, and not getting stoned. They may have useful self-talk, which we can encourage them to use as their mantras for making good choices. Each responsible or courageous step reported in the session can be punctuated and responded to with the therapist's asking, "Wow! Are you aware of how you did that? What did you tell yourself to pull that off?" In this way, we gain valuable information about what works for the client and how resourceful and creative he or she is. At the end of the first family session, the therapist can again compliment the teen, gently encouraging him or her to do more of what is working to keep him or her out of further trouble. Do not offer the client any therapeutic experiment to do because precontemplators more than likely will not implement the recommended change strategy.

Contemplation Stage

Once the high-risk adolescents advance to the *contemplation stage*, they have begun to recognize that there is a problem worth looking at; however, they are ambivalent and not ready to take active steps to resolve the problem. They may have long-term careers of self-injury or other self-destructive habits that have helped them to effectively cope with emotional distress. Nothing else may have worked to provide rapid emotional relief. They may not be able to count on their parents to soothe and comfort them. One of the most effective strategies for helping any client in contemplation get unstuck or less ambivalent about change is the *decisional balancing scale* (Prochaska et al., 2006; Velasquez, Crouch, Stephens, & DiClemente, 2016; see Form 2.1 at the end of the chapter). When beginning the decisional balancing inquiry with the adolescent, we can ask him or her to reflect on the *advantages* and *disadvantages* of continuing to engage in risky behaviors or use unproductive coping strategies by responding to the following questions: "In what ways has [risky behavior/unproductive coping strategies] benefitted you?"; "OK, on the flip side, in what ways has [risky behavior/unproductive coping strategies] backfired on you or cost you in some way?" Next, the adolescent is to write down all of the advantages and the disadvantages of continuing to engage in his or her choice self-destructive behavior or other unproductive coping strategies in the designated columns. Last, he or she is to rate each one in the order of importance from 1 to 4, with 4 being most important. This highly practical and effective tool offers the adolescent the opportunity to see and critically reflect on the advantages and disadvantages of continuing to rely on problematic coping strategies. Many adolescents will see how their disadvantages are outweighing the advantages, be more open to exploring alternative coping strategies, and will move into the next stage of readiness for change: *preparation*.

Preparation Stage

Upon entering the preparation stage, clients are more committed to abandoning unproductive attempted solutions and problematic behaviors. However, they will report specific barriers that might get in the way of trying to change. For example, a single mother is afraid that if she no longer gives in to her explosive, tyrannical son and set limits on him, he will try to hurt her. In these situations, the therapist needs to problem solve with the mother and co-generate action steps to be put in place should violence erupt. For example, she might have her brother, who has a close relationship with his nephew, present when she attempts to enforce a consequence. In similar cases, I have brought in the son's male adult inspirational other to help support the mother's position of authority. The adult inspirational other can be a coach, teacher, spiritual leader, a close cousin, and so forth—any adult who has a strong and meaningful connection with the adolescent.

Action Stage

The next stage of change is the *action stage*. At this point, the adolescent or family members are ready to partner with the therapist to set realistic goals and implement change strategies. They are highly motivated, ready, and willing to do anything to improve their situations. Typically, the parent caller who initiated the family therapy is in this stage.

Maintenance Stage

Adolescents and family members in the *maintenance stage* have already abandoned unproductive coping strategies but could slip back into their former problematic behaviors. Therefore, the important therapeutic work we need to do is arm them with relapse prevention tools to help them stay on track. In addition, we need to cover the back door by doing worst-case scenario planning with the family and key resource people from their social networks.

Termination Stage

Once an adolescent or family member makes it to the *termination stage*, they are totally confident that they have conquered their problems for good and are on a solid pathway for future success. These individuals can serve as expert guest consultants for adolescents who are experiencing difficulties the consultants used to have and offer valuable wisdom about what works and how they conquered their problematic behaviors.

Client Psychological Reactance Levels

Another critical area family therapists need to assess and accommodate is family members' *psychological reactance levels* (Beutler et al., 2011; Norcross & Wampold, 2013). Clients who have grown up in highly controlling environments or have been physically or sexually abused are going to have high levels of psychological reactance. They will have their guards up and are not likely to comply with any direct attempts to change them until a safe, trusting therapeutic alliance has been developed. This is not resistance or noncompliance; it is about client self-protection. The majority of high-risk adolescents are highly reactive to their parents, social control agents, and therapists brought in to try and change their problematic behaviors. Adolescents by nature can be highly oppositional. Therefore, direct logical reasoning and straightforward therapeutic intervention strategies should be avoided. Instead, indirect questions and therapeutic strategies should be employed. The following questions are inviting to highly reactive adolescents because they give them the power to be the experts:

> "If you were the program director of this adolescent inpatient program, how would you change it to make it better?"
> "What special activities would you add to the program?"
> "If I were to work with another teen just like you, what advice would you give me to help her out?"
> "If I were to work with another family just like yours, what would I need to change first that would make a big difference for that teen in that family?"

The other strategy that works well with highly reactive adolescents and family members is to give them plenty of room to choose from a wide range of coping tools and therapeutic experiments which suits them best to try out.

Clients with low levels of psychological reaction are in the action stage of readiness for change. They are eager to set goals and go to work. They are fired up to experiment with new coping tools and change strategies.

Strategies for Engaging
Reluctant Nuclear and Extended Family Members

With more challenging and complex high-risk adolescent cases, key nuclear and extended family members may be reluctant to participate in family therapy. These may include powerful adolescents ruling the roost at home; fathers who are reluctant to attend for various reasons; antagonizing older and younger siblings; an overinvolved grandparent in or outside the home who is protective of or undermines the parents' or legal guardians' authority; and aunts or uncles also protecting or undermining parents. If, after a session or two, change is not occurring with the attending family members, engage in *persistent outreach* efforts with these other key individuals. With families of adolescent substance abusers, research has indicated that therapists' persistent outreach to engage reluctant family members increased engagement rates from 20 to 75% over more passive efforts (Santisteban et al., 1996). Persistent outreach efforts can include sending texts and letters to key immediate and extended family members who may need to be engaged for family therapy. They may have attended one session and not returned. Your willingness to go the extra mile with them conveys that you strongly care and consider them important members of the family team.

One way to find out who the most powerful absent individuals are in the clients' systems is to ask the following questions to the attending adolescent, his or her attending sibling, or the most concerned parent:

> "On a scale from 1 to 10, with 10 most concerned about you/stressing you [the adolescent identified client] out the most, your brother or sister [the attending sibling], your son or daughter [the parents], what numbers would you give to absent family members?"
>
> "What specifically are they [absent family members] doing to try to help you/him or her out?"
>
> "What specifically are they doing that you would like us to work on changing?"
>
> "What specifically do you think would have to change with your family situation so that [these absent family members] would be less compelled to be overly involved and concerned?"

Once we secure this important information from attending family members, we can send invitation texts or letters, offer to meet with them alone in your office, in their homes, or in another neutral setting. As with new clients, we need to build solid alliances with these individuals and come to know their stories of involvement, particularly the driving forces for their attempted solutions. We need to respectfully find out about the history behind their attempted solutions and try to gain their allegiance in the change effort. In some cases, there may be an axe to grind from unresolved family-of-origin conflicts. If this is the case, we can attempt to resolve these issues between the immediate and extended family members in future family therapy sessions if they wish to do so. Two common engagement dilemmas that many family therapists struggle with are engaging powerful adolescents and fathers in treatment. Below, I discuss effective strategies for engaging and retaining challenging adolescents and reluctant fathers in family therapy.

Engaging Powerful Reluctant Adolescents

Coaching Parents to Facilitate Engagement

Whether you are seeing one or both parents or legal guardians of a powerful, reluctant adolescent, the first step we need to take is to explore all of their unsuccessful attempted solutions to try to get the teen to join them. Their attempted solutions usually take the form of the following parental actions: pleading, bribery, threats of imposing extreme consequences, kicking the adolescent out of the house, or institutionalizing him or her. Ideally, we need to get the parents to abandon all of their unproductive solutions. It is helpful first to find out about any past successes they have had at getting the adolescent to cooperate with them. We need to find out all of the details about what worked, such as being calm, having a nonthreatening tone of voice, not nagging, not making demands or threats, giving ample options and choices in decision making, and so forth. Serving as the parents' coach, the therapist should begin by trying out strategies that worked in the past to gain the adolescent's cooperation to attend the next family session. We need to have plan B, C, and D as backup strategies just in case. Sometimes having the more laid-back parent take over as the lead parent can successfully gain the adolescent's cooperation with attending family therapy. Another parental strategy that can work is offering to take the adolescent, after the family session, to a favorite restaurant the family has not been to in a long time.

Texts and Letters

One highly effective intervention with challenging and powerful adolescents refusing to come in for family therapy is the use of a paradoxical letter (Weeks, 1991; Weeks and L'Abate, 1982). It has long been said that there is nothing more powerful than the written word. Texts or letters written by the therapist and delivered to adolescents by their parents convey the importance of not budging from their positions of nonattendance and of digging in more despite their parents planning their futures for them, such as considering residential treatment for them. The empathic recommendations in such a letter can elicit rebellion against it, as in the case below.

Sean, a white 16-year-old, had been heavily abusing a wide range of substances since age 13. He also was failing most of his subjects at school and had a truancy problem. I had seen the parents twice. They were totally burned out with Sean's multiple outpatient and inpatient treatment experiences and frequent phone calls at their workplaces from staff at his therapeutic day school for behavioral problems and not completing his schoolwork. Well before I saw Sean's parents for the first time, they were already looking into finding him a residential treatment center or a special boarding school. In fact, in both of our sessions they had brought this up as a possible plan for the near future if he continued to refuse coming to see me with them. Apparently, Sean was unaware of the parents' plan. So, in finding out from the parents Sean's preferred way of communicating with them and his friends, they thought I should text my provocative paradoxical letter to him. I sent him the following text letter:

Dear Sean,

As you may know, I am the therapist who has met with your parents a few times. I must say I miss not having you here and getting to know you by hearing how you see yourself and learning about what you want for yourself in the future, rather than hearing only what your parents think about you and what they want. However, they have made it quite clear to me that therapy has been a real drag for you and you really hate it. So I think you should not put yourself through yet another downer of a therapy situation. In fact, I don't blame you for not wanting any more stress in your life . . . who needs that, really! My guess is if you did come in for a session with your parents you would probably sit slouched in a chair with your head down and not say a word. There was one thing I did want to make you aware of that your parents have brought to my attention, and it has to do with future plans for you. Now, I truly believe in a democratic process when it comes to family-related future planning, but maybe you are the kind of kid who feels OK with his parents deciding his future for him. You could just chill at home and adopt a wait and see mind-set with what your parents are planning for you. Although something tells me you are not that kind of person and that when you really believe in a cause or something that is important to you, you draw the line and refuse to budge. Well, I have to go now but I would like you to ask yourself, "Would I like to be in charge of my future, or do I want my parents to take charge of my future for me?"

Best wishes,
Matthew

The parents and I had scheduled another family session for 2 days later with the hope that Sean would show up to take charge of his future. The parents were instructed not to make any mention of what their future plans were for him until he agreed to come with them for family therapy. Apparently, Sean had been asking his parents a lot of questions about what their "future plans" were for him, and he was quite eager for us to meet as a family group. The parents did a fine job of keeping their lips sealed about their plans to increase Sean's motivation to attend family therapy with them. In addition, they prepared a list of expectations and guidelines for Sean to take steps to eliminate his problematic behaviors both at home and at school, and a realistic date for these changes to happen in order to prevent his being shipped off to a residential treatment center or boarding school. One bargaining chip that the parents did hold was Sean's strong desire to get his driver's license. Their position was that he had to maintain abstinence from drugs and stay away from his "stoner friends." Not only was Sean an active participant in our next family session but also he desperately wanted to avoid being shipped off to a residential treatment center or boarding school. In addition, he now had a girlfriend and needed "wheels to take her out." The parents also told Sean that they would do random drug screens using hair follicle analysis to keep him honest and to help uphold his commitment to change. They warned him "three dirty screens" would result in his being sent to a residential drug rehabilitation center. I ended up building a strong alliance with Sean due to the parents' tough stance with him and the family and I worked on relapse prevention together.

Home Visits and/or Meeting in Neutral Safe Places

In spite of the parents' and therapist's best efforts to engage the adolescent for family therapy, he or she may still refuse to attend. The therapist can then offer to do a home visit or meet with the adolescent in some location where he or she would feel most comfortable. To help ensure that the adolescent is at home or at the agreed location, the parents can attach a highly desired privilege to cooperating and taking responsibility. Once you have the opportunity to finally meet the adolescent, you need to try your best to build good rapport. Keeping this first meeting as nonthreatening and light as possible, I invite adolescents to share with me their hobbies, interests, talents, and life passions. As part of this conversation, I have them play for me their favorite music on their iPods, smartphones, or on their instruments, show me their artwork, rap songs, poetry, and so forth. Adolescents tend to warm up to therapists who take a deep and sincere interest in their natural talents and meaningful interests.

If it appears an alliance is developing, you can explore with the adolescent what he or she would like you to change first about the parents to make home life less stressful. You also can find out what privileges the teen would like you to fight for with the parents. Next, you can point out how your work schedules are a bit crazy to be able to continue meeting at the adolescent's house, and would he or she be willing to give a family therapy session a try. The adolescent might point out that therapy has not worked in the past and how he or she greatly dislikes it. You can then explore what specifically former therapists did that really turned him or her off. Once you have this valuable information, you can commit to avoid making the same mistakes and strive to be the kind of therapist the adolescent would like you to be. You also can tell him or her that you will make it safe, honor his or her voice in sessions, and make sure he or she will have an adequate amount of individual session time. By this time, reluctant adolescents are often on board with attending the next family session. If they get cold feet or something negative transpires over the week with their parents and they are hesitant to go to my office, I will offer to do the family session in their homes.

Involving Adult Inspirational Others and Peers of the Adolescent

One resiliency protective factor high-risk adolescents often possess is to have meaningful relationships with adults outside of their homes (Anthony, 1987; Kauffman, Grunebaum, Cohler, & Gamer, 1979). These adults serve as caring *inspirational others*. They have made themselves consistently available to provide support and advice to high-risk adolescents when they needed it. They can be extended family members, teachers, coaches, spiritual leaders, adult neighbors, and community leaders. These important adults can assist in getting and retaining high-risk adolescents in counseling. In addition, if approved by the adolescent and his or her parents, adult inspirational others can participate in family therapy sessions.

Other key individuals in high-risk adolescents' lives are their closest friends. Friends can be recruited and pair up with their adult inspirational others to aid in engagement and change efforts in the social contexts where adolescents are having difficulties (Selekman, 1995, 2005, 2009; Selekman & Beyebach, 2013). In the first family sessions, I often ask adolescents, "When you are really stressed out, which friends do you turn to first for advice and support?" It is these friends who really care about the client. You want to secure written consent to involve them in collaborative meetings at school and family sessions if the parents approve. These allies can strengthen our alliances with adolescent clients—co-constructing solutions, helping them stay on track between sessions, and reducing the likelihood of relapses. This provides a support system in school to prevent and curtail bullying and fighting with peers. The case example below illustrates how adult inspirational others can pair with the high-risk adolescents' closest friends.

Cedric, an African American 15-year-old, had a long history of fighting with peers, disrupting his classes, getting suspended for swearing at teachers, and bullying. His aggressive behavior dated all the way back to his elementary school years. According to Samantha, Cedric's single mother, her ex-husband was very abusive both physically and verbally toward her and Cedric. Cedric had witnessed a lot of domestic battery and at times would get hit trying to protect his mother. At this point, the parents were divorced, and Samantha's ex-husband was in jail for murder. In spite of all of the traumatic life events Cedric had endured, he was a talented running back and was starting on the varsity football team at his high school. Cedric and his football coach, Mr. Smith, formed a very strong bond, and the latter worked hard with his star athlete to cultivate his natural gifts. They would have lunch together, and Mr. Smith would try and impress upon Cedric the importance of "taking pride and joy in your accomplishments," "having good character," and to "treat others with respect and dignity." These valuable words of wisdom emotionally resonated with Cedric. The coach also had shared with Cedric that he thought the team could go far in postseason playoffs and that it would not happen with him getting suspended or, worse yet, expelled for bullying and fighting. I got Samantha's permission to contact Mr. Smith and ask him to try and engage Cedric for family therapy, which could include his participating in sessions if he was OK with that and if her son would agree to try that out. I warmed up to Mr. Smith right away and could tell that he cared a lot about Cedric and believed strongly that he would be heavily recruited by top college football teams and offered numerous scholarships. We set up a meeting in his office with Cedric. With the help of Mr. Smith, I was able to establish rapport with Cedric and start talking about what ideas he had at school for helping him not cave in to swearing at teachers, fighting with, or bullying peers. Cedric thought it would be a great idea to try getting passes from his teachers to go meet with Mr. Smith or go to the main office to "chill out" when he was starting to lose his temper or peers were pushing his buttons. He also thought it would be helpful if two of his closest friends on the football team could be involved to provide added support. A week later, we met again with Mr. Smith and two of Cedric's football friends, Warren and Jackson, the fullback and the quarterback, respectively. They agreed to be available to provide support at school, working closely with Mr. Smith and Carmen, the school social worker. After trying out this new support team approach at school for a few weeks, Cedric dramatically decreased his verbal and physical aggression, was no longer bullying and fighting, received no suspensions, and he had not been kicked out of one class for disruptive behavior. Cedric agreed to attend family therapy with his mother, as long as Mr. Smith, Warren, and Jackson could participate. I had Samantha, Cedric, Mr. Smith, Warren, Jackson, and their mothers sign off on my *significant other consent form* (Form 4.1) in order for these key resource people from Cedric's social network to participate in our family sessions. With the support team's and Cedric's hard work over the ensuing months, he not only continued to soar as a star on the football team (averaging 150 yards on the ground per game and scoring multiple touchdowns), but his grades improved as well. I continued to tap the expertise of the support team members to help consolidate Cedric's gains and prevent relapses.

Secret Mission Projects with Key Members from the Adolescent's Extended Family

When efforts to bring the adolescent in for family therapy proves futile, we can explore with parents if there are any key resource people from their extended family who have a very close relationship with their son or daughter. Once this grandparent, uncle, aunt, or cousin is identified, the parents or legal guardians can give us written consent to contact this relative and invite him or her in for a planning session. During this session time, we can find out from this key resource person what the adolescent has enjoyed doing and talking about with him or her. A well thought out *secret mission project* can be devised with the relative and the parents to engage the adolescent for the next family session, which the relative will participate in (Selekman & Beyebach, 2013). While the relative is spending quality time with the adolescent, he or she can gently introduce the idea of attending the next family therapy session with the teen, serving as his or her advocate to better get the adolescent's needs met. The following case example demonstrates how tapping a relative's strong connection with a reluctant high-risk adolescent can engage him or her in family therapy.

Raquel, a Puerto Rican 16-year-old, had a long history with bulimia, self-injury, having toxic boyfriends, arguing with her parents, and multiple inpatient and outpatient treatment experiences. Also, she had refused to attend family therapy with her parents. According to her parents, she "despised therapy with a passion." I had explored with the parents whether she had an extremely close relationship with a relative whom we might call upon to assist in the engagement process. Apparently, Raquel had a very close relationship with the mother's younger sister, who was in her 30s. In the past, they would have lunch and go shopping together. Fairly consistently, the mother pointed out how Raquel would come home after seeing Sandra (the maternal aunt) raving about what a fun time they had together and how they could talk about anything. In the next meeting with the parents, we met with Sandra and explained the difficulty we were having getting Raquel to attend family therapy sessions. Sandra confidently stated, "Leave it to me. . . . I will get her here." Sandra set up a date with Raquel to have lunch and go shopping. Raquel had opened up to Sandra at lunch about her cutting and bingeing and purging more lately due to rejection by a popular boy at school whom she had liked who was now "running around with a girl" she greatly disliked. Sandra provided a lot of support to Raquel and had encouraged her to accompany her to the next scheduled family therapy session to begin addressing the "rejection issue" and to stop hurting herself. Sandra gave me good press about being "a nice man" and that I like to give teens their own "individual space time" to confidentially share private details they don't want their parents to know. Raquel agreed to go to family therapy on the condition that Sandra would join us in sessions. Thanks to Sandra's leverage with Raquel and this very successful *secret mission project*, I was better able to engage Raquel. I worked with her to steer clear from toxic relationships and learn alternative coping strategies for dealing with emotional distress. Sandra made a commitment to make herself available both in and out of sessions to further support Raquel.

Involving Alumni Guest Consultants

Alumni guest consultants can be invaluable in engaging new reluctant adolescents, particularly when the alumni recruited used to have the same difficulties the teen is currently struggling with and they are very close in age. These valuable resource people have conquered their former self-destructive behavioral difficulties and are functioning well in all areas of their life. After meeting the alumni and giving written consent, the parents can escort the alumni and therapist home to meet the reluctant adolescent and attempt to engage him or her. If the adolescent would like to have the alumni participate in separate sessions with him or her or in future family sessions, we should accommodate their request.

With reluctant adolescents actively involved with gangs or struggling to exit from a gang, bringing in former gang members just out of adolescence (19 to 20 years old) can be most advantageous. They lived the reality of being shot, stabbed, watching their best friends being killed on the streets, and spent time in the juvenile detention center. Their stories of resilience can be quite inspirational for a young gang member to hear how they worked their way out of the gang lifestyle to a GED, perhaps going to community college, and getting jobs. These young adults also can share their stories about how they broke free from gangs and how not to fall back into this lifestyle. Some of the gang-involved youth I have worked with are ambivalent about giving up their gang affiliations. They feel a strong sense of connection, respect, and empowerment with this second family that they have not received in their families at home. In addition, they are growing up in extremely violent communities where being in a gang is about protection and survival. The former gang member consultants you recruit need to be able to address how they dealt with these dilemmas. The case example below illustrates the tremendous benefits of using former client gang member alumni not only to help engage a reluctant gang-involved adolescent for family therapy but also to contribute to transforming his or her life.

Pedro, a Mexican American 17-year-old, had been in a Latino street gang for 3 years. In spite of all of the parents' efforts, including trying to get him to counseling and to meet with their priest, Pedro had refused to cooperate. In addition to running with his gang, Pedro was smoking more marijuana, drinking, and getting failing grades in school. Because of his truancy problem, his major academic decline, and being at risk for expulsion from high school, the school social worker had referred the family to me. After two family sessions, unsuccessful at getting Pedro to come with his parents, I presented the idea of introducing them to two former gang members, 19 and 20 years old, respectively, who were now working and going to a community college. My former clients met with the parents in the next session and told their stories and how they were now turning their lives around. We found out from the parents the days and times when Pedro might be around the house. When Pedro greeted us at the front door, he was not as rough and tough as the parents had described him to be. In fact, my having seen his parents twice did not threaten him. He actually warmed up to both my former clients and me. My alumni did a great job of engaging Pedro and offered to help him to get a job at one of their workplaces, support him while he tried to get out of his gang, and if he felt OK with it, join us in a few of the family sessions. Although there was a strong pull to stay in the gang and it took a couple of months, Pedro drummed up the courage with the support of my alumni to break free from the gang and turn his life around. Another bonus was that Pedro landed a part-time job at one of my former client's workplaces. They also agreed to get together with Pedro a few times a month to continue to support his efforts to do better in school and stay substance free. By this time, the parents and Pedro were getting along much better.

Effective Alliance-Building and Retention Strategies with Challenging Adolescents

Once parents have succeeded in bringing in their reluctant adolescents for family therapy, we can employ the following alliance-building strategies to increase the likelihood of the adolescents' ongoing retention in treatment.

Strengths and Talents

Take a strong interest in and have adolescents converse about their key strengths, talents, meaningful life passions, and solicit examples of their personal achievements, which can be utilized for co-constructing solutions.

Stories of Courage, Grit, and Resilience

Invite adolescents to share their personal stories of courage, grit, and resilience, which can be tapped as future models for resolving or overcoming present difficulties and life challenges.

Dreams and Visions

Invite them to share their future dreams and visions. What do they want to accomplish and be known for? This can be tapped for co-creating compelling future realities with them.

Goal Definers

Ask adolescents what they wish to change first, even if it has nothing to do with the reason for the referral and what the parents want for them. Going with whatever adolescents want for themselves is a great way to foster cooperative relationships with them.

The Big Three Questions

There are three important questions we need to ask adolescents in the first session:

"How can I be helpful to you?"
"What is the number-one thing that your parents do that makes you the most upset and that you wish for me to change?"
"What privilege do you really want me to fight for with your parents?"

When therapists deliver for their adolescent clients by changing the parents' problem-maintaining interactions and successfully negotiating the privileges they strongly desire, they will be more likely to attend future family therapy sessions and be active participants in the change effort.

Use Humor, Absurdity, and Surprise

Beginning with the first encounter with adolescents and throughout the treatment process, use playfulness, humor, absurdity, and surprise. It makes them eager to attend sessions to hear and see what is going to happen next. The case below illustrates how humor, absurdity, and surprise can spark a therapeutic breakthrough with a reluctant adolescent. These helped to elicit the adolescent's goal and a clear and solid work project to collaborate on.

Jillian, a 17-year-old white girl, was referred to me for an emergency family assessment session by her high school dean after she carved a deep cut into her arm with a sharp object. Jillian had had several inpatient and outpatient treatment experiences for self-injury, substance abuse, bulimia, and family conflicts dating back to age 13. In addition, she had been diagnosed with borderline personality disorder and bipolar disorder due to her intense mood swings, according to her mother, Sylvia. I also had learned from Sylvia that, prior to this incident, Jillian had not cut herself for over a year. Once we began the session, Sylvia did most of the talking and Jillian would respond to my questions by turning her back to me in her swivel chair. Sylvia pointed out to me that Jillian "really hates therapy." I had noticed that Jillian had been swiveling a lot in her chair since the beginning of the session, so I saw this as a great opportunity to seize and foster a cooperative relationship with her. I had Sylvia go to the waiting room lobby so I could meet alone with Jillian. I shared with Jillian an idea that just popped into my head. I said to her, "How about we swivel four times to the right and four times to the left in our chairs and when we are done, we can meet face-to-face and we can talk about anything you wish to talk about." Prior to the two of us swiveling together in perfect sync, I caught a half-smile on Jillian's face. When we met in the center face to face, Jillian had said to me, smiling and chuckling, "Dude, you are crazy!" After a good laugh, I asked Jillian what had precipitated her self-injuring episode and she said, "Well, my best friend, Cindy, and I had a big argument and it seemed like she didn't want to be friends with me anymore. I was really worried about that. We have known each other for years." She went on to tell me that the cutting episode occurred both as a form of self-punishment and to "numb out" her anxious feelings. I asked her if she wanted help to try and reconcile her relationship with Cindy and she loudly proclaimed, "Yes!" In honoring her preferences, I asked Jillian which she would prefer as a plan of action: my offering her some tools and strategies for resolving her conflict with Cindy or inviting Cindy in so I could directly help the two of them to resolve their differences. Jillian opted to pursue the first option and to work on this goal alone with me. At the end of the session, when asked what the family meeting was like for her, Jillian said, "That was fun!" Jillian attended future family sessions and also was an active participant in collaborative meetings at the school. Those focused on better grades and safety plans for support at school to help prevent future self-injuring episodes. The great news was that Jillian was able to resolve her conflicts with Cindy and better solidify their relationship.

Intergenerational Negotiators

Once we find out what privileges adolescents desire, we have to serve as intergenerational negotiators, representing them with their parents. We can negotiate something-for-something contracts with both parties. By agreeing to pursue and achieve a negotiated small behavioral goal that the parents would like to see happen, the adolescent can earn the privilege he or she strongly desires. It is important that we let them know that it will be hard work, and they may encounter bumps in the road in trying to achieve their contracted work project. As part of worst-case-scenario planning, we can co-construct solution steps for getting back on track to successfully manage any surprises that may try to derail them.

Engaging Reluctant Fathers

Being Mindful of and Sensitive to the Role of Fathers from Different Cultural Backgrounds

Be sensitive to the fact that in some cultures fathers wield all the power in the home. They may not feel they need to be as central as the mothers in their children's lives. In fact, they may expect their wives to take care of all responsibilities for children and domestic affairs. Fathers may view their sole role as being the main breadwinners. In addition, for many cultural groups, seeking psychotherapy or family therapy runs counter to beliefs that personal affairs and difficulties should be kept in the family. They may seek emotional consolation and consultation from their spiritual leaders or extended family. This is not to say that we should discourage mothers from inviting their husbands to attend family therapy with them, but fathers may balk at the idea. Sometimes, these fathers will agree to give it a try, and it is our job to make them as comfortable as possible and explain what family therapy is about and its potential benefits. Finally, it is important to make them feel like highly valued participants in family meetings.

Coaching an Attending Parent to Facilitate Engagement with a Nonattending Parent

The attending parent first has to abandon unproductive attempted solutions for getting the nonattending parent to attend family therapy. With each attempted solution, therapists can map out the circular pattern of interaction on paper so the attending parent can see how the other partner becomes defensive, blames them for the kids' problems, or just plain balks at the idea of going for family therapy. Next, explore any past successes the attending parent has had in getting his or her partner to cooperate. We have the parent experiment over the next week with these past successful strategies to see if they succeed in bringing the reluctant partner to the next family session.

All is not lost if the attending partner has exhausted all of his or her options and can't get the other to attend. The attending parent can still be the main agent for change in the family system. Szapocznik and his colleagues (1989, 2003) have demonstrated that it is possible to change entire family systems through one family member. Through the attending parents' perseverance and grit they were able not only to produce significant changes with their adolescents' behaviors but also to disrupt negative interactions in their marital or couple relationships. If the attending parent requests that I attempt to directly engage the absent parent, I am happy to do so and will employ the persistent outreach methods discussed below.

Texts and Letters

If texting is the nonattending partner's preferred way of communicating, I will text about my strong desire to meet and discuss what has the best shot of working with the challenging adolescent. Otherwise, I will send a very nice letter with same requests. With reluctant fathers, I let them know the following: "You are like the captain of the ship, and without your strong leadership and expertise, we will be lost at sea or may crash into a rocky reef, where the situation will get much worse. It may be difficult for your crew to survive." Since many of these fathers like to be in charge, using words like *captain, king, leader, expertise, guidance, wisdom,* and so forth, often helps them warm up. It may be beneficial to point out in the text or letter the following: "What a great team you and [your partner] can make, like Superman and Wonder Woman, combining the mother's sensitivity with the father's power and toughness, a real dynamic duo!"

Home Visits and/or Meeting in Neutral, Safe Places

In some cases, texts or letters will get reluctant fathers to attend the next scheduled family meetings or be willing to meet alone with the therapist in their homes or neutral, safe places. Therapists need to be open to meeting with reluctant fathers in a wide range of places where they feel most comfortable or that works with their tight work schedules, such as their workplaces or at a coffee shop, preferably away from other people. As we should do with all new clients, we first want to come to know reluctant fathers by their strengths, talents, hobbies, interest areas, and life passions. Ask fathers, "How can I help you with your family situation?" We may learn the parents are divided in their management of their adolescents due to different parenting styles, marital discord, postdivorce conflicts, and so forth. The first step is to attempt more parental unity around the management of their adolescent's problematic behaviors. It is risky to deal with the emotionally charged marital and postdivorce conflicts too early in family treatment. Next, if fathers are on board with improving parental teamwork, we can find out where things break down and what specifically they think has to change to resolve the division. If they appear to be receptive to the idea of joining the next family sessions, we can strengthen that commitment by reiterating that their leadership abilities and toughness can help turn their family situations around.

With separated and divorced parents who can't tolerate being in the same room with each other, it may be most advantageous initially to see each parent separately with the children. Establishing separate goals and work projects designed to resolve their adolescent's behavioral difficulties can strengthen the teen's relationships with each parent. Once these changes occur, partners are sometimes more willing to attend together and be civil. I make strategic use of research with divorced parents by letting them know that when parents work together civilly, uphold mutually agreed-upon household rules and consequences in both homes, and consistently stick to the visitation schedules in their divorce decrees, it provides their children with a strong sense of emotional security. This greatly aids children in coping better with this difficult and stressful family transition process (Wallerstein, Lewis, & Blakeslee, 2001). In situations where one parent is inconsistent with parental teamwork or resists it, I continue to work with the most committed parent, support his or her position of authority in the family, and encourage him or her not to give up. Even with one parent or legal guardian, we can use a harm-reduction approach to decrease the adolescent's problematic behaviors, which can greatly reduce the consequences of his or her poor choices.

Effective Alliance-Building and Retention Strategies Once in the Door

There are three major alliance-building and retention-enhancing strategies that can be pursued with reluctant fathers who agree to attend family therapy for the first time.

Strengths and Talents

Strive to build solid working alliances with reluctant fathers in the initial sessions with them. Begin by coming to know them by their top strengths, talents, interest areas, life passions, and key competencies in their work roles. These can be can be utilized in the parenting department.

Balancing Relationships and Meeting Individual Needs

In honoring the father's preferences, we ask him if he would like to have some individual session time so we can learn about what his perspectives, theories of change, and best hopes are regarding the adolescent's presenting problems. If we have seen the mother a few times alone and/ or with the adolescent, to help balance things out, it can be helpful to see the father alone for part of or as much of the session time as he wants. This individual session with father's strategy can continue if he would like more time alone, if we still have a weak alliance with, or inadvertently something was said in sessions that may have upset him and caused ruptures in our nascent alliance.

Repairing Alliance Ruptures

When alliance ruptures occur with fathers, it is critical to meet with them alone to find out specifically what we said or did in sessions that offended them, made them feel disrespected, or misunderstood. In response to fathers' blaming their partners, attempting to silence their voices with their anger, or treating them in some other disrespectful way in front of their children, rather than asking the kids to go to the waiting room right away, we can make the tactical blunder of abruptly cutting them off or, worse yet, ganging up on them. This only serves to further fuel their anger toward both of you. When this happens, we need to offer fathers individual session time to let them air their frustrations, for us to apologize for offending them, and to explore with them how best to get back on track. This may entail their desire to work with their partner on better teamwork, improving their communications and conflict-resolution skills, or wanting to have more individual session time.

Key Findings from Empirically Supported Family Therapy Research on Effective Engagement and Retention Strategies

In this section, I discuss *emotional safety, multipartiality, validating all family members' perspectives, structuring skills, establishing systemic treatment goals and a mutual sense of purpose,* and *reframing*—five important empirically supported findings from family therapy research studies that play a major role in the alliance-building process, help prevent premature dropout from occurring, and greatly contribute to create a therapeutic climate ripe for change.

Emotional Safety

Friedlander and her colleagues (Friedlander, Escudero, & Heatherington, 2006; Friedlander et al., 2011) have found that one of the most important therapist-facilitated activities that must occur for alliance building with families to occur is providing a therapeutic climate that is emotionally safe for family members to allow themselves to be vulnerable and share with one another their thoughts, feelings, needs, concerns, and even secrets, without any fear of being invalidated, yelled at, shamed, blamed, rejected, or physically threatened or harmed. In the first session, therapists can share with families a house rule that everyone's voice will be heard and celebrated throughout the therapeutic process and this will be actively enforced. Emotional bonding between the therapist and each family member is encouraged through the use of relationship skills like warmth, genuineness, validation, empathy, and conveying understanding.

Multipartiality: Validating All Family Members' Perspectives

Along with feeling emotional safety, the family therapist needs to simultaneously honor and embrace each family member's unique perspective, theory of change, expectations, and best hopes for what they would like to get out of family therapy. This means that each family member feels like the family therapist takes his or her side without privileging any one family member's views or desires over other members' positions and needs (Escudero, Heatherington, & Friedlander, 2010; Friedlander et al., 2006, 2011). One of the true master family therapists and trainers who modeled *multipartiality* at its best was Harry Goolishian (Goolishian & Anderson, 1988). Not only would Harry create an emotionally warm and safe dialogical space in the therapy room, but the gentle way he would carry himself vis-à-vis the consulting therapist and each family member made everyone feel felt and heard. This would open up space for family members to courageously share the previously unexpressed secrets, taboo subjects, catastrophic fears, or other unspoken concerns with one another. In addition to his tremendous warmth, Goolishian used both the curiosity of a cultural anthropologist visiting an indigenous tribe's village for the first time and *generous listening*. He listened deeply and respectfully to family members' stories and avoided being a narrative editor. Hoffman (2002) has cited the works of Ludwig Wittgenstein (1953) and Jean-François Lyotard (1996) as being the first to write about "listening generously." She quotes Lyotard commenting on Wittgenstein's *language games* concept, which is a self-contained linguistic system that creates meanings through negotiation between two or more people: "For us, a language is first and foremost someone talking. But there are language games in which the important thing is to listen. Such a game is a game of the just. And in this game, one speaks only inasmuch as one listens, that is, one speaks as a listener, and not as an author" (p. 71).

This quote captures the essence of how Goolishian validated families as being the true experts of their stories. It is how all of us should conduct our conversations with families, particularly in initial sessions with therapy-veteran clients, using not knowing, curiosity, generous listening, and multipartiality. It is critical across the course of family therapy to maintain strong therapeutic alliances with each family member and honor their unique perspectives on their family's story.

Structuring Skills

Alexander and his colleagues (2013) have found in their functional family therapy research that the therapist's *structuring skills* play a major role in ensuring emotional safety for families, help strengthen therapeutic alliances, and increase clients' hope and expectations in their therapist's ability to help them to resolve their difficulties. Structuring skills include taking charge in sessions when things get heated and out of hand, showing good timing with knowing when to split up family members and meet with individuals or subgroups, displaying good timing with intervention selection, and conveying a high level of confidence and competence to families. At treatment outcome, clients who had had positive treatment experiences rated therapists' structuring skills as being critical to their success.

Establishing Systemic Treatment Goals and a Mutual Sense of Purpose

Another way we can establish alliances with all family members is to have them identify a systemic goal they all agree on. After carefully listening to all family members' concerns and what they would like to change, any commonality or consensus about a pressing difficulty that needs to be resolved first can be negotiated as their initial treatment goal. For example, if all family members are complaining about their constant arguing with one another, we can ask if they would like to work on resolving this difficulty first. By agreeing as a group to do so, they are conveying to one another, "We are in this together and it has to be a team effort." Having systemic goals and a sense of purpose have been identified as critical alliance-building factors that contribute to positive treatment outcomes (Escudero et al., 2010; Friedlander et al., 2006, 2011).

Reframing

The majority of empirically supported family therapy approaches discussed in Chapter 1 employ *reframing* as both an effective way to reduce client defensiveness and offer family members positive alternative ways of viewing their problem situations (Alexander et al., 2013; Diamond et al., 2014; Henggeler & Schaeffer, 2010; Liddle, 2010; Robbins et al., 2010; Robin & Le Grange, 2010). Reframing consists of relabeling or co-constructing a negative behavior, pattern, life situation, or dilemma into something positive. Transforming something negative into something positive increases clients' hope and expectation, which in turn increases their motivation to change. Some examples of reframing include: an adolescent with attention deficit disorder (ADD) is an *active–dynamic–determined* adolescent; an angry parent is a *concerned parent*; a strong-willed adolescent is *assertive*; an adolescent problem is a *family problem*. The narrative therapy strategy of *externalizing the problem* also is a form of reframing in that it can dramatically change family members' view of the problem situation as residing inside the adolescent (White, 2007; White & Epston, 1990). This nonblaming and playful strategy also can successfully foster family teamwork to conquer the oppressive problem that had been getting the best of all of them, including the adolescent client and involved helping professionals from larger systems, for a long time. Once family members' view of the problem situation changes, often their interactions with one another change as well.

Reframing should be used sparingly, and we must carefully observe and listen to family members' responses after trying this strategy out. The danger in reframing too much is that clients may think you are being sarcastic or trying to talk them out of their problems, which can lead to them feeling invalidated because you are not taking their difficulties seriously enough.

Troubled Alliances, Relationship Ruptures, and Premature Dropouts

By soliciting session-by-session client feedback regarding the quality of our therapeutic relationships and their perceptions of the change process, we will be more likely to establish strong alliances with them and prevent or quickly repair relationship ruptures and prevent premature dropout situations. When we fail to solicit regular feedback from or don't take family members' reported concerns or expectations seriously and commit to remedying these difficulties, they may feel invalidated. It can weaken and/or rupture our therapeutic alliances with them and cause one or more family members to drop out.

Signals of Weak Therapeutic Alliances and Ruptures

A number of studies have identified signs of weak therapeutic alliances and ruptures (Eubanks-Carter, Muran, & Safran, 2010; Friedlander et al., 2006, 2011; Lambert, 2010; Lambert & Shimokawa, 2011; Safran, Muran, & Eubanks-Carter, 2011; Swift & Greenberg, 2015). Weak therapeutic alliances and festering unrepaired ruptures in our relationships with certain family members can lead to their eventually dropping out. Therefore, therapists need to be on the lookout for the following warning signs that require their immediate attention:

- The therapeutic climate feels unsafe due to the therapist allowing blaming and other negative interactions to go on far too long.
- A family member does not respond to the therapist or other family members when spoken to.
- The therapist invalidates a family member by not genuinely listening or responding to his or her concerns.
- Family members may experience the therapist as not being gender, or culturally sensitive or gay affirmative.
- One or more family members perceive the therapist as taking sides or splitting alliances.
- The therapist has failed to invite family members to share their treatment preferences, theories of change, expectations, and concerns.
- Therapist mismatch with questions asked and therapeutic tools

and strategies offered and family members' unique stages of readiness for change.

- After a relationship ruptured occurred, the therapist failed to take responsibility for his or her actions and take constructive client-informed steps to repair it.
- The therapist makes too many statements and gives too much advice.
- The therapist has an interrogative interviewing style.

Strategies for Repairing Alliance Ruptures

When something we said or did has silenced certain family members or made them upset and dissatisfied with their treatment experience, it behooves us to do the following:

- Immediately explore what upset a particular family member if you are not aware of what triggered the relationship rupture.
- Listen generously and adopt an open and nondefensive therapeutic stance.
- Once you are aware of what upset the family members, you need to validate them, clarify any misunderstandings, accept responsibility for your unhelpful actions, and make a commitment to not allow it to happen again.
- New treatment goals may need to be negotiated. Carefully match what you do therapeutically with the stages of change that the family members are presently in (Norcross et al., 2011).
- Successful rupture resolution can be an opportunity for client growth and change and can be alliance enhancing.

Research indicates that when therapists fail to immediately take the above steps to repair or rigidly adhere to their choice therapy models as the best way to resolve those ruptures, poor treatment outcomes or premature termination from therapy become more likely (Eubanks-Carter et al., 2010; Safran et al., 2011).

Major Reasons Why Clients Drop Out of Treatment

In their extensive meta-analysis research on client *premature termination*, Swift and Greenberg (2015) found clients are most likely to drop out when the costs of continuing therapy outweigh its benefits. Beyebach and Carranza (1997) found that the therapist's interviewing style plays a major role in why clients drop out of treatment. Some other major reasons include:

- Dissatisfaction with the type of therapy used.
- Clients' preferences and treatment expectations were either not discussed or were not honored.
- Lack of choice or input in clinical decision making.
- Failure to elevate clients' hope early in treatment.
- Unrealistic expectations regarding change not happening fast enough.
- Environmental obstacles including financial limitations, transportation, child care, scheduling conflicts.
- Stigma and negative opinions from family and friends about attending therapy.
- Anxiety and discomfort with the therapeutic process, including being vulnerable, fear of addressing emotionally painful issues, fears about losing control, being yelled at, or blamed after sessions by other family members.
- Significant other does not approve of partner's attending therapy.
- Client setbacks and deterioration had a demoralizing affect and led to client drop out.
- Unrepaired alliance ruptures.

Several studies have indicated that clients who had dropped out of treatment only expected to attend a few therapy sessions (Mueller & Pekarik, 2000; Swift & Callahan, 2008). This is a good reason for therapists to educate clients in initial family sessions about their treatment approach, which includes the mechanics of sessions and therapist expectations for clients, letting them know about the frequency of sessions and typical duration of treatment. Based on this important information, clients can then decide whether there is good fit with their unique needs and difficulties. Research also indicates that if clients feel their situation is not changing by the third session they can become demoralized and lose their faith in the therapist's ability to help. This can set the stage for their prematurely leaving treatment (Duncan, 2010).

The Decisional Balancing Scale

Directions: List all of the *advantages* and *disadvantages* of attempting your choice solution to cope with or resolve your difficulty. Rate each advantage and disadvantage on a scale from 1 to 4.

1 = Slightly important, **2** = Moderately important, **3** = Very important, **4** = Extremely important.

Advantages	Disadvantages

CHAPTER 3

Building Strong Partnerships with Pessimistic Helping Professionals and Members from Families' Social Networks

> When you turn walls sideways, you build bridges.
> —ANGELA DAVIS

With community mental health clinics and residential treatment centers closing due to state and federal funding problems, more adolescent state wards are being placed into foster homes, and they have much shorter lengths of stay in hospital-based programs. As a result, we are going to see many more challenging high-risk adolescent family cases presenting with multiple problems, extensive treatment histories, and failures. In some cases, the same helping professionals from larger systems had been previously involved with the siblings and parents of our current high-risk adolescents. When we attempt to collaborate with these professionals, we are met with strong reactions of skepticism, frustration with the clients' inability to change, and burnout over having to deal with them again. The parents or legal guardians may equally feel frustrated and have long-standing conflicts with these helping professionals and the larger systems they represent. This can lead to some professionals not being invested in partnering with us in family therapy sessions or serving as key members of the solution-determined collaborative team, or following up with our requests for advocacy for the clients in their respective larger systems and communities.

Another major dilemma may develop while hosting collaborative meetings with helping professionals. Intense conflicts between helping professionals may occur regarding problem explanations, the adolescent's diagnoses, the treatment goals, and the *best* treatment approaches for the family's presenting problems. We need to avoid taking sides or parading our own positions and make it possible for all meeting participants to feel safe to voice their diverse perspectives and opinions. This can be a difficult task to pull off, particularly when some helping professionals are rigid in their positions and disputing other participants' ideas about what to do.

Finally, a third major dilemma we may face involves clinical situations where key resource people from the clients' social networks wield a tremendous amount of power with the client families and who may have a long history of undermining the parents' or legal guardians' authority and thwarting previous therapists' change efforts. Contributing to these fierce family politics may be long-standing unresolved intergenerational conflicts among the parents' adult siblings or the grandparents. The high-risk adolescents may have become either pawns for one or both parties or forces with them against the parents.

In this chapter, I address all three of these collaborative meeting dilemmas and present the latest empirically supported research on resolving disputes and difficult negotiations. I also provide a wide range of collaborative tools and strategies for resolving conflicts, split alignments, and groupthink that can prevent collaborative participants from dropping out.

The Many Sides of Conflict: Harnessing the Power and Opportunities in Disagreements

In complex conflict dispute situations, the parties involved get stuck and polarized in either/or thinking, which keeps the situation deadlocked. Mayer (2015, pp. 4–5) contends that conflicts are embedded in seven polarities, which he refers to as the *conflict paradox*:

1. *Competition and cooperation*: We tend to view these as opposite strategies that opposing factions need to choose between, when in reality, competition requires cooperation, and without competition the impetus to cooperate is absent. Therefore, a more nuanced mixed approach is in order, which combines both cooperative and competitive moves.
2. *Optimism and realism*: A constructive approach to conflict can only occur when both optimism and realism are at play. We are motivated by optimism and guided by what is realistic.

3. *Avoidance and engagement*: We cannot avoid or address all conflicts. All conflicts involve a combination of conscious and unconscious decisions about what to engage and avoid. When we choose to address one conflict area we inevitably have to avoid another.
4. *Principle and compromise*: Many people believe compromising on important issues indicates a lack of principle and is cowardly. We have to decide whether we want to attempt to resolve the conflict in line with our most important values or beliefs or compromise on something that is essential to us.
5. *Emotions and logic*: Many experts believe that the key to being effective in resolving conflicts and conducting successful negotiations is being rational and controlling our emotions. However, emotions are an important source of power and an essential tool for moving through conflict constructively.
6. *Neutrality and advocacy*: It is critical for facilitative interveners of group conflict to juggle being effective advocates for the disputing parties and for the collaborative group process and simultaneously bringing as neutral or impartial a perspective as possible to the group.
7. *Community and autonomy*: The dynamic tension between our need for community and autonomy infuses our thinking and action throughout our attempts to resolve conflicts.

It is Mayer's (2015) contention that all parties involved in the conflict have to deal with these polarities, and the facilitative interveners (we) must skillfully find a way to model and help them embrace both elements rather than seeing them as contradictory. The bottom line is that conflict is not a bad thing. It can be a wake-up call for us to be realistic with our thinking, and a reminder to us to avoid *groupthink* (Sunstein & Hastie, 2015)—that is, getting too wedded to any one or two particular ways of view of the clients' situations. Our job is to create a collaborative, safe climate where everyone's voice is heard and where conversational flow is strong. This optimizes the co-generation of multiple ideas and high-quality solutions worth trying out.

Mary Parker Follett, one of the major management pioneers on leadership, conflict, and power, found in her research that the best leaders adopt a "power with" others mind-set. This was a collaborative and mutually beneficial type of power. She also believed that, without conflict, there is probably a lack of purposeful engagement in the group or organization (Brisken, Erickson, Ott, & Callanan, 2009). According to Coleman and Ferguson (2014), "Researchers have found that when people have a sense of efficacy and inclusion at work and view their tasks, rewards, and other outcome goals as shared and cooperative, it greatly increases the odds of the constructive use of power between them and of positive outcomes from conflict" (p. 56).

We need to adopt a benevolent leadership role when hosting collaborative meetings. Empowering and supporting the participants even when they have disagreements can foster solid teamwork and innovative thinking. Furthermore, we can reframe for the participants that having different perspectives is welcomed and a source of strength for our collaborative team.

Resolving Destructive Conflicts and Disagreements among the Helping Professionals in Collaborative Meetings

When destructive conflicts erupt in our collaborative meetings, we need to actively take charge and not allow them to spiral out of control. Caspersen (2014) contends that it is critical that we determine with all parties involved in the destructive conflict what specifically each of them has chosen to listen to and how they hear what they each have said. She recommends asking them, "If this were said without mutual attack, what would it sound like?" Next, after listening to each party's response to this question, we can ask, "How will that make a big difference in your being able to resolve this disagreement or agree to disagree in a more constructive way?" In addition, after these intense conflicts are resolved, the parties might still want further assurance that their concerns will be addressed. In response to their concerns, it can be quite advantageous to tap the expertise of the other collaborative group members, including the parties involved in the conflict, to prepare a written action plan. By tapping the collective wisdom of the collaborative group in the form of an action plan, we are optimizing for a *higher order of conflict resolution*. Brisken and his colleagues (2009) have observed through their extensive years of organizational consulting work and research that conflict can be an invitation for a higher order of resolution. They write:

> This means listening, deciphering, and unlocking new alternatives. It means achieving new understanding of the situation and grasping the basic needs of those involved. Conflict has the potential of drawing us into new areas of introspection and reveal the hidden complexity of the situation. It often entails grappling with paradox and allowing all the different layers of history to come into a new alignment. (p. 157)

Shapiro (2016) approaches complex, emotionally charged conflict dispute situations from a different angle. Rather than allowing the group to fall prey to "you" versus "me" or "us" versus "them" thinking, he believes

conflict resolution can only occur in "the spaces between the relationships" of the disputants and recommends that we reframe for the group
the conflict as being "a quest for harmonious coexistence" (p. 193). He
contends that in emotionally charged conflict dispute situations, all parties involved truly want the same thing—to feel safe, to be listened to, to
be respected, and so forth. In this spirit, group members can be asked to
visualize what harmonious coexistence would like for each of them. Next,
they can evaluate together which of their visualized scenarios, looking at
the pros and cons of each, would be most likely to foster harmony in their
collaborative relationships. As a group, they can come up with concrete
action steps that they can take to achieve harmonious coexistence and
conflict resolution without compromise. Later in this chapter, I discuss
other collaborative tools and strategies that can be used in collaborative
meetings for constructively managing disagreements and destructive conflict situations.

Resolving Long-Standing Conflicts among Families, Helping Professionals, and the Larger Systems They Represent

Throughout my professional career, I have worked with numerous therapy-
veteran high-risk adolescent family cases with many years of antagonistic
relationships with helping systems where they felt mismanaged and misunderstood, and where their presenting difficulties got much worse. Some
of my former clients of color felt that the helping professionals they had
to deal with were racist and insensitive to their cultural values and practices. These professionals often had previous involvement with my adolescent clients, their siblings, and their parents and were feeling burned out
and frustrated with their crises, defensiveness, failure to keep the lines of
communication open, and noncompliance with the treatment recommendations of their doctors, therapists, juvenile justice, and child protection
systems. Needless to say, in such circumstances, neither party is eager to
sit down and resolve their differences. However, unless we make a valiant
attempt to resolving the long-standing conflicts between the helping professionals and the family, a cooperative relationship will not develop, the
clients will remain hopelessly entangled in the larger systems the helpers
represent, particularly if the latter are alarmed and concerned.

    With these challenging clinical dilemmas, I have found it to be most
advantageous to have the family take the lead in determining which
helper or helpers they would like to begin the conflict resolution process
with. We can have a family session prior to inviting the helpers to join us.
The family session is used to co-construct a nonblaming written agenda
consisting of their most pressing questions, concerns, expectations, and

current needs. Our job is to help the family write their agenda in such a way that does not put the helpers on the defensive, helps foster coopera- tive relationships with them, and helps us move as a group from "what was" (past negative antagonistic relationships) to "what is" (the family's new relationships with the helpers and the helpers' receptivity to best meeting the family's current needs). In the context of these reconciliatory meetings, we need to make it as emotionally safe as possible for all parties and try and accomplish the following:

- Make room for each participant's unique stories and accounts of past events and interactions with one another.
- Underscore in the participants' responses when they may have mis- construed what the other party had said or done.
- Point out that there are many ways to view stressful or negative events and that our survivalist brains are hardwired to view stress- ful and life events through a negative or pessimistic lens (Hanson & Mendius, 2009).
- Make room for the helpers to share their expectations with the family and how they would like their interactions to be different now.
- Actively cut off accusatory and blaming attacks, and move the con- versation in a positive, future-oriented direction toward "what can be."

It may take a few meetings to accomplish this. Once the family and helpers succeed, they can begin as a team co-creating a compelling future reality, eventually liberating families from all of the larger systems they had been ensnared in for years.

Resolving Long-Standing Family Disputes and Conflicts with Powerful Members from Their Extended Family and Social Network

With some complex high-risk adolescent families, the intensity of the fam- ily feuds and conflicts is like a hornets' nest. There may be grandparents who wield all of the power, constantly overindulging the adolescents, res- cuing them, and undermining their sons' or daughters' authority. In some cases, adult siblings of the parents may have had long-standing conflicts with the parents, undermine them, or use the adolescents as pawns to even the score with their siblings. The following case example illustrates how adult siblings can undermine their siblings' parenting roles and greatly contribute to maintaining the adolescent's difficulties.

I once worked with a Caucasian family where the older unmarried maternal aunt, Leslie, had long-standing sibling rivalry issues with her younger sibling, Lucy, who was "happily married." Leslie always been envious of Lucy's looks and popularity with peers in the schools they attended. Leslie had thought for years that Lucy was their parents' "favorite daughter," so Leslie would get even with her younger sister by feeding her 15-year-old nephew, Tom, with negatives about his mother, encouraging him not to listen to her, and buttering him up with gifts to reinforce his allegiance with her. Once this family dynamic was brought to my attention by both Lucy and Tom, I got consent to meet with Leslie and involve her in sessions alone with Lucy. Not only did Lucy want to have a better relationship with her only sibling, but also she was concerned about Tom's increased temper flare-ups, oppositional behaviors, fighting at school with peers, and swearing at her. Tom felt caught in the middle of her mother's and his aunt's battles with each other, even though he did like getting showered with gifts. However, he was getting tired of being "stressed out" and "fighting Aunt Leslie's battles for her." After meeting alone with Leslie and coming to know her perspective on the rivalry with her sister, I asked if she would be willing to do some sessions with Lucy and me. By the end of our third conjoint session, not only was I able to de-triangulate Tom out of their long-standing battle but also both women were able to share things with each other that they had never expressed before. For example, Leslie did not know that Lucy had always been jealous of her having been a better student. Lucy also pointed out that she had been upset that their parents had sent Leslie to her first choice college and she had to settle for a "much lower-grade college." Another high point in this session was Leslie's apologizing to Lucy for dragging Tom into their unresolved conflicts and for undermining her parental authority. Finally, I asked them separately to hop into my imaginary time machine and go back to a time when they were closer and got along better. They both went back to their junior high days, when they did a lot of fun things together and used to compare notes about boys. Lucy reminisced about how when she was in seventh grade they had gone to their favorite ice cream store and shared an enormous banana split. I could visibly tell that the time traveling and reliving good times was triggering a lot of positive emotion for them; that they were both smiling and laughing a lot together, which they had not done in years. The two sisters made a commitment to continue healing their relationship and getting together more often. In fact, one of the outings they had together was to go to their favorite ice cream shop and devour a banana split together. Shortly after this third session, Leslie went over to Lucy's house to apologize to Tom for bringing him into the middle of her battles with his mother and that she would no longer do this.

In clinical situations where the adolescents are sitting on the shoulders of one or both grandparents in coalitions against their "incompetent" or "irresponsible" adult son or daughter, we need to first meet alone with the grandparents in an attempt build solid alliances with them. Next, we need to give them plenty of room to share their stories of concern about their adult son or daughter as a parent and solicit from them what their ideal outcome goals and best hopes are for him or her once they change.

I also like to know from the grandparents what small signs of progress would look like over a week's time with their son's or daughter's parenting role. I also ask how they will know when they can serve as consultants from the sidelines or from afar to their son or daughter, rather than being compelled to take over parenting their grandson or granddaughter. Once we have solid working relationships with the grandparents and family, we can begin conjoint family sessions with the parents and grandparents to attempt to resolve their conflicts, which may date back to the parent's childhood or adolescence. If this can be accomplished, the following steps can be pursued:

1. Renegotiate their relationship so it is a more balanced and mutually respectful adult relationship.
2. The grandparents can assume a consultant-like relationship to the parent.
3. Grandparents support the parents' authority by enforcing their rules and consequences.
4. Grandparents stop the excessive gift giving to their grandson or granddaughter.
5. Be a unified team—grandparents and parents—in holding their grandson or granddaughter accountable for his or her actions.
6. Have the grandparents support and positively reinforce parental growth steps.

Two other challenging family social network dilemmas may disempower parents: when friends' parents or powerful peer groups undermine parental authority. When there is a lot of conflict or a major emotional disconnect between the parents and their adolescents, teens are more likely to try to get their needs met elsewhere. They can adopt their friends' "cool" and "ultra-liberal" parents, to whom they may complain about how awful their own parents are. Not only may these parents allow them to drink, smoke weed, and play video games for excessive amounts of time but also they make the adolescents' visit so cozy that they may choose to spend all of their free time there because it is like a fun country club. The friends' parents become big time enablers and end up greatly disempowering the adolescents' parents. In these case situations, I have the parents contact the friend's parents to arrange a meeting that I can mediate. It is important that they let their sons or daughters know that they are intending to do this and their rationale for it. The adolescent's parents then have the opportunity to voice their concerns and reach out to the friend's parents for support, which is likely once the friend's parents learn how poorly the adolescent may be doing in school or with other behavioral concerns. In addition, the adolescent's parents can establish an agreement with the friend's parents about what the adolescent cannot do, such as any drug or alcohol use. They can also agree to keep communication open between them, particularly if they have heard through the grapevine that the party on Friday night will be in an empty house with no parental supervision. I have heard from my adolescent clients that it is much more anxiety provoking when the parent squad "busts the party" than when the police do.

In situations where the adolescents' peer groups wield all of the power, I get written consent to bring in their friends to our sessions. This strategy can be quite effective at infiltrating adolescents' peer groups in a positive way, in that we gain an insider's perspective of their social lives and have an opportunity to build rapport and gain leverage with their closest friends. Once their friends discover that we are "cool," "nice," and "caring," they will respect and work for us between sessions in helping our clients steer clear from risky situations. It is like harm-reduction therapy. They don't want to see their close friend (the client) end up in the juvenile detention center, psychiatric hospital, or drug rehab. This peer group intervention strategy does not always work, but when it does it can help turn a very difficult situation around. Including the peers of the adolescent client in family sessions can be very helpful for rebuilding trust with their parents and tapping his or her friends' creativity for fresh ideas for resolving their family difficulties. With written consent, I also have had adolescents' closest friends sit in on meetings with family members and helping professionals from larger systems to share their creative expertise.

Major Collaborative Tools and Strategies

In this section of the chapter, I present 15 collaborative tools and strategies that we can employ to help create a cooperative climate ripe for co-constructing multiple high-quality solutions with involved helping professionals from larger systems, family members, and with key members from their social networks. Each collaborative tool and strategy is described below.

Keeping an Open Mind-Set

Although it is true that no theory can truly be objective, we need to strive to keep our minds as open as possible. We play with and reflect on the multiple ideas our collaborators are contributing in our meetings, without getting too attached to any one idea. At the same time, we need to avoid elevating our own inner thoughts and voices above those of our collaborators. We need to model for the collaborative team that there are many ways to look at families' problem situations; there is always more to their stories. Therefore, as facilitators of collaborative meetings we need to ask open-ended questions and invite participants to elaborate further on their different perspectives.

Presence

Although we may have some great ideas about what we would like to do with our collaborators, we need to keep an open mind to what they might like to do. We may need to quickly shift gears, particularly if they do not appear excited about what we had in mind for them. This is the crux of what *presence* is all about. Presence is all about what's happening right now in the moment, aware of our thoughts, unsupported assumptions, and feelings. Presence is generously listening to each member of our collaborative group as a consistent practice at each meeting. Gerzon (2006), quoting Susan Skjei's poignant words on presence, says, "Presence is about the alignment of heart, mind, and soul. It's about developing the capacity to use the tools in the right context and for the right reason" (p. 104).

According to Scharmer (2007, 2013), what we pay attention to and how we attend to fellow members of the collaborative group is at the heart of what we can create together. He contends that our "blind spots" prevent us from fully attending to what group members are saying. They are the inner places that we typically operate from, that comprise our beliefs, values, worldview, and so forth. Increasing our awareness of our blind spots to help us listen generously, with an open mind, open heart, and open will is critical for bringing forth and co-creating important systemic changes.

Using Respectful Curiosity

When operating from a position of respectful curiosity, even the most pessimistic, hostile, or historically uncooperative helping professionals and key members of our clients' social networks will have grave difficulty resisting our questions. It is hard to rebel against nonthreatening, curious people. If anything, they will want to help us know the facts or the story as they see it. In this facilitative stance we become like cultural anthropologists enthusiastically wanting to come to know an indigenous tribe's customs, values, rituals, and lifestyle. Along the way, we can ask open-ended questions for clarification, further elaboration, or to help us with our confusion about something they had said.

Honoring Each Helper's Commitments

It is important to remember that there are no villains in the client's story. The referral source or another helping professional may have mishandled the client's situation in some way or failed to team up with others who had sought their support, but we still need to give them the benefit of doubt. We need to come to know what drove their thinking and actions. The helper's thinking and actions I am referring to here is called a *commitment* (Kegan & Lahey, 2001). A commitment consists of an individual's beliefs and values that drive his or her attempted solutions, particularly how he or she approaches and tries to resolve difficulties. If in any way the high-risk adolescent's intimidating, aggressive, or potentially life-threatening behaviors are similar to a helping professional's former clients who caused harm to themselves or others, this may elevate the professional's anxiety level. The professional may feel compelled to try to independently control the situation before something dire happens. Cynthia, a 17-year-old Caucasian self-injurer with bulimia, was referred to me by her school social worker. Her case helps illustrate how commitments can drive a helping professional's attempted solutions.

In spite of my seeing Cynthia and her mother for family therapy and actively collaborating with the school social worker, the social worker insisted on seeing my client three to four times per week in her office. The daughter had complained about this situation to me and to her mother, which in turn led to the client's high school dean getting involved. I called for a collaborative meeting at the school. Sitting around the circle were the mother, daughter, the social worker, the dean, and a teacher Cynthia had confided in about her bulimia and self-injuring difficulties. Using respectful curiosity, I asked the school social worker, "Is there something you are seeing or hearing with Cynthia that is really worrying you that you think we need to immediately attend to?" In response to my question, the social worker suddenly became quite emotional and explained that she had "lost a student to suicide who had had a long history of self-injury" at a former high school where she had worked. Not only did the family, the social worker's colleagues, and I rally around her to comfort her but also after this meeting, she no longer felt compelled to see my client for individual sessions.

Providing a Climate Ripe For Creative Abrasion, Agility, and Resolution

When hosting collaborative meetings, we can optimize the co-generation of multiple high-quality ideas and solutions by striving to provide a safe and ripe climate for the following three critical processes to occur: *creative abrasion, creative agility,* and *creative resolution* (Brandeau, 2014; Coughran, 2014; Justus, 2014). Creative abrasion captures the essence of what happens when we bring together family members, people from their social networks, and professionals from different practice settings. They have quite diverse or disparate ideas, which can set the stage for intense debate, disagreement, and conflict. As facilitators, our job is to use curiosity to explore how the participants' seemingly disparate ideas can be woven together in such a way that multiple high-quality solutions can be co-generated.

With creative agility, families can choose which of the collaborative group's "experiments" they would like to try out over the next week. At the next scheduled collaborative meeting, the family can share the outcome results, have the lead voice in deciding what worked and why, whether any modifications are needed to improve upon certain experiments, or whether to abandon one or all of them.

Creative resolution occurs when the members of the collaborative team are able to hold opposite views in their minds and two or more different avenues for problem resolution. This leads to integrative decision making—that is, the ability to combine disparate ideas and create something new and special together. Solutions emerge through trial and error with their co-constructed solutions or experiments. Thus all members of the collaborative group are generous with sharing their creative ideas, with power and control, and credit for the positive outcomes they co-produced (Hill, Brandeau, Truelove, & Lineback, 2014).

Being a Beacon of Positivity and Hope

One powerful way we help co-create a collaborative context is by serving as *beacons of positivity and hope*. As hosts of collaborative meetings, we need to adopt the mind-set that not only do the attending family members have the strengths and resources to conquer their difficulties, but so do the helping professionals and key resource people from their social networks. They possess the creative expertise to help empower the clients to achieve their desired outcomes. We can find out from the helping professionals and adult social network participants what their past successes have been with similar adolescent and family difficulties or with their own children. These professionals and social network participants often possess certain skills and talents outside of their work or parenting roles, which also can be tapped for co-constructing solutions. Using compliments and cheerleading in collaborative meetings to acknowledge the helpers' and social network participants' support and advocacy between meetings encourages them to persist. Cramer (2014) contends that when we think, speak, and act out of the positive side of the ledger, collaborative meeting participants will feel more hopeful and confident.

Even when there are client setbacks or heated disagreements in our collaborative meetings, we need to help group members see the light in and opportunities these inevitable situations provide for learning and wisdom. In addition, we need to reframe setbacks as an indication that headway had already been made and that disagreements and conflicts among participants indicate how highly committed and invested they are in trying to resolve the adolescent's difficulties. The bottom line is that people do not dig in and fight with one another unless they are invested in the resolution of the dilemma. Branzei (2014) contends that cultivating hope helps imprint and sustain forward momentum in groups.

Encouraging Everyone to Contribute

As the facilitators of collaborative meetings, we need to create an emotionally safe conversational sanctuary that optimizes for group members' risk taking and encourages everyone to have their voices heard. When we or our collaborators pose questions, we should try to solicit as many responses from the group members as possible to keep the conversation going. The more ideas co-generated, the more likely we will come up with multiple high-quality solutions. Research indicates that groups generate many more innovative ideas and make better decisions when their members participate equally in the conversations (Galinsky & Schweitzer, 2015). Ultimately, we need to create a collaborative context where it is all about teamwork and a strong sense of we-ness to achieve desired outcomes that give the group a noble cause to commit to.

Using Multipartiality

Another way we create an emotional safe and trusting climate in collaborative meetings is by using *multipartiality* (Anderson, 1997; Goolishian & Anderson, 1988). Multipartiality consists of validating and honoring everyone's unique perspectives unconditionally, without challenging or privileging our own viewpoints above theirs. When we model this, other members of the group often will listen more intently and treat each other with respect when they have the floor. It also can help loosen up narrow, rigid beliefs some group members may be clinging to about the high-risk adolescent's and family's presenting problems. They may discover that there are multiple ways to view the client's difficulties and none are "more correct" than others.

Persuadability and Reversing Your Position

We need to demonstrate to meeting participants a high level of openness to being persuaded by them to let go of our views, reverse our positions, and to play with and adopt other participants' ideas. According to Pittampalli (2016),

> Being persuadable requires rejecting absolute certainty, treating your beliefs as temporary, and acknowledge the possibility that no matter how confident you are about any particular opinion—you could be wrong. It involves actively seeking out criticism and counterarguments against even your most long-standing favored beliefs. Most importantly, persuadability

entails evaluating those arguments as objectively as possible and updating your beliefs accordingly. (pp. 3–4)

More negative, pessimistic, and pathology-minded meeting participants are often quite surprised when we are willing to embrace their views and recommendations and reverse our original beliefs about the client's situation. Doing so can loosen up their rigid and narrow beliefs about the client's situation and lead to their becoming much more open to combining their ideas with or entertaining the views of other meeting participants.

"Yes . . . And"

Often with complex high-risk adolescent family cases with extensive treatment histories, involved helping professionals, people from the clients' social networks, and even family members can fall prey to either/or thinking about what the problems are and what the solutions should be. This black-and-white way of thinking can set the stage for heated debate and intense conflict over who's right and who's wrong. As facilitators, we need to move group members from their polarized views and positions and model for them the benefits of adopting a *"yes . . . and"* position. This entails inviting group members to think about constructive ways their diverse viewpoints and ideas can be connected to create something special together.

Crafting and Asking Bold and Intriguing Questions

The linguistic construction of the questions we ask can make a big difference in either opening or narrowing the possibilities our collaborators can consider. Therefore, we should avoid questions that produce "either/or" or "yes/no" responses that back listeners into a corner. Instead, ask questions that promote reflective thinking and deeper, more meaningful conversations. Such questions begin with *what, what if, how,* and *why.* Some examples of bold and intriguing questions are as follows:

> (*to the family*) "What are your best hopes from our work together?"
>
> (*to the family*) "What resources and capabilities do you think we need to have in place to empower you to successfully achieve your best hopes?"
>
> (*to the family*) "What if, as a collaborative team, we could pull off a major change you strongly desire beyond your wildest dreams? What would that be and how would it make a big difference with your situation?"

(*to the family*) "What question, if answered, could make the most difference to the future of your situation?"

(*to the family*) "If there was one thing we haven't yet talked about that
you think would give us a better understanding about your family
situation, what would that be?"

(*to the family*) "What would you like to say that has never been said
before to any other providers you have worked with in the past?"

"What needs our attention going forward?"

"What are the advantages and disadvantages of our pursuing that
strategy?"

"How can we support each other in taking the next steps?"

"How can we better stand united as a collaborative team and not
allow tension and conflict to divide us?"

"How can we empower you as a family in the best way possible so that
you know you can always count on us?"

"What obstacles or challenges might come our way, and how will we
tackle them?"

"What are the missing pieces of this problem puzzle that would give
us more clarity and better understanding about this situation?"

"If 'anorexia' could talk to us and join our next meeting, what do you
think it would say about Debbie, her family, and us in general as a
collaborative team?"

"What steps do you think we can take as a collaborative team to
empower Debbie to break free from the clutches of 'anorexia' and
take back control of her life again?"

"Why this problem and what is it a solution for?"

"Why do you think it feels so strained and uncomfortable in our
meeting today?"

"Why do you think we get stuck rehashing the same issues every
meeting? Is there something else more pressing that demands our
attention right now?"

(*to the family*) "What's not being talked about that needs to be talked
about?"

Presenting Your Ideas in a Tentative Way

When hosting collaborative meetings, we need to avoid at all costs presenting our ideas as if they are the TRUTH. By doing so, other members
of the collaborative meeting will be turned off by our ignorance; they
will think we are "know-it-alls" and decide not to attend future meetings
because they will think their views are meaningless to us. Once we have
heard from all members of the collaborative team, we can revisit some
of the earlier shared ideas that resonated with us. We need to share our

thoughts in a tentative way, beginning with qualifiers like: "I wonder if . . ."; "Could it be . . ."; or "I was struck by . . . ."

Employing Suspension

In some collaborative meetings, we are going to have strong emotional reactions to certain group members. This often occurs when the adolescents and their families have made considerable progress but some of the involved helping professionals or even overinvolved extended family members question the changes or still view the high-risk adolescents as "manipulators," "borderlines," and the parents as "incompetent." As we observe these members directly challenging or downplaying family members' progress, our upset feelings will start to rise; negative thoughts will flash like neon signs in our minds toward these group members. We will be tempted to come to our clients' rescue and defend them, but this is a dangerous facilitative move. It can lead group members to feeling that we are hostile and that the collaborative context is not safe. Some members may stop attending, and the conversational flow will come to a screeching halt. Instead, we need to employ *suspension* when these situations occur in our collaborative meetings (Bohm,1996). Suspension consists of first pretending to create a cartoon cloud over our heads and filling it with all of the negative thoughts and feelings we are experiencing. Next, we are to reflect on those thoughts and feelings and what their real source may be ("My clinical knowledge and skills are being questioned," "You don't have as much experience as I have," "I'm right, and you're wrong," etc.). Once we have paused for reflection, we can attempt to formulate questions to ask these more skeptical members of the group, such as:

> "Help me understand how you came to that conclusion. Have you been involved with similar case situations in the past?"
> (*turning to other members of the group to solicit their input*) "Do you have similar concerns as Mr. Hawkins [skeptical group member], or do you currently view Timmy's [identified client] situation differently now?"
> "Is there something specific that you think we have missed in my sessions with the Smiths that you think is critical for us to address?"
> "How will you know when you are less concerned with Timmy's situation?"
> "Now that you [concerned high school dean] discovered that Julia is cutting herself at school again, what would you like me to address with her first?"
> "Do you think this might be related to some negative peer interactions

Julia's encountering or something going on with her family situation?"

Questions like these can open up space for us to find out from even the most negative, pessimistic, and pathology-minded team members important areas that we may never have thought of that need to be addressed to enhance clients' progress and solidify their changes.

Suspension helps us adopt a position of empathic curiosity vis-à-vis other collaborative group members, conveying to them that we are genuinely interested in their views, concerns, and topics to address with mutual clients.

As facilitators, by taking the time to gain a better understanding of negative, pessimistic, and pathology-minded group members' problem explanations and concerns, the more receptive they will be to entertaining alternative viewpoints and co-generating solutions with us.

Using Possibility and Transformational Scenario Planning

With some highly complex, challenging, high-risk adolescent cases, the current collaborative team of professionals involved may be at a loss for what to do. These families may be presenting with *wicked problems* (Camillus, 2015; Weisbord & Janoff, 2007). According to Camillus (2015, p. 53), there are five essential characteristics of wicked problems that render traditional problem solving methods useless:

1. The perceived "problem" is difficult to define.
2. There are multiple, significant stakeholders with conflicting values and priorities who are affected by the perceived problem and responses to it.
3. There are many apparent causes of the perceived problem, and they are inextricably tangled.
4. It is not possible to be sure when you have the correct or best solution; there is no "stopping" rule.
5. The understanding of *what the problem is* changes when reviewed in the context of alternative proposed solutions.[*]

One of the most effective strategies for addressing wicked problems is the future-oriented feed-forward technique of *possibility scenario planning*. This involves having the collaborative team and the family walk

---

[*]Some of my thinking in this chapter was inspired by an article in *Rotman Management Magazine,* published by the University of Toronto's Rotman School of Management (*www.rotmanmagazine.ca*).

backwards from multiple future scenarios of success (see Form 3.1 at the end of the chapter). Since the future has not yet happened, the family–multiple helper system is liberated from a dark, problem-saturated past, mired in conflicts and treatment impasses, and the sky becomes the limit. For Camillus (2015, p. 54), there are two different types of wicked problem scenarios: *multiple possible futures* and *chaotic ambiguity*. With the first wicked problem scenario, he would most likely recommend the following steps to us:

1. The collaborative team and family identify the uncertainties that can affect the future of the adolescent and his or her family.
2. Juxtapose possible future outcomes for each of the uncertainties, preferably two different outcomes for each uncertainty to describe alternative future scenarios that may emerge.
3. As a group, co-develop strategies and action plans for each of the identified scenarios.

The second wicked problem scenario involves having no clarity about what the future may be like and that the best way to predict the future is to create it together. Tormala, Jia, and Norton (2012) found that the potential for a brighter, much-preferred future reality outshines the clients' present state of affairs in that it produces higher levels of arousal in, attention, and commitment from all parties to taking steps to achieving their desired outcomes. A *transformational scenario planning approach* can be employed to help us clearly define the vision of *what* and *where* the family and providers wish for them to be and together identify the key resource people who can serve as catalysts for helping them to achieve their desired outcome (see Form 3.2 at the end of the chapter; Camillus, 2015). The three-step process Camillus (2015, p. 56) recommends is as follows:

1. Visualize and describe together the desired future state the family would like to have.
2. Identify the key resource people or catalysts that can bring about the desired future state.
3. Develop a plan for supporting the key resource people or catalysts to be able to create the desired future state.

It is important to note that catalysts selected for this transformational planning process can be from outside our clients' social networks and be known in their communities as possessors of special knowledge and expertise for resolving the types of difficulties our clients are struggling with.

Making Room for Celebrating What We Have Appreciated in Our Work Together

Throughout the course of our work with the collaborative team, we need to make room for sharing with one another what we have appreciated about our working together. Family members can be invited to share the memorable things they greatly appreciated the involved helpers saying or doing for them within and outside the meetings. Research indicates that we are hardwired to remember being acknowledged, which helps to further strengthen the cooperative relationships of the members of a collaborative group and retain their continued and committed investment in the ongoing problem-solving effort (Galinsky & Schweitzer, 2015). The case example below nicely illustrates this.

I once worked with an adopted highly oppositional African American 14-year-old girl and her single mother. In our initial family therapy session, the mother described giving her daughter a harsh whipping with her belt and leaving visible marks on her body. Not only did this mother courageously agree to report herself to child protective services but also she committed to learning new parenting strategies and attending future sessions with me. When the child protective worker came to our third family session, she gave the mother a glorious review about how "responsible" she was and "working so hard to be an even better parent." She further added how my client was a "refreshing change" for her in that she frequently had to "chase after other parents to go to counseling." The mother had a big smile on her face and thanked the worker for being "so kind, considerate, and caring" both on the telephone with her and in this family session. She went on to say that the worker had given her hope that she could be a much better parent. The mother also thanked the worker for periodically checking up on her daughter's school performance and behavior. She had attributed the worker's school monitoring to her daughter's doing better in school. The worker gave the mother all of the credit for her daughter's dramatic school turnaround.

We can amplify and solidify everything that is mutually shared and all of the positive outcomes due to hard work together. We can use future-vision questions to have group members speculate what the families' compelling future realities will look like as they continue to make progress.

Possibility Scenario Planning

Directions: As a team, collaborate on listing three positive and three negative future scenarios for the problem situation. In the second column, write corresponding alternative positive outcomes for each scenario. In the third column, write the steps family members, key social network resources, and involved helping professionals will take to help you achieve a positive outcome.

Future Uncertainties (Positive and Negative)	Alternative Possible Future Outcomes	Steps to Be Taken by (Family Members and the Collaborative Team Members)

Based on Camillus (2015).

Transformational Scenario Planning and Action Steps

Directions: As a team, collaborate on listing four to five outcomes that the family would like to achieve. In the second column, write down what key catalysts (possessors of special knowledge and expertise) should be recruited to help you accomplish these goals. In the last column, write the steps the team and catalysts will take to help your family achieve its desired outcomes.

Desired Future Outcomes	Identified Key Catalysts Needed for Desired Future Outcomes	Steps Taken to Support Family and Catalysts to Achieve Desired Future Outcomes

Based on Camillus (2015).

CHAPTER 4

Collaborative Treatment Team Planning and Goal Setting

The strength of the team is each individual member.
The strength of each member is the team.

—PHIL JACKSON

Often, high-risk adolescents and their families have had extensive treatment histories. In many of these past treatments, providers were the privileged experts who decided what was *best* when it came to goal setting and treatment planning. As a result, the clients either dropped out of treatment or experienced one negative treatment outcome after another, becoming demoralized and highly pessimistic. Placing these therapy veterans in the expert position is at the heart of families' positive treatment outcomes. They have the lead voices in co-constructing well-crafted, *solution-determined collaborative treatment plans* with us. These plans honor their preferences, theories of change, stages of change, their expectations, treatment goals, and empowers them to choose among therapeutic tools and strategy options that suit them best. In addition, as part of the collaborative treatment planning process, families can decide who participates in sessions. This might include key resource people from their social networks and involved helping professionals from larger systems. Families can decide the frequency of visits and when they feel satisfied and ready to complete treatment. The collaborative treatment plan is fluid and evolves across the course of family therapy. As clients' goals are achieved, new goals and team members may be added as needed. Family members are strongly encouraged to let their therapists and their helpers from larger systems and social networks know how to help at any point in the treatment process.

Depending on a family's preferences and comfort levels, it can be quite advantageous to have the referring person, helpers from larger systems, and people from their social network participate in the treatment process. This offers the family and the therapist a great opportunity to hear from these important individuals their problem explanations, their concerns, attempted solutions, and what their best hopes and ideal outcome pictures are. Most important, they bring to the table added expertise and creativity for co-generating multiple high-quality solutions with the family and the therapist. Finally, they can aid and support family members between sessions with implementation of change strategies to consolidate their gains.

Since well-formulated, small, doable behavioral treatment goals play such a central role in clients' treatment success, I next discuss all aspects of the goal-setting process.

The Art of Well-Formulated Treatment Goals

The most important components of a well-crafted solution-determined collaborative treatment plan are well-formulated, client-defined treatment goals. Well-formulated behavioral treatment goals are small, realistic, doable, and salient. They are the start of something new, not the end of something. As part of the goal-setting process, therapists need to solicit a clear picture from each family member of the *what, how, where, when,* and *who* of goal attainment. This should also include specific action steps and how they will be thinking and feeling differently when they achieve their goals. The more detailed their descriptions are, the more we empower them to get to their desired goal destinations.

An often-neglected part of the goal-setting process is preparing family members for unexpected speed bumps and major obstacles that could prevent them from achieving their goals. Oettingen (2014) has done extensive research on the benefits of *mental contrasting* when it comes to goal setting. This entails having clients focus on the joys and excitement of achieving their goals and having them identify potential obstacles. Next, the clients are asked to spell out the specific concrete steps they will take to successfully manage any obstacles. Oettingen (2014) has developed a four-step mental contrasting model called *WOOP* (Wish, Outcome, Obstacle, Plan).

Below I discuss four categories of solution-based questions that assist clients in establishing well-formulated treatment goals. I cover how to negotiate solvable goals with angry, frustrated, highly pessimistic, and demoralized parents. I also address how to formulate harm reduction goals with adolescents and parents who may be in the precontemplation or contemplation stages of change.

Key Questions for Establishing Client-Generated Small, Realistic Treatment Outcome Goals

The four question categories discussed in this section were developed by Steve de Shazer and his colleagues at the Brief Family Therapy Center (BFTC) in Milwaukee, Wisconsin (de Shazer, 1985, 1988, 1991; de Shazer et al., 2007; Lipchik, 1988). The BFTC team was strongly influenced by the psychotherapeutic wizardry and effective treatment methods of the great hypnotist Milton H. Erickson (O'Hanlon, 1987; O'Hanlon & Weiner-Davis, 1989; Short et al., 2005; Zeig, 1980). Erickson skillfully listened for and embedded in his questions clients' key words, matched word tenses they used, and used their metaphors and belief system material in his conversations with them to rapidly foster cooperative partnerships. He believed that all clients, no matter how disturbing their behaviors or how extensive their treatment histories, strongly desired relief from their difficulties and possessed the necessary strengths and resources to change (Erickson & Keeney, 2006; Havens, 2003; Zeig, 1980).

The Miracle Question

In the spirit of Erickson's playful use of an imaginary crystal ball with clients, de Shazer and his colleagues created the *miracle question* (de Shazer, 1985, 1988, 1991; de Shazer et al., 2007). This is the first question in the list below. The follow-up questions elicit in great detail family members' ideal outcomes in key relationships and all other areas of their lives.

"Suppose all of you go to bed tonight and while you are sound asleep a miracle happened, and all of your difficulties and concerns are completely solved. When you wake up tomorrow, what will each of you notice that is different? How will each of you be able to tell that things are better?"
"How will that make a difference in your relationship with your father?"
"What effect would that change have on you [the father]?"
"What will you be the most surprised with that changed in your daughter's relationship with her mother?"
"What will you [the mother] notice first that is different with Cindy?"
"If your sister were sitting in that empty chair over there, what would

she be the most surprised with that changed in your relationship with her?"

"When you have a 'better attitude' about school, which one of your teachers will faint first?"

"What about you will Mrs. Smith be the most surprised by the day after the miracle happened in her class?"

"What will your friends be the most surprised with that changed with you after the miracle happened?"

"I'm curious, are any pieces of the miracle already happening a little bit now?"

"Wow! Are you aware of how you got that to happen?"

"What else is a little bit better?"

Presuppositional Questions

Presuppositional questions are rooted in the work of Milton H. Erickson (de Shazer et al., 2007; Havens, 2003; O'Hanlon, 1987; O'Hanlon & Weiner-Davis, 1989; Zeig, 1980). This category of questions embeds presuppositional words like *when, will, going,* and *did* to raise family members' confidence, expectancy, optimism, and hope. For example, Erickson once consulted with a client deemed schizophrenic with an extensive treatment history. With a strong sense of confidence, he looked into the client's eyes and said, "How surprised *will* you be *when* you completely change in one week's time?" The client was surprised and empowered by such an uplifting prognosis, which dramatically countered everything he had heard from past psychiatrists and therapists. Erickson's powerful words propelled him into actively turning his life around and committing to staying out of psychiatric hospitals (Havens, 2003). Presuppositional questions are quite versatile and can be used as an alternative to using the miracle question for goal setting; for consolidating family members' gains; to get unstuck when treatment is at a standstill; and for goal maintenance and relapse prevention purposes. Below are examples of presuppositional questions that can be used to establish clients' treatment goals.

"In the first part of our session I want to get to know you all better and learn more about what brought you here today. After that, we're going to talk about solutions and change, where you want to be when we have a successful outcome here. Tell me, what will be the first sign that will tell each of you we're on the road to success?"

"Let's say our session today turns out to be beyond each of your wildest dreams. When you leave my office today, what will each of you notice that has changed and is much better with your situation?"

"Let's say I handed each of you my trusty imaginary crystal ball and you are gazing into it over the next week. What steps will we see each of you take that will make your situation better?"

"How will you be viewing yourself and feeling differently about your situation when you pull that off?"

"What else are you going to do over the next week to further improve your situation?"

"Tommy, which will you straighten up first in your bedroom—your desktop or under your bed?"

"Let's say we were to run into one another 6 months down the road at the shopping mall, after we successfully completed counseling together. The three of you notice me from a distance and run up to me to share the great news about how well you are doing together as a family. What will I be the most surprised to hear? What next? What specifically will the three of you tell me you had done to pull that off?"

"Let's say I asked you to walk back with me from the future to help me better understand the steps you took to have a better relationship with your mother. What specifically will you tell me you did to get your relationship with her to such a great place?"

"Steve, what if your former probation officer and high school dean were to see us talking together at the mall and joined us in our nice conversation? What great news will you share with each of them that will really blow their minds?"

"Tammy, slips are like great teachers. Tell me, what did you learn from that slip on Tuesday that you will put to good use the next time you are faced with a similar stressful situation?"

Best Hope Questions

Best hope questions can be used in combination with the miracle question when setting goals with families (George, Iveson, & Ratner, 1999; Iveson, 2003; Ratner et al., 2012). The question according to Iveson (2003) is, "What are your best hopes out of our work together?" He adds, "To the client, come several important messages: the therapist's belief that the client's agenda is paramount, that the client has agreed to the meeting for a purpose and, perhaps most important of all, the therapist has put him or herself entirely in the hands of the client since no one else in the entire universe can answer this question" (p. 62).

Often, families respond to best hope questions in a similar fashion to the miracle question. They move forward in their chairs, may smile, and appear eager to share what they really want for themselves and their key relationships. Some examples of best hope questions are the following:

"What are your best hopes from our work together?"
"What will your everyday lives be like when your best hopes happen?"
"What are you already doing or have done in the past that in some
    way contributes to making your best hopes happen?"
"How will each of you know that you have taken further steps toward
    making your best hopes happen?"

Scaling Questions

Steve de Shazer and his colleagues developed *scaling questions* to aid clients in identifying small, realistic behavioral goals they wish to achieve
(de Shazer, 1988, 1991; de Shazer et al., 2007; Ratner et al., 2012). We
can use scaling questions to rate the following with our clients: whether
their situations are better enough compared with past points in time or
an imagined future point; specific behaviors and interactions they wish to
see changed compared to time periods in the past; and their hope, confidence, commitment, and readiness to terminate therapy. Some examples
of scaling questions are presented below.

"On a scale of 1 to 10, where would you rate your situation today,
    with 10 being better enough and 1 being a need for a little more
    fine-tuning?"
"At a 7! Wow! Are you aware of how you got up to a lucky 7?"
"Is that different for your son to do that?"
"Are you aware of what you did that helped pave the way for him not
    to lose his temper with you?"
"Billy, what are you telling yourself to not blow up with your mother?"
"Can you think of anything that she is doing differently that is help-
    ing the two of you get along better?"
"Billy, you rated your situation at an 8 and Carolyn [the mother], you
    rated things at a 7. What will each of you do over the next week to
    get up to a 9 and 8, respectively?"
"So, on a scale from 1 to 10—where 1 means when you decided to seek
    help and 10 means the day after the miracle—where would you say
    you're at today?"
"At a 3, 4 [the parents], and 6 [the adolescent], respectively. (*to the
    parents*) Why not lower ratings?"
"So your son's cleaning his bedroom was a personal first for him! Are
    you aware of how you got him to do that?"
"Is that different for you to go a few days without nagging him?"
"Tim [the father], what specifically have you been doing to prevent
    Tommy [the son] from slipping below a 4?"
"Over the next week, when the three of you take steps upward to a 4,

5, and 7, respectively, on your scales, what specifically will each of you tell me you did to make that happen?"

"So, 4 weeks ago, you and Camille were at a 1 and 2, respectively, with your arguing. Where were you on that scale 2 weeks ago?"

"Wow! At a 5 and 6. What steps did each of you take to make that happen?"

Negotiating Solvable Treatment Goals with Angry, Frustrated, Demoralized, and Highly Pessimistic Parents

Often, parents or legal guardians of high-risk adolescents come to us with extensive treatment histories of feeling misunderstood and mismanaged by past therapists and treatment program providers. Some of these parents or legal guardians and their families would not have made it to our offices if it were not for powerful larger systems representatives that can enforce compliance with treatment by threatening dire consequences. I discuss below how to build rapport and negotiate solvable goals with angry, frustrated, demoralized, and highly pessimistic parents.

Angry and Frustrated Parents

Angry and frustrated parents or legal guardians need plenty of floor time to share their long, problem-saturated stories on the treatment circuit with their challenging adolescents. They may test our patience by being hostile or defensive with us. It is important not to personalize their verbal assaults or get defensive with them, but instead to be a generous listener and validate them. We also need to find out from them the details regarding what former therapists and treatment program providers did that upset them, as well as what they had missed or failed to resolve that we need to attend to. One of the major challenges with angry and frustrated parents is their strong desire to see multiple problematic adolescent behaviors changed all at once. Family therapists get into trouble with these parents by trying to convince them that it is only possible to change one behavior at a time. We need to adopt a compromising position and see if we can reduce the number of problematic behaviors down to three or four. We can establish multiple scales with them when initiating the goal-setting process (George et al., 1999).

The case example below illustrates how to collaboratively establish multiple scales with Barbara, an angry and frustrated African American single parent of Don, a 16-year-old male juvenile offender with an extensive treatment history. Barbara had grave difficulties entertaining the likelihood of miracles happening or thinking her best hopes would ever be realized. Even when asked how she had prevented the situation from getting much worse with Don and what kept her from seeking help for him, she could not identify anything that was working for her or her son. In addition, Don was boycotting our first family session, despite my outreach efforts to get him to come.

BARBARA: I really can't take this much more! He is a nightmare to live with!

THERAPIST: What specifically would you like to change first with him?

BARBARA: He's got to stop smoking weed, swearing at me all of the time, coming in at 2 or 3 A.M., get his homework done because his teachers are calling me all of the time about his missing assignments, his bedroom looks like a pig sty, and I am sick of all of his lying bullshit!!!!

THERAPIST: Out of Don's six upsetting behaviors are there three or four that you think are most pressing to change first?

BARBARA: Yes. What I want to see changed first are his smoking weed, incessant swearing at me . . . I am going to crack him in the mouth if he keeps doing it . . . respecting my midnight curfew time for him on the weekends, and staying on top of his homework. His teachers are constantly calling me about this.

THERAPIST: So, let me get this straight with you: you would like to see Don stop smoking weed, stop swearing at you, respect his curfew time, and stay on top of his homework. Am I correct?

BARBARA: Yes. I am so sick and tired of him not respecting me and putting up with all of his crap! If he doesn't start immediately to turn it around, I am sending him to his father's house to live!

THERAPIST: OK, so what I would like us to do is create four scales so I have a better sense of where these behaviors have been in the past and ideally what small signs of progress in these problem areas over the next week will look like. So let us call Scale A "Not Smoking Weed," with 10 being not at all and 1 being all of the time; Scale B "Not Swearing at Me," with 10 being not at all and 1 being all of the time; Scale C "Respecting My Curfew Rule," with 10 being all of the time and 1 being not at all; and Scale D "Staying on Top of His Homework," with 10 being all of the time and 1 being not at all. How does that sound?

BARBARA: Great.

THERAPIST: So a month ago, where would you have rated his smoking weed, swearing at you, respecting your curfew time, and staying on top of his homework?

BARBARA: I would say they were all at 1 a month ago.

THERAPIST: How about 2 weeks ago on all of the scales?

BARBARA: I would say with the weed he moved up to an 8.

THERAPIST: Are you aware of how you got him up to an 8?

BARBARA: Well, he just spent a week in the juvenile detention center for violating his probation after I let his probation officer know that he was still smoking weed.

THERAPIST: Is that different for you to take a tough stance with him and notify his probation officer like that?

BARBARA: Well, yes. I just decided that enough is enough and he needs to take responsibility for his poor judgment.

THERAPIST: Did that surprise him that you took such a tough stance with him?

BARBARA: Yes, he told me he was pissed off at me, but I told him I'm not going to mess around anymore.

THERAPIST: (*Reaches over to feel Barbara's bicep muscle.*) Wow! What is your consultation fee? I work with a lot of single mothers who could benefit from a consultation with you about how to be tough with their kids and flex their muscles.

BARBARA: (*Laughs and smiles.*) Yes, I felt good about what I did.

THERAPIST: How about with his swearing, respecting his curfew time, and staying on top of his homework—where would you have rated his improvement in those areas 2 weeks ago?

BARBARA: At 4 with the swearing, at 6 with the curfew situation, and at 5 with the homework.

THERAPIST: Are you aware of how you got him up to 4, 6, and 5, respectively?

BARBARA: Well, as you put it, I have been "flexing my muscles" more lately with him and enforcing his probation contract and my household rules. In fact, last weekend he was grounded for sneaking out of his bedroom window and going to a rave party late on a school night. He is afraid if he gets busted with the weed, he will go back into the juvenile detention center. With the homework, he knows that his probation officer will be visiting his school to check up on his grades and behavior there. It seems like he is thinking more about this.

THERAPIST: I love the way you are "flexing your muscles" in all of these important areas by holding him accountable for his actions. What is your secret to maintaining your toughness and consistency with him lately?

BARBARA: Well, I know that if I sent him to live with his dad it would be really awful. His dad has never been there for him. He's a real loser! He's a drunk and used to be violent toward me; that is why I divorced him. I guess I want to see if I can spare him from having to face that.

THERAPIST: Wow! What a loving and caring mother you are to realize you could provide a much better reality for Don in your home. You also have come to the realization that consistently setting limits and being tough with your son is good for him and a loving parental act. So let me ask you this, over the next week, what affect would Don's taking steps upward on scales A to a 9, C to a 7, and D to a 6 have on scale B?

BARBARA: Well, I think the swearing problem will improve the more I continue to be tough with him by taking away privileges and grounding him. Oh, I forgot to mention watching my own swearing at him.

THERAPIST: Anything else you are going to do to help pave the way for him to get up to that 9, 7, 6, and a 5 with the swearing?

BARBARA: No.

THERAPIST: I forgot to ask do you anticipate any bumps in the road or obstacles that might get in the way of your achieving your goal over the next week?

BARBARA: Well, if I find weed in the house or if I get multiple calls from his teachers about missing assignments, it will be hard for me to remain calm with him, to say the least.

THERAPIST: So what steps will you take to stay on track heading upward on the scales with Don even if these upsetting unexpected speed bumps or obstacles attempt to derail you?

BARBARA: Well, like I said before, "be tough, flex my muscles," and hold him accountable for his actions by enforcing my consequences and letting his probation officer know.

As readers can see, it is possible to work on multiple goals simultaneously with parents who have difficulty picking one goal to work on at a time. By using multiple scales we were able to identify some important sparkling moments of Barbara's parental toughness and consistent limit setting. The scales made her much more aware of her ability to positively influence and change her son's problematic behaviors. Although her son's problematic behaviors initially appeared to be separate issues, she also could see they were interconnected. A change in one or more of these behaviors could change the others. I used mental contrasting with Barbara to cover the back door if unexpected obstacles to goal attainment cropped up (Oettingen, 2014). This provided her with a great opportunity to identify what specific action steps she planned to use if Don should choose to push her buttons with flare-ups of problematic behaviors. The good news was that Barbara eventually succeeded in changing all of these behaviors with her son and he was spared from having to live with his father.

Demoralized and Highly Pessimistic Parents

Demoralized and highly pessimistic parents or legal guardians experience a strong sense of hopelessness and despair after years of unsuccessful treatment for their adolescents. Often, these parents have difficulty responding to the miracle, presuppositional, and best hope questions. As an attempt to cooperate better with their pessimism, it can be helpful to ask them *coping questions* (Berg & Miller, 1992; de Shazer et al., 2007). The case example below illustrates how to use coping questions with the demoralized and highly pessimistic white parents of their 14-year-old adopted daughter, Mary, with a long treatment history of explosive and out-of-control behaviors.

THERAPIST: It sounds like Mary can really drain the life out of you with her challenging behaviors, but tell me, what steps have you taken to prevent this situation from getting much worse?

JILL: Well, I've been walking away lately and not allowing myself to get sucked into power struggles with her.

THERAPIST: Is that different for you to "walk away" and not "get sucked into power struggles" with her?

JILL: Yes, typically I cave in and allow her to walk all over me.

THERAPIST: How did Mary respond?

JILL: She looked really surprised that I refused to be her verbal punching bag.

THERAPIST: What else are you doing to prevent the situation with Mary from really escalating and getting much worse?

JILL: Well, Chip [Jill's husband] and I are getting a little bit better at backing one another up when dealing with Mary's meltdowns.

THERAPIST: What effect has your parental teamwork had on reducing the frequency of Mary's meltdowns?

CHIP: Well, they are happening a little less and with shorter durations when she sees that we stand united. However, when they do occur they are really intense!

THERAPIST: It sounds like the two of you are a dynamic duo! We should anticipate that there would be tests to see just how strong your parental teamwork is, so keep standing united! Of those two parenting areas where you appear to be making some good headway, which one or would you want to work on? Or do you want to work on both simultaneously?

JILL: Both. If I can learn additional ways to not to get lead-footed with Mary when she pushes my buttons that would be great.

CHIP: I don't have that problem with Mary, but I think having better teamwork with Jill could help.

THERAPIST: Do either of you anticipate any bumps in the road or other major challenges that Mary might pull that could derail you in achieving your goals?

JILL: Well, I can imagine her catching me off guard and trying to drag me into a power struggle with her.

THERAPIST: So, what are two things you can do to not let that happen?

JILL: I can walk away or lock myself up in my room and read my book until it is time to get dinner together.

THERAPIST: Chip, what bumps in the road or obstacles do you think might try and trip the two of you up?

CHIP: Well, I can imagine that Mary will attempt to divide us when we are standing united. She is very clever in picking up on any differing opinions regarding how to manage her.

THERAPIST: So, what are two things you and Jill can do to not let that happen?

CHIP: Go in a separate room to deliberate until we agree on the best strategy to pursue with or consequence to give Mary. Also, I guess if Jill gets hooked and lead-footed with Mary, I can take over as the main disciplinarian.

Once I shifted gears and better cooperated with the parents' pessimism by asking coping questions, I learned about some of their very effective parenting moves. It gave the parents hope to realize that they have more control over the situation than they originally thought. Earlier in the session, when asked about pretreatment changes, the parents had not mentioned new parenting strategies or as part of their ideal miracle scenarios. The parents decided that the goals they wanted to pursue were to get even more proficient at doing what they found was working and do it more often. Finally, using mental contrasting, I had the parents identify possible bumps and obstacles that might derail and how to manage them if they should crop up (Oettingen, 2014). The couple did a nice job of identifying the concrete steps they will take to stay on track.

Some demoralized and highly pessimistic parents do not respond well to coping questions and we must shift gears again and use *pessimistic questions* (Berg & Miller, 1992; de Shazer et al., 2007). Pessimistic questions exaggerate the parents' pessimistic position and can increase the intensity of parents' need to take action to prevent the dire from happening to their kids. Treatment goals can take the form of preventive action steps. Examples of pessimistic questions are as follows:

"Let's say a police officer rings your doorbell at 4 A.M. Sunday morning to tell you that your daughter is no longer alive. What effect would that have on both of you individually?"

"How about on your marital relationship?"

"What would you miss the most not having Cara around anymore?"

"Who will attend her funeral?"

"What would the eulogies be?"

"If we could help prevent this tragic situation from happening, what is one step that you have never taken before that may be worth trying and possibly could help at least a little bit?"

"Some parents in your situation would have thrown in the towel with counseling a long time ago. What keeps you going?"

"What else keeps you hanging in there?"

"Some parents in your situation may have put their son in a group home or military school, tried to make him a ward of the state, or better yet, put him up for adoption. What has stopped you from pursuing those options?"

"You say that you love him and you could not do that to him. In what ways have the two of you conveyed your love to him lately?"

"How else?"

"What would be a tiny baby step he could take over the next week that would give you a glimmer of hope?"

"How about with the two of you—is there a tiny step the two of you could take over the next week that you think could help a little bit?"

Another category of goal-setting questions to ask demoralized and highly pessimistic parents is *subzero scaling questions* (Selekman, 2005, 2009; Selekman & Beyebach, 2013). These illogical questions are quite effective with depressed and suicidal veteran therapy clients. They help increase awareness of their coping abilities, resourcefulness, and resilience. The case example below illustrates how to increase hope using subzero scaling questions with Olivia, the highly pessimistic mother of Melanie, a 16-year-old with an extensive treatment history for depression, self-injury, and bulimia.

THERAPIST: Where would you have rated your situation a month ago on a scale from –1 to –10 with –10 being your situation is totally hopeless and irresolvable and –1 being that you have an inkling of hope your situation can improve a little bit?

OLIVIA: At –10.

THERAPIST: How about 2 weeks ago?

OLIVIA: At a –7.

THERAPIST: Are you aware of how you got her three steps up higher on that scale?

OLIVIA: Well, lately I have been telling myself not to give up on Melanie.

THERAPIST: Anything else you started doing 2 weeks ago that has also been helping a little bit more?

OLIVIA: I got Melanie to talk to me about her boyfriend breaking up with her.

THERAPIST: Is that different for her to open up to you about things like that?

OLIVIA: Yes, she never tells me about her private matters.

THERAPIST: Are you aware of how you opened up the lines of communications with her?

OLIVIA: Well, I left her a nice loving note in her bedroom expressing my desire to be there to listen to and support her.

THERAPIST: Is that different for you to do that?

OLIVIA: Yes. Typically, I ask her 20 questions and she blows me off.

THERAPIST: Where would you rate your situation with Melanie today?

OLIVIA: I would say at –4.

THERAPIST: Are you aware of how you helped get her up to a –4?

OLIVIA: Well, we have been talking a lot more. I even got her into the kitchen with me and we have been cooking different global cuisines together!

THERAPIST: So, when do you plan to open up your restaurant?

OLIVIA: Ha! We are not that good yet!

THERAPIST: What are you going to do over the next week to get you and Melanie one step higher up to a –3?

OLIVIA: Keep leaving her nice notes around the house, have relaxing conversations with her, and cooking up a storm together!

THERAPIST: Do you anticipate any possible bumps in the road or obstacles to achieving your goal?

OLIVIA: Well, sometimes Melanie will shut down and resist talking with me or hanging out in the kitchen.

THERAPIST: Can you think of anything you did in the past that seemed to help a little bit when she shuts down and stops communicating with you?

OLIVIA: Yes. I need to be patient and give her breathing room when she shuns contact with me. After a few hours, I can check in with her to see if she might like to hang out together doing something she might like to do, like going shopping. Typically that works.

THERAPIST: The way you skillfully handle that situation reminded me about how teenagers are like cats. If we are patient and wait for them to decide to come to us, they will snuggle up in an affectionate way. Conversely, when we force ourselves on them, they will hiss, scratch, or bite.

OLIVIA: So true!

Through the use of subzero scaling questions, I was able to open up space for Olivia to identify how she was already taking positive steps to turn her situation around with her chronically depressed daughter. In addition, using mental contrasting, I explored with Olivia what potential bumps or obstacles could get in the way of her achieving her treatment goal (Oettingen, 2014). After identifying what they were, I explored with Olivia whether she had any past successful strategies that she might use to move the obstacles out of the way. She came up with a few great ideas to try that had worked in the past.

Strategies for Managing Lack of Goal Consensus among Parents, Adolescents, and Involved Helping Professionals from Larger Systems

In this section, I discuss how to manage clinical situations where there is a lack of consensus goals among parents, their adolescents, the referring person, and other involved helping professionals from larger systems. First, I discuss how to negotiate separate treatment goals with parents and their adolescents in a way that is acceptable to both parties. Second, I discuss how to negotiate realistic and solvable goals with the referring person and other involved helping professionals from larger systems.

Lack of Goal Consensus between Parents and Their Adolescents

High-risk adolescents with extensive treatment histories are notorious for not agreeing to pursue their parents' goals for them. Therapists often needlessly antagonize adolescents by pushing them to commit to their parents' goals for them. This can prevent an alliance from developing with adolescents and leave us little leverage for retaining them in treatment. Therefore, it is most advantageous to establish separate treatment goals and go with whatever the adolescents wish for help with, even if it has nothing to do with the reason for their referral to us. This could be helping get social control agents off their backs; helping them deal with relationship difficulties, including romantic relationships; requesting our help in changing annoying parental behaviors; changing their relationships with their annoying siblings; and fighting for privileges they really want from their parents. A variety of scaling questions can be used to negotiate a small behavioral goal for them to pursue over the next week in line with what they want. We also can explore what positive steps they may be willing to take over the next week that would really blow their parents' minds and make them more open to giving them desired privileges. This has to be done in a delicate, non-pushy way, particularly when adolescents are still in the precontemplation stage of change.

More often than not, parents understand why they and their adolescents don't see eye to eye on the initial treatment goals. Parents may still demand that their adolescents *must* immediately change their most problematic behaviors, even if separate goals are negotiated. In these situations, we can make a commitment to address their concerns during our individual family session time with their adolescents. During this time, we would explore what small sign of progress over the next week would please the parents. In addition, we can explore with the parents whether they have particular behaviors they would like to reduce or eliminate, such as nagging, yelling, making threats, and so forth. Using scaling questions, we can have parents rate these unproductive parenting behaviors currently and prior to entering treatment. Along the way, we can listen for constructive coping and problem-solving strategies they are already using that help even a little bit in curtailing their adolescents' problematic behaviors. Next, we can negotiate a goal with the parents for increasing what works over the next week. Scaling questions can be used to provide a quantitative measurement of one of their parental behaviors both past and present that they are tired of falling prey to and they contend their kids find annoying. The Romeros, a Puerto Rican couple, had brought their highly oppositional 16-year-old daughter, Tanya, in for family therapy for her incessant verbal abuse, temper outbursts, academic decline, marijuana abuse, and breaking of household rules. It proved counterproductive early in the session to see the whole family together due to an intense blame–counterblame interaction pattern between the parents and Tanya. I split them up and met with the parents alone first. Below I demonstrate how to use scaling questions to measure a chronic yelling pattern over time to aid in the goal-setting process. I asked the Romeros to pretend that Tanya was in the empty chair rating their yelling at present and at different times.

THERAPIST: Let's say Tanya was sitting in that empty chair over there and I asked her, "What is the number one behavior your parents engage in that really annoys you the most?" What would she say?

CARLITA: Our constantly yelling at her.

THERAPIST: If we asked her, "Where would you have rated your parents yelling 4 weeks ago on a scale from 1 to 10, with 10 being once in a while and 1 being all of the time?" what would she say?

TOMAS: Probably at a 1.

THERAPIST: How about 2 weeks ago?

TOMAS: I think we have made some progress. I would say maybe at a 4.

THERAPIST: Are you aware of how you got three steps up on that scale?

TOMAS: Well, what would you say honey, I think we have been better at catching ourselves before we speak and trying to regroup with our tempers.

THERAPIST: That's great! Can you think of what specifically you are telling yourselves that helps you not to cave in verbally to blasting Tanya?

CARLITA: Well, I tell myself, "I don't want it to be World War III tonight, I really want peace and quiet after work."

THERAPIST: Wow, I love your thinking there, parental damage control at its best! Anything else the two of you have been telling yourselves or doing differently when Tanya pushes your buttons?

TOMAS: Sometimes I walk away instead of blowing my stack and getting into it with her.

THERAPIST: Just out of curiosity, has Tanya indicated to either one of you that she has noticed, even a little bit, a reduction in your yelling behavior?

TOMAS: No. But she has been more reasonable over the past 2 weeks.

THERAPIST: When you say "more reasonable," what do you mean by that?

CARLITA: Well, she has been a little more cooperative with doing her homework minus the power struggles. Not as nasty with her mouth.

THERAPIST: Where would Tanya rate your yelling behavior today?

TOMAS: Probably at a 6.

THERAPIST: Wow! What do you think is telling her that you are doing much better and got up to a 6?

CARLITA: Well, we have been trying to be more mindful of thinking before responding and sidestepping clashes with her.

THERAPIST: If Tanya were really sitting in that chair over there, what do you think she would say she appreciates the most about what you are doing differently with her now?

TOMAS: Probably not riding her about doing her homework and getting into battles with her about it.

THERAPIST: What are you doing instead with the homework situation?

CARLITA: We are now not saying a word about homework to see if she starts taking charge of it.

THERAPIST: Is that working?

CARLITA: Surprisingly, yes.

THERAPIST: What's your hunch about why it is working?

TOMAS: Probably because when there is no tension and stress, she does better and can be more responsible.

THERAPIST: Good deduction, Tomas. People in general are much better problem solvers and much more creative when not stressed out. So, what do you think Tanya will need to see the two of you do over the next week to rate you one step higher up to a 7?

TOMAS: Probably increasing what we have already told you should get us up to that 7.

THERAPIST: Yes, I was going to share with you the old adage, "If it works, don't fix it." Do more of it! I look forward to hearing next week about what further progress you made and how you got up to that lucky 7!

Once conflicts in their relationships have greatly decreased and the family's emotional climate has become more positive, we can highlight and consolidate their gains. If families wish to establish new mutually agreed-upon treatment goals, we can do it at that stage in the treatment process. This was the case for the Romero family. As the parents greatly reduced their yelling and sidestepped getting into power struggles with Tanya, she became much more cooperative about following their rules, staying on top of homework, and staying away from drug-using friends.

Lack of Goal Consensus between the Referring Person and/or Other Involved Helping Professionals and Families

With many high-risk adolescent cases, the referring person and other involved helping professionals may have highly unrealistic goals for the clients. If not negotiated down into solvable terms, we are setting the stage for these families to experience yet another treatment failure. It is critical that we establish strong partnerships with the referring person and the involved helpers so that it is possible to negotiate more realistic goals and treatment objectives with them. Once family members give verbal or written consent to collaborate with the referring person and other larger system professionals, we need to initiate relationship building and face-to-face meetings with them either individually or as a group. Operating from a position of curiosity, we need learn their stories of involvement with the family, their concerns, expectations, attempted solutions, and best hopes for them. If their goals seem highly unrealistic, too monolithic, or too vague, we need to negotiate more realistic goals. In some cases, this may not be difficult once the referring persons and involved helpers experience with us a strong sense of team, mutual purpose, and commitment to helping out the family in the best way possible. Ultimately, the best way to negotiate more realistic treatment objectives is for the referral sources and involved helping professionals to attend collaborative team meetings with families present. Family members then have the opportunity to give feedback on whether their goals are highly unrealistic. They can also share what specifically they want help with and what their personal goals and needs are.

Negotiating Realistic Harm Reduction Goals

High-risk adolescents who have had long careers of self-injury, eating disorders, substance abuse, video gaming, and consuming cyber-porn often report in initial sessions grave difficulty with pursuing total abstinence treatment goals. Their self-destructive habits have served them well as resources for coping with multiple stressors. They may be in the precontemplation or contemplation stages of change in the very beginning of treatment; they are not in a place to identify their goals and an action plan to conquer their self-destructive habits. These adolescents also may tell us up front that they have been engaging in their self-destructive habits for so long on a daily basis that it would be absolutely impossible for them to go cold turkey. It is a much more realistic goal-setting strategy to adopt a *harm reduction* approach (Marlatt, 1998; Selekman & Beyebach, 2013; Tatarsky, 2007). By reducing the frequency of their self-destructive habits, they and concerned others will concurrently observe a reduction in the physiological, psychological, social, and life consequences as a result of their habits. The biggest challenges are negotiating this with the adolescents, their parents, and also with larger systems professionals like probation officers and actively involved school administrators. Most high-risk adolescents view tapering down or cutting back as a realistic initial goal and much more doable than the total abstinence demanded by parents and involved social control agents. It is helpful to pursue harm reduction goals with adolescents when they report they have lost control and there have been consequences as a result of their habits. We can still help them in other ways they might request while concurrently pursuing harm reduction goals.

One effective way to gently move adolescents toward harm reduction is the *two-step tango* engagement strategy discussed in Chapter 2. With this strategy, we alternate between restraining them from changing, highlighting the benefits of their habits, and planting seeds about the potential costs of continuing their habits. This strategy may move them in the first session from precontemplation to contemplation or even to the preparation stage of change.

We need to go with whatever unique quitting style the adolescents choose to pursue. With heavy to severe self-destructive habits, such as engaging in their habits multiple times per day, a teen might be willing to experiment with include limiting the activity to once or twice a day or even trying to be totally abstinent one day out of seven. Some adolescents who engage in self-destructive habits on a random basis shoot for two or three days of total abstinence. We should encourage them to increase the self-generated coping and problem-solving strategies they are already using on their days of abstinence to experiment with on their goal days. It is important to cover the back door prior to sending them out to pursue their harm-reduction goals. Explore with them potential obstacles that might undermine or derail them. This could include certain people, places, school stress, conflicts with their parents, and other triggers. We can do worst-case scenario planning by writing down each of these major triggers and the steps they can take to stay on track for their harm reduction goals.

We may encounter high-risk adolescents who are cutting themselves and abusing alcohol and other substances—a potentially life-threatening situation! If the adolescents contend that it will be impossible for them to achieve total abstinence at the beginning of treatment and they have long careers of engaging in these self-destructive habits, have them experiment with separating self-injuring from substance abuse. Together with the adolescent, come up with a daily schedule, with different times each day when they can cut themselves and when they use substances. Although this sounds counterintuitive and quite radical, adolescents can discover that they have more self-control over their habits than they originally thought. It helps move them to a place of wanting to pursue harm reduction goals and to begin addressing habit-maintaining stressors.

Identifying and Mobilizing the Collaborative Team for Treatment Planning

The family has the lead voice in determining who the *right* people are to serve on the team, and what the team's priorities are. Families need to regularly give us feedback on whether our teamwork with them is delivering the results they desire. Whenever possible, have the referring person, involved helping professionals, and key members from the family's social networks attend the initial family therapy session. Key people from the social networks can include adult inspirational others of the adolescent (caring teachers and coaches, clergy, a community leader, a very close older cousin or aunt or uncle, an adult friend of the family); one to two close, concerned friends of the adolescent; and other actively involved relatives. In order to involve any of these other people, we must secure signatures from the clients, the friends' parents, the friends, and the adult inspirational others on the significant other consent form (see Form 4.1 at the end of the chapter). Once the team members have been identified, contacted, and have agreed to participate, we will need to be as flexible as possible to accommodate everyone's schedules when scheduling team meetings. Sometimes, it may be necessary to schedule these meetings at other helping professionals' offices in order to ensure their participation, particularly if they wield a great deal of power and play major roles in ensuring that the family is in treatment.

In some cases, families may feel more comfortable meeting alone with their new therapists once or twice before agreeing to have a collaborative team meeting. If this is the case, we can do the legwork and, with their written consent, contact the key individuals they wish to have participating in future scheduled collaborative team meetings. Outside of family meetings, we can try to meet with their identified helping professionals from larger systems and key resource people from their social networks to establish rapport with them, solicit their concerns, and hear their theories of change and best hopes for our individual family therapy work with the clients. I put their parents and adolescents in charge of contacting the adolescent's close friends, their parents, and inspirational others, and securing signatures on the consent forms.

Since collaborative treatment plans are fluid and evolve across the course of treatment, families can have us add other people such as concerned friends to the team. Such people might serve as advocates for them in dealing with oppressive larger systems and with certain challenges they may face in their communities. Including all these important and resourceful others from clients' social ecologies in the treatment process facilitates the rapid co-generation of high-quality solutions. It can also greatly reduce clients' lengths of stay in treatment. Family therapists who work solo and do not have access to an in-house team of colleagues no longer have to be isolated with these challenging, high-risk adolescent cases. We can have solution-determined team members working for us in a variety of social contexts that we don't have regular access to support clients' efforts to conquer their difficulties.

The Mechanics of Hosting and Facilitating Treatment Team Planning Meetings

When hosting and facilitating treatment team planning meetings, it is critical that we provide a comfortable and safe conversational space where everyone's voices are honored. It is best to conduct these meetings in a circle rather than crunched together around a rectangular table where some participants can barely see one another. Indigenous groups around the world conduct their important meetings in circles, which respectfully conveys that all participants are equals and everyone's voice is honored and respected. Research indicates that circle seating in meetings activates people's need to belong, tends to focus them on the group's collective objectives, and persuades them to favor messages and proposals that highlight group benefits rather than the benefits to any one individual (Zhu & Argo, 2013). The type of sacred conversational space we need to strive to provide is a *collaboratory* (Muff, 2015). According to Muff (2015), "A collaboratory is a facilitated space open to everybody, and in particular to concerned stakeholders, to meet on an equal basis to co-create new solutions by drawing on the emergent future. It is a place where people can think, work, and learn together to invent their common futures" (p. 12).

We must be gracious hosts and hostesses and treat the team members like they are our own relatives or close friends making them feel warmly welcomed and comfortable. Let them know how much you appreciate their willingness to set aside time in their busy schedules to come to the meeting and support the adolescent and his or her family. We also need to let them know that they should feel free to chime in when they have ideas, questions, need clarification, and have any specific concerns. The more positive and upbeat we keep the meeting climate, the more likely family members will feel comfortable taking risks and sharing important events and life stories. These will often elicit empathy and compassion, and intensify the desire of other team members to help the family. The other team members might also take risks and share related stories that they or similar clients have encountered and how they dealt with those situations. Social psychology research has indicated that when the positive emotion and optimism in a team meeting is at a moderate level, it opens up the group's minds to alternative views of problems. This helps us to come up with more high-quality, novel solutions for complex problem situations. In fact, working groups with positive emotional climates are three times more likely to find solutions than groups that experience negative emotions when working together (De Dreu, Baas, & Nijstad, 2008; Isen, Daubman, & Nowicki, 1987; Morgan & Barden, 2015).

How we should conduct our first gathering depends on whether the team meeting is also the initial family therapy session. If this is a combined initial family therapy session and team meeting, first establish rapport with everybody around the circle. Then it is most respectful to invite the family members to share their stories of how and why they think they were referred for family therapy. They can explain their problem views, past attempted solutions, their concerns and expectations, and their best hopes for treatment outcomes. The other team members can share their stories of involvement, concerns, and best hopes for the family. If treatment goals have not been set, we can ask the miracle, presuppositional, best hopes, and scaling questions to expand the possibilities. The other members of the team can chime in, including what they will be most pleased and surprised by. We can explore whether any team members have noticed pieces of the miracle already happening. Each pretreatment change can be celebrated, amplified, and consolidated, including how these changes can be increased.

For more pessimistic family and team members, we can cooperate with their pessimism by asking them coping and/or pessimistic sequence questions if necessary. Once this produces something useful to the goal-setting process, we can return back to scaling questions to negotiate small behavioral treatment goals with the family and the other team members.

With more chronic situations, where larger systems professionals are highly pessimistic, frustrated, and have had a long history of involvement with the adolescent and family, it may be helpful to *externalize the problem* (Durrant & Coles, 1991; White, 2007; White & Epston, 1990). Carefully derived from family and team members' descriptions, the adolescent's major presenting problem can be externalized into an oppressive entity that is the real culprit. Once there is consensus about what the group wants to call the externalized problem, we can get the family and other team members fired up to join forces to conquer the problem once and for all! The adolescent can come up with a team name for them. A *habit control ritual* (Durrant & Coles, 1991) can be put in place at home and in every social context where the externalized problem brainwashes the adolescent to get into trouble. Charts can be set up at home, school, or in any other social contexts where the problem preys on the adolescent and his or her relationships with team members and others involved. As a team they are to keep track of their victories over the problem (useful self-talk and coping and problem-solving strategies), as well as the problem's victories over them. It is helpful for the adolescent and team members to get together daily in their respective contexts to reflect on their progress and where they may need to tighten up with the structure, so as to outsmart and weaken the problem. Similar to scaling questions, percentage questions can be used to measure how the family and team currently rate their situation, for example, what percentage out of 100% are they in charge of the problem versus the problem being in charge of them? A goal can be set over the next week or two, along with what steps they will take to be 10% more in charge of the problem. We can continue to monitor all social contexts where the problem typically strikes. The habit control ritual can be a playful and fun therapeutic experiment that not only successfully stabilizes the adolescent's difficulties, but also changes the view of the original problem.

The beauty of hosting these solution-determined collaborative treatment team-planning meetings is hearing all of the creative ideas that members of the team come up with. Often they dovetail nicely into the adolescents' learning styles, key strengths, and talents. For example, a school social worker came up with the idea of having 15-year-old Kim, a white girl with a long history of treatment for bulimia and self-injury, put together an eating disorder prevention project curriculum at their high school. At this particular high school there had been a rash of eating disorders among the female students. Since Kim was a talented writer, interested in psychology, and quite popular with her peers, the school social worker could not think of a better coauthor and more knowledgeable cofacilitator for groups. Kim was thrilled, and her parents and the other participants on our solution-determined collaborative treatment planning team thought this was a great idea.

As facilitators of these team meetings, we should model "yes . . . and" mind-sets and encourage family and fellow team members to look for ways to connect their ideas, coming up with innovative high quality solutions. The case below nicely illustrates the positive cascading effect of encouraging "yes . . . and" in connecting team members' ideas.

The high school football coach was an adult inspirational other of Willie's, a 16-year-old African American gang-involved youth and talented former defensive end for his football team. The coach came up with the idea of having Willie serve as an assistant coach for his summer football camp for elementary school-age children. Coach Spencer shared with all of us that Willie's size, strength, and speed will make him an excellent college football scholarship recruit if he could get back on the team his senior year, break free from the gang, and improve his grades. The probation officer chimed in that by taking the summer job, Willie could fulfill his community service hours that the judge had ordered after Willie had violated his probation. Willie had smiled and said, "That would be sweet working and playing ball again!" Willie's parents thanked Coach Spencer and Mr.

Chandler (the probation officer) for trying to help their son turn his life around and for not giving up on him. Since Willie had a greatly outdated IEP (individualized education plan) with highly unrealistic learning goals and objectives, the attending psychologist, Dr. Flores, who had referred him and his family to me, chimed in that they should have a meeting very soon to update his IEP and put resources in place prior to his senior year to better his chances for academic success and help him to be eligible to play football. Both Willie and his parents thought this would be very helpful and they thanked Dr. Flores for finally doing something about the school situation. What was so beautiful about this whole exchange was that all I did was to help create a safe conversational space for members to adopt a respectful "yes . . . and" position vis-à-vis one another. They spontaneously strung together their wonderful ideas to help Willie get out of the gang and have a brighter future.

The case example of Willie illustrates the transformative power of actively involving the most concerned helping professionals from larger systems and key members from the clients' social network at the very beginning of family therapy. Pentland (2014) has found that the following three factors contribute to successful teamwork and collective intelligence as a group:

1. They co-generated a large number of ideas that were presented in a clear and concise manner.
2. They engaged in "dense interactions," that is, group members constantly were alternating between advancing their ideas and responding to their colleagues' ideas with words like *good, right,* and *tell me more,* which signaled to them consensus on an idea's value, good or bad.
3. All members of the team had equal time to contribute their ideas and reactions to them, respectfully listened to one another, and took turns, which ensured the co-production of a variety of high-quality ideas.

The family has the lead voice in deciding how often the team meets. On average, these 60- to 90-minute meetings typically occur once or twice per month initially. Over time, the team might meet every other month or quarterly, depending on the unique needs of the adolescent and his or her family. If unexpected crises should occur, we may decide to meet more frequently for a time. During periods between team meetings, it is helpful to update team members, particularly the helping professionals from larger systems, on how the adolescent and his or her family are progressing.

Team meetings always begin with highlighting and celebrating clients' positive changes and the pivotal roles played by team members in contributing to the clients' success. As hosting facilitators of the team meetings, it is important that we provide ample space for the family members to share what specifically they appreciated team members doing for them since the previous meeting. It is also nice to invite the team members to share what they appreciate most about the clients' efforts and progress.

With complex, high-risk adolescents who have long-standing, intractable difficulties, we can begin by asking *propelling questions,* such as the miracle or similar *what-if* future-oriented questions. The propelling questions move the team conversation forward into a preferred future and can increase hope and optimism among the team members. Then we can introduce *can–if* inquiry with them (de Shazer et al., 2007; Morgan & Barden, 2015). This consists of inviting team members to act as if the ideas they come up with are possible. Can–if thinking helps the team find solutions for each constraint the clients and they are faced with. Morgan and Barden (2015, pp. 87–96) identify seven different types of can–ifs as frameworks that can empower teams to generate breakthrough solutions:

1. We *can if* we think of it as . . .
2. We *can if* we use other people . . .
3. We *can if* we remove *x* to allow us to *y* . . .
4. We *can if* we access the knowledge of . . .
5. We *can if* we introduce a . . .
6. We *can if* we substitute *x* for *y* . . .
7. We *can if* we resource it by . . .*

Once team members generate a wide range of practical and doable can–if ideas, we can create a *can–if map* that can be put on a flipchart or marker board for all team members to see. They can then develop goals and an action plan together (Morgan & Barden, 2015, p. 98; see Form 4.2 at the end of the chapter).

Working with Families Who Initially Don't Wish to Pursue the Collaborative Team Format

All is not lost if the family wishes to meet a few times without including others. We need to respect their concerns and move forward with the goal-setting and treatment-planning process with them alone. Consent forms can be signed to give us permission to separately collaborate with

---

*Reprinted with permission from *A Beautiful Constraint: How to Transform Your Limitations Into Advantages, and Why It's Everyone's Business.* Copyright ©2015 John Wiley & Sons. All rights reserved.

the referring person and other involved helping professionals. This way we can build relationships with them, hear their stories of involvement, and develop best hope goals for the adolescent and the family. The family has to determine who in their social networks they would feel comfortable having us collaborate with and who can be most helpful with the change effort.

Sometimes, families feel more comfortable after a few family therapy sessions and are willing to include an involved helper or two and possibly a key resource member from their social network in our meetings. Adolescents particularly like having their adult inspirational others and even a few of their closest friends come in and support them.

Some families of high-risk adolescents do not wish to have other involved helping professionals and concerned members from their social networks participate in their family sessions. One of the major reasons is due to long-standing antagonistic relationships with them. In spite of our best efforts in explaining why it is helpful to include these powerful people, families may still balk at the idea. In Chapter 3, I discussed effective strategies for how to resolve these long-standing conflicts.

The Solution-Determined Collaborative Treatment Plan: The Bishops

I next present the Bishop family case to illustrate how to co-construct a solution-determined collaborative treatment plan.

DeSean, a 14-year-old African American youth, had been court-ordered for family therapy after having spent 3 months in a juvenile detention facility for armed robbery and repeated assault and battery charges. While in the juvenile detention center, DeSean had gotten into a few fights, which he contended were in self-defense. He claimed it was "really awful in there" and declared to all of us that he plans "never to go back there again!" I underscored his conviction and stressed that we were all at this meeting to empower him to move forward with his life and not have to go back to places like that. DeSean had been in and out of treatment since age 8 for anger management difficulties, fighting, and gang involvement. His father was in jail for murder and his mother had lost custody of DeSean and his 12-year-old brother, Wallace, due to physical abuse and chronic difficulties with heroin abuse. The boys' aunt and uncle, Mr. and Mrs. Bishop (the mother's older sister), had assumed legal guardianship of them. The Bishops have had custody for 3 years.

Present on the Bishops' hand-picked team were the following individuals: Mr. Knight, DeSean's probation officer; Pastor Livingston, their spiritual leader; Carolyn, DeSean's favorite 25-year-old cousin; Ms. Cortez, DeSean's middle school social worker; and DeSean's favorite teacher, basketball coach, and adult inspirational other, Mr. Stinson. After getting acquainted, all members of the team, including the Bishops and DeSean, shared their problem stories, obstacles for change they were faced with, and their desired outcomes. Some team members asked, "How do we keep DeSean away from his gang and prevent further police involvement when some of his friends are gang members? What steps can be taken to help DeSean get caught up in school and do better academically?" DeSean asked, "How can I control my anger better when it has always been a problem for me?"

Later in the meeting, these constraint questions were revisited in a can–if action map (see Figure 4.1). The team members then responded to best hopes and miracle propelling questions. Mrs. Bishop shared that in her miracle for DeSean he would be staying out of trouble with the law, not getting into fights, going to church with them on Sunday mornings, and doing better in school by studying for tests and completing his homework. Mr. Bishop wanted the same and was looking forward to seeing DeSean be the starting point guard this coming season and on his high school varsity basketball team in the future. DeSean's current middle school basketball coach and inspirational other, Mr. Stinson, shared with him and the group that he was friendly with Mr. Bridgewater, the high school basketball coach and had already put in the good word for him about his star potential. DeSean perked up and asked, "What did he say?" Mr. Stinson responded, "Mr. Bridgewater said he planned to check you out this season and watch some of your games because he needs a good point guard on the varsity team next year." DeSean had a big smile on his face and all members around the circle smiled and some cheered him on with encouragement about this being a great goal for him to strive for. Again, Mr. Bishop shared enthusiastically, "I can't wait to see you out there! I will grab courtside seats!" DeSean started laughing and told his uncle to "chill" because he felt he was embarrassing him. Mr. Stinson added that he would always be there with support for DeSean and that before this year's basketball season had begun he would be willing to work with him at least three times per week after school on his basketball fundamentals and "further fine-tuning" his "field goal shooting" to help him to score more 3-point baskets. DeSean voiced a strong desire to do this with him. Mr. Knight's miracles for DeSean were for him to steer clear from his gang, no more arrests, stop the fighting with his peers, do better in school, and follow the Bishops' house rules. He also shared his desire to see him continue to excel as a basketball player this season and next year at the high school. DeSean openly admitted that he had a "short fuse" with his anger and felt it was difficult for him to maintain self-control. When asked how he saw himself successfully managing his anger in his miracle picture, he couldn't imagine this happening. Ms. Cortez, his school social worker, chimed in she could teach him some mindfulness meditations and related practices to help him to stay calm and not react to his anger. DeSean agreed to try that out with her. She also planned to offer him additional counseling support and arrange a school collaborative meeting with all of DeSean's teachers. They would come up with a catch-up plan, since he had fallen way behind and was failing some of his classes. All team members were invited to attend the school meeting once it was scheduled. For Pastor Livingston, the miracle question sparked some highly practical solutions for keeping DeSean off the streets and away from the gang during his free time. Five elderly congregation members needed some help with their yard work. Apparently, they were willing to pay whomever the pastor lined up to do

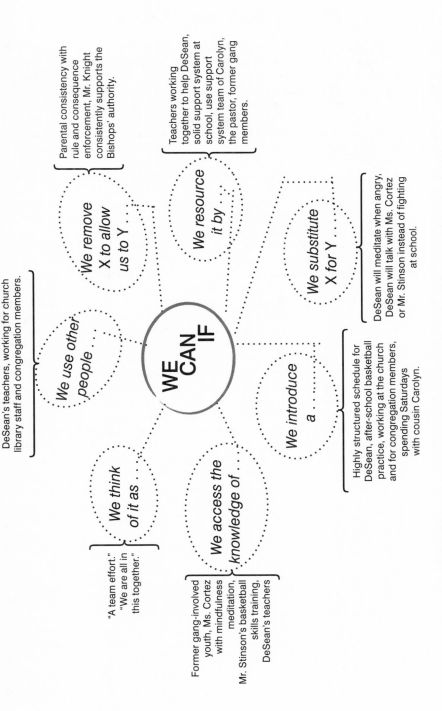

FIGURE 4.1. The Bishop family can-if map. Based on Morgan and Barden (2015).

the job. The pastor also needed help with straightening up the church library, for which he could pay DeSean. DeSean liked the idea of being able to earn money. Mr. Knight chimed in, "That sounds great! You will learn how to earn money legally. By the way, the judge likes to hear that his people are taking responsibility like this, particularly when it comes to helping out the elderly in the community." DeSean smiled. Finally, Carolyn shared that in her ideal miracle picture she and DeSean would reinstate their Saturday morning breakfasts again and either go to a movie or shop together in the afternoons. She added how much she had missed hanging out with DeSean and that he could always text her if he needed support with anything. Apparently, they had not done this for a year. DeSean made a commitment to Carolyn in our meeting to reestablish their tradition.

For additional support with helping DeSean steer clear from his gang, I presented the idea to him and the team of bringing two former gang-involved clients from his neighborhood to one of our family sessions or an individual session with him. They were 18 and 19 years old, respectively, now working and going to a junior college. DeSean, the Bishops, and the other team members thought this was a great idea. After we reviewed team members' and the family's goals, the Bishops and DeSean requested that I help them out with parenting skills, improving their family communications, and help him to better manage his anger, stop the fighting, and steer clear from his gang. Prior to adjourning, we briefly discussed concretely with team members how they would constructively manage any obstacles they might encounter to achieving their goals. Following this discussion, I shared with the team members that I would be checking in weekly with them to hear about what further progress they were making toward achieving their mutually agreed-upon goals and assist with any unexpected challenges. These may occur while implementing their action steps and/or plans. DeSean had the final words. He thanked everyone around the circle for coming and being there for him. I put our team's can–if action map up on a white marker board, which visually captured the team members' ideal miracles and paved the way for my writing up the solution-determined collaborative treatment plan.

By putting clients in charge of who should comprise solution-determined collaborative team membership and by using a team approach, a dynamic and synergistic effect occurs among team members, which leads to the co-generation of novel ideas and multiple high-quality solutions. In DeSean's case, our caring and creative team members were able to come up with a highly structured plan that filled up his free time and helped steer him away from the gang and from making poor choices in and outside of school. There was excellent representation on the team from every larger system he interfaced with. Because of this we were able to cover all the bases for optimizing DeSean's future success. An added bonus provided by Pastor Livingston was scheduling DeSean to help elderly people with their yard work, with the hope that he would find meaning and purpose in caring for others. An integrative family therapy approach was used that blended together the best elements of multisystemic, functional, multidimensional, and collaborative strengths-based family therapies. This enhanced the Bishops' parental unity and consistency with rule and consequence enforcement, improved family communications, and helped strengthen their parental bonds with DeSean. Individual session time in our family meetings strengthened my alliance with DeSean and increased his motivation and commitment to further hone his use of mindfulness, visualization, and other emotional distress tolerance skills to resolve his anger management and fighting difficulties. When DeSean was living with his heroin-addicted mother, the family situation was chaotic, she and her multiple transient boyfriends were physically abusive toward him, there were no rules, and he had experienced a great deal of emotional invalidation and disconnection in their relationship, which eventually led to DeSean's joining his gang to feel a strong sense of belonging, validation, and empowerment. When DeSean began living with the Bishops there was initially much limit testing because he was not used to rules, structure, or being nurtured by parental figures. It was like a roller coaster ride. There were times when DeSean displayed tremendous impulse control and walked away from potential fights or invitations to hang out with gang members. Then there would be an occasional fight at school or he would sneak out at night and rendezvous with his gang "homies" after a rumble with a rival gang led to a police arrest and a weekend in the juvenile detention center. Mr. Knight wanted DeSean to know that he would enforce his probation contract and would back up the Bishops' rules with hard consequences.

Once everyone's goals and action plans are clearly and concretely articulated, we write them up as a solution-determined collaborative treatment plan (see Figure 4.2). All team members sign and date it to make it into an official contract. Each team member receives a copy. Since the team members had come up with so many great ideas, there was no need to add therapeutic tools or strategies to the Bishops' solution-determined collaborative treatment plan. In future family therapy sessions, the Bishops are offered a wide range of therapeutic tools and strategies to assist them in achieving their goals. Over time, DeSean eventually broke free from his gang, since he now had a healthy family environment and had the drive and the strong determination to create a better future.

In the next chapter, I present a transtheoretical comprehensive resource guide for selecting specific therapeutic interventions for specific types of adolescent, parental, and family difficulties. This classification system of therapeutic interventions can help family therapists hosting team meetings select appropriate interventions to recommend and build into the co-developed treatment plan.

Parents' Goals:

1. Consistently enforce our household rules with DeSean.
2. Consistently impose and enforce our consequences for violation of our rules, not doing homework, getting into trouble at school for fighting, and for any gang and police involvement.
3. Will report to Mr. Knight problems with DeSean's household rule compliance, completion of schoolwork, fighting problems, and any gang and police involvement.
4. DeSean will attend church services with us every Sunday morning.

DeSean's Goals:

1. I will commit to respecting my uncle and aunt's household rules, regularly doing my schoolwork, avoid getting into fights, and stay away from my gang and police involvement.
2. I will accept any consequences I should receive for violation of any rules, for not doing my homework, for fighting, and any gang or police involvement.
3. I will commit to learning and practicing the mindfulness meditations and other coping tools that Ms. Cortez and Matthew teach me to better manage my anger and not fight with my peers.
4. I will seek out Ms. Cortez or Mr. Stinson to talk instead of losing my temper or when provoked to fight by peers at school.
5. I will commit to having Saturday morning breakfasts and spending afternoon time with cousin Carolyn.

Ms. Cortez's Goals:

1. Teach DeSean mindfulness meditations and related practices to help him better manage his anger and reduce the likelihood of him getting into fights.
2. I will make myself available daily when DeSean would like to talk or needs additional support with provoking peers and teachers he is having problems with.
3. Regularly collaborate with DeSean's teachers to come up with a manageable assignment catch-up plan and ensure that he gets additional help he may require with any of his subjects.

Pastor Livingston's Goals:

1. I will make myself available to DeSean if he needs additional support and wishes to talk.
2. Employ and monitor DeSean's working in the church library and will arrange with elderly congregation members for him to do yardwork for them.

Mr. Knight's Goals:

1. I will weekly monitor that DeSean is following the Bishops' household rules, not getting into trouble with his gang or the police, and performing better academically.

(continued)

FIGURE 4.2. The Bishops' solution-determined collaborative treatment plan: Team members' goals and implementation action steps.

2. I will let DeSean's public defender and the judge know about his new work responsibilities at his church and regularly check in with Pastor Livingston to find out how the job situation was going.

Mr. Stinson's Goals:
1. I will commit daily to make myself available to DeSean if he would like to talk or if he needs additional support.
2. I will commit at least three times per week to meet with DeSean after school to work on further honing his basketball fundamentals, particularly his field goal shooting.

Carolyn's Goals:
1. I will commit to having weekly Saturday morning breakfasts with DeSean and spending some high-quality afternoon time together.
2. I will make myself available via texting, phone calls, or impromptu meetings if DeSean needs to talk or wants added support.

Matthew's Goals:
1. I will provide weekly family therapy to the Bishops to improve their family communications, conflict-resolution skills, and strengthen their parental bonds with DeSean.
2. Teach the Bishops effective parenting skills, particularly the importance of parental unity with rule and consequence enforcement.
3. Provide individual session time in the context of family therapy to further hone DeSean's mindfulness and emotional distress tolerance skills and address any additional difficulties he needs help with.
4. I will involve Charles and Les, two former gang-involved clients, to share their expertise and wisdom regarding how they gave up gang life, turned their lives around, and to provide additional support to DeSean in his efforts to steer clear from his gang and further police involvement.
5. I will regularly communicate with all members of the team to ensure that agreed-upon goals and action steps are being achieved, address any concerns, and to resolve any glitches or obstacles with the implementation of our treatment plan.

Signatures of Team Members:

Parent: _____ Date: _____

Parent: _____ Date: _____

Client: _____ Date: _____

Name: _____ Date: _____

Name: _____ Date: _____

Name: _____ Date: _____

Name: _____ Date: _____

Name: _____ Date: _____

Therapist: _____ Date: _____

FIGURE 4.2. *(continued)*

Significant Other Consent Form

I/We _____ give my/our therapist _____
permission to include in my/our counseling sessions the following two friends/adult
significant others: _____ and

for the purpose of providing additional support in my/our treatment. I will explain to
my friends, their parents, and adult significant others that confidential information will
be shared in our counseling sessions and that it is *not* to be disclosed outside of our
meetings. I will obtain signatures from my friends, their parents, and any adult significant
others I wish to include in my/our counseling sessions.

_____   _____
Signature of Client   Date

_____   _____
Signature of Parent/Guardian   Date

_____   _____
Signature of Friend's Parent   Date

_____   _____
Signature of Friend   Date

_____   _____
Signature of Friend's Parent   Date

_____   _____
Signature of Friend   Date

_____   _____
Signature of Adult Significant Other   Date

_____   _____
Signature of Adult Significant Other   Date

_____   _____
Witness   Date

Notice to client/significant others: I/We understand that this consent shall expire in 1
year from the date of our signature(s) or until the calendar date _____.
I/We understand that I/we may revoke this consent at any time during my/our treatment.
I/We also agree not to hold my/our therapist responsible for any violation of my/our
confidentiality by participating friends or adult significant others. I/We (friend's parents)
agree not to hold the therapist responsible for any possible negative effects of having my/
our teen participating in his/her friend's counseling sessions.

Can–If Map

Directions: In each of the bubbles, write down your collaborative team's ideas for: We use other people . . . , We remove X to allow us to Y . . . , We resource it by . . . , We substitute X for Y . . . , We introduce a . . . , We access the knowledge of . . . , and We think of it as . . . for resolving the problem situation.

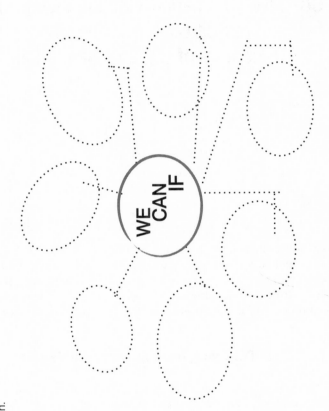

CHAPTER 5

Co-Developing and Selecting Interventions to Suit Clients' Strengths, Theories of Change, and Goals

> Imagination is everything. It is a preview
> of life's coming attractions.
> —ALBERT EINSTEIN

In this chapter, I present practical guidelines for co-developing therapeutic experiments with families. When treatment is at a standstill, these helpful idea-generating strategies often produce high-quality solutions. The chapter includes a transtheoretical compendium of therapeutic experiments and rituals for the adolescent, parents, and their whole families.

Co-Developing Novel Solutions with Families

As the great hypnotist Milton H. Erickson discovered, the most efficient way to empower our clients to resolve their difficulties is to utilize as much as possible their strengths, resourcefulness, meaningful metaphors, theories of change, life passions, talents, key interests, and inventiveness (Duncan et al., 2010; Havens, 2003; Zeig, 1980). This is why it is so beneficial to give families the pretreatment change experiment discussed in Chapter 1 prior to their initial family therapy sessions. It is a way to increase their awareness of self-generated coping and problem-solving ideas and give them flashes of insight about what works. We can then tap their expertise to see what they can continue doing that is already working and utilize their creative ideas to generate novel solutions for unresolved presenting problems the clients still wish to change. If we listen intently to our clients, they will not only tell us how to best establish cooperative partnerships with them but also provide us with ripe opportunities worth seizing for co-constructing solutions. The following case example illustrates how listening carefully for and seizing an important family exception to conflict led to our co-developing a pattern intervention strategy for disrupting the parents' entrenched and long-standing arguing problem.

Hilda, a 17-year-old Norwegian girl, and her parents were brought in for a family consultation for her long history of hashish abuse and running away from home. She also had been locked into the role of marital therapist to her recovering heroin-addicted parents, who constantly argued with each other. In the past, Hilda had served as their referee when they would get into heated arguments. She was a confidante for the mother when she wished to complain about her father. For Hilda, smoking hash and running away from home were coping strategies for dealing with her stressful family situation. Prior to the consultation, Hilda had landed a job, stopped smoking hash, and had joined her friend's band, which gave her a reprieve from the family stress. I amplified and consolidated all of Hilda's gains and shared with her that she had done a fine job of bringing her parents in for family therapy and that she could now hand over her family marital therapist role to Kerstin, the consulting therapist. The parents took responsibility in the session for their incessant arguing and for wrongly involving Hilda in their marital conflicts. I explored with the couple what was different when they did not argue with each other and the specifics about what happened instead. The family lived on a large farm, and it turned out that the one daily activity they jointly engaged in there with no arguments and excellent teamwork was when they "fetched the hens" together. I seized this important exception and recommended they make strategic use of fetching the hens as a way to disrupt a potential argument. After having the parents and Hilda identify triggers that often sparked their arguments, the couple was told that if one partner senses an argument is about to happen, he or she is to cry out, "It's time to fetch the hens!" The family and Kerstin laughed and thought this was a great idea and were eager to try it out. In following up with Kerstin, the strategic use of "fetching the hens" helped the couple to greatly reduce the frequency of their arguing. They eventually contracted to work on what turned out to be the underlying "real problem," which was their sexual intimacy difficulties. Since Hilda was doing much better and Kerstin had taken over as the official marital therapist, she no longer had to have family therapy sessions.

The following are nine practical guidelines for co-developing therapeutic experiments with families.

1. Explore with family members what self-generated pretreatment changes may help them to resolve their unresolved presenting difficulties, such as creative ideas, flashes of insight, or strategies

they had thought about or had already begun to experiment with that were working.

2. If there have been specific ideas that family members had found useful and wish to develop further, brainstorm with them what needs to be added to make them even more effective solutions.

3. Once families' self-generated solution strategies have been further refined, determine the *when, where,* and with *whom* they need to be tested out.

4. In the next family session, evaluate the outcome of implementing their therapeutic experiment(s). If they are effective, encourage them to do more of what works. If they report that it helped a little, explore if one or two therapeutic experiments need further fine-tuning or should be discarded.

5. Other client resource areas to tap for co-constructing therapeutic experiments are their life passions; key interest areas; hobbies; recent epiphanies; certain serendipitous practices they regularly engage in; skill competencies they have with music, drama, dance, art, sports; their favorite authors and characters and celebrities from books, TV shows, and movies.

6. Ask parents, "Have you had any solution strategy idea for changing your kids' behaviors, maybe something really crazy, but you held back from trying it because you were not sure it would work?"

7. If the parents respond to the question in 6 above by warming up to the idea of trying an off-the-wall strategy, determine with them the *when, where, how,* and with *whom* it will be implemented.

8. Follow guideline 4, to evaluate the outcome of this therapeutic experiment and what to do next.

9. If you and the family are feeling at a loss for what known therapeutic interventions may work best with their main presenting difficulty or if previously tested therapeutic tools or strategies were not helpful, use the idea-generating strategies discussed after the case example below.

In the case example below, Constance is a British single mother with three chronically fighting adolescent daughters. The case illustrates the positive outcome results parents can achieve when we ask them the question in guideline 6: "Have you had any solution strategy idea for changing your kids' behaviors, maybe something really crazy but you held back from trying it because you were not sure it would work?"

Constance had been divorced for 3 years from her abusive alcoholic husband, Samuel. For years Claire, Constance's 15-year-old daughter, tried to protect her mother from being hit by her father and occasionally would also get hit, which was why Samuel had lost his rights for joint custody and visitations with the children. The situation had taken its toll on Claire and led to her self-injuring for 4 years and problems with depression and anxiety. On top of those difficulties, her 13-year-old sister, Sarah, and her 11-year-old sister, Elizabeth, were constantly pushing Claire's buttons behind the scenes, trying to set her up to be yelled at by their mother. According to Constance, several times a week the daughters got into intense verbal clashes, which occasionally resulted in hitting and tears shed. While meeting alone with the mother in the session, I learned from that Constance had tried just about everything to change her daughters' behaviors, including seven past treatment experiences, and nothing had worked. I asked her the crazy idea question. Suddenly, a light bulb lit up over Constance's head and she had a flash of creative insight. Since all the girls liked rap music, she had this crazy idea that if she came up with a fun rap song called "More Lovin' and Less Fisticuffin'" and fun lines to go with it she could sing instead of yelling at her daughters all of the time—maybe they would start to cooperate with doing their chores and homework, get along better, and Claire would stop cutting herself. Constance came up with the following rap lines to surprise her daughters with:

> "When there's more lovin' and less fisticuffin' you have a chillin' mom."
> "When there's more chorin' [chores getting done] and homework done, the
>   privileges will be a happenin'."
> "Yo! Yo! Yo! More lovin' and less fisticuffin' that's what it's all about!"

When I reconvened the daughters, I had Constance sing for her daughters. They all laughed because Constance not only was singing her great lines but she added all of the classic rapper dance movements and head bobbing. I soon learned from the daughters that they had missed this fun and playful side of their mother and were so tired of her nagging and yelling. I asked the daughters if they thought their mother could get a recording contract as the next new hot rapper and they laughed again. I also asked them to think of additional rap song lines for their mother to add or even serving as her chorus. What grew out of the Constance's crazy idea was a playful pattern intervention strategy that ended years of nagging and yelling and had a dramatic effect not only on changing the emotional climate at home but also, most important, on her daughters' problematic behaviors. To help counter Claire's depressive and anxious moods and self-injuring behaviors, she learned a variety of mindfulness and disputation tools and strategies.

Idea-Generating Strategies
for Co-Developing Solutions with Families

There are a number of playful and out-of-the-box idea-generating strategies we can use with families when treatment is at a standstill. The strategies also can be useful when we pick up on innuendos of unsaid secrets, which may be contributing to the maintenance of families' presenting difficulties. It is important to equip all family members with paper and pencils so that they can write down their ideas, doodle, and draw any images that enter their minds while doing these exercises. For the sake of brevity, I limit my discussion to four effective idea-generating strategies we can pursue with families: *changing perspectives, synesthesia questions, question storming,* and *crazy and absurd ideas.*

Changing Perspectives

Sometimes when we view problems or difficulties from a different angle or perspective it triggers associations and novel ideas (Michalko, 2006). In fact, Marguc, Forster, and Van Cleef (2011) found in their research on global processing and grit that when we are faced with a difficult task or complex situation, we need to step back until we see the big picture and opportunities worth pursuing. We can have family members respond to the following questions to see if they spark novel ideas worth developing into potential solutions for their presenting difficulties:

> "If you were to hop into an imaginary helicopter and gain a good aerial view of your family, what would you see that may be hard for us to see at ground level that we have missed addressing, but definitely needs to be resolved?"
>
> "If you were to look at the problem upside down, what do you think you would see?"
>
> "If you were to look at the problem through a microscope, what do you think you would see that we are missing that we need to address?"
>
> "If you were to see a *Godzilla*-size version of the problem, what would you be the most scared of, and what steps would you take as a family team to defend yourselves and attempt to conquer it?"
>
> "If you were given special X-ray goggles and you could see through the problem, what do you see that you think we need to address?"

After responding to these questions, the family members are invited to share what ideas were sparked for them. Decide together which ones might be worthwhile pursuing for solution construction and testing out as experiments.

Synesthesia Questions

Synesthesia is a neurological phenomenon in which stimulation of one sensory cognitive pathway leads to automatic, involuntary experiences in a different sensory or cognitive pathway (Cytowic, 2002; Michalko, 2006).

Synesthesia often occurs with individuals using hallucinogenic drugs. The great Russian Abrstract Expressionist artist Wassily Kandinski was heavily inspired by music, such as symphonies and the use of improvisation, which is quite apparent in some of his best artworks. In fact, some of his paintings looked very similar to musical scores with varying movements of the objects on the canvases (Fisher & Rainbird, 2006). Synesthesia questions tap into family members' inventiveness and imagination to produce some intriguing and creative ideas. Some examples of these types of questions are as follows:

> "What type of music would this problem sound like if we could hear it?"
> "Ask yourself, 'If this problem were to come to me for therapy, what would be the first thing it would share with me?'"
> "What else is the problem trying to tell us?"
> "If this problem were edible, what would it taste like?"
> "If this problem had an aroma, what would it smell like?"
> "If this problem were a sculpture, what would be its shape, and what would its texture be?"
> "If this problem were a painting, what major school of art would it represent and what famous artist might have painted it?"

In addition to sparking creative ideas, this fun activity also separates the problem from being connected to the adolescent, in a similar fashion to externalization of the problem (White, 2007). Furthermore, the synesthesia questions can dramatically alter family members' rigid and unproductive ways of viewing the problem.

Question Storming

When keeping treatment progress at a standstill and we are picking up on innuendos of secrets or something that is not being said, *question storming* can be a great therapeutic option to pursue (Dyer, Gregersen, & Christensen, 2011; Roland, 1985). We can tell clients that some families may have unspoken rules about subjects that are not supposed to be talked about or for some reason it may feel unsafe or scary to talk about certain subjects in the company of other family members. In addition, there may be certain unresolved conflicts, unexpressed family member concerns, or family politics keeping the treatment situation at a standstill. Rothstein (2011) has found that "question asking" can have a positive cascading effect in empowering parents, improving the quality of parent–child relationships, and empowering children to be more curious and improve their academic performance.

To begin kicking off this intellectually stimulating activity, the family is first asked to respond to the following question: "What are the important questions we have not yet asked about our family problem situation?" Next, they are to co-generate a list of six to seven questions in response to your central question, beginning with the following qualifiers:

"What?"
"What if . . . ?"
"How?"
"Why?"

After they co-construct their list of questions, they are to circle those questions that they found most helpful in sparking new ways of viewing their problem. We can explore with family members which questions resonated with them the most, in what ways, and how they will put their new ideas to use over the next week. As part of this discussion, family secrets may be revealed and constructive action steps can be planned for how to remedy those situations so the secret keepers feel safe and supported.

Crazy and Absurd Ideas

The *crazy and absurd* idea-generating strategy has been my client families' favorite exercise to do together. As a group, they are to decide what problem they wish to change first. If the parents and the adolescents do not come to an agreement, we can do two separate rounds of this exercise. If they do agree, they are to co-generate as many outrageous and wild and crazy ideas they can think of for resolving the problem. After generating at least five or six outrageous ideas, they need to circle the ones they think have the best shot of working. Next, they are to further refine their circled ideas and figure out how to implement them. This exercise injects more playfulness and fun into the family relationships, enhancing their solution construction abilities, and makes family change an enjoyable team effort.

The Transtheoretical Compendium of Therapeutic Interventions for Specific Adolescent, Parental, and Family Difficulties

I now present below a comprehensive transtheoretical compendium of therapeutic interventions for specific adolescent, parental, and family difficulties. By targeting our interventions at multiple systems levels within the family, we can neutralize adolescents' painful negative emotions and oppressive thinking patterns through the use of mindfulness mediation and related practices, and we can give them cognitive skills training. We can also offer them engaging and fun therapeutic experiments that play into their key strengths and best ways of expressing themselves. At the parents' level, we can transform their negative, outmoded beliefs, disrupt their unproductive and destructive interactions, and strengthen their relational bonds with their adolescents. On the family level, we can improve families' communications, problem solving, conflict resolution skills, and establish stronger and more meaningful family relationships.

Adolescent Coping Tools and Therapeutic Experiments

Many high-risk youth are struggling to cope on a regular basis with oppressive thoughts and powerful negative emotions. For these young people, simply changing outmoded family beliefs and problem-maintaining patterns of interaction often is not enough to provide them with relief from their inner emotional turmoil. We need to arm them with an arsenal of effective coping tools and strategies. Seven major sets of skills are presented below that can help high-risk adolescents better manage their negative emotions and oppressive thoughts, maintain self-control when faced with powerful triggers and cues, and improve their relationship skill effectiveness.

Mindfulness Meditations and Related Practices

According to the cognitive and positive psychology guru Martin Seligman, one of the most important life skills we need to teach young people is *mindfulness meditation* (Seligman 2002). By teaching young people how to detach from and become disciplined observers of their strong negative emotions and oppressive thoughts without caving in to their choice self-destructive behaviors, they will develop the capacities to maintain self-control and better regulate their moods. We also need to teach them that those thoughts and feelings are not solid but fluid, temporary visitors in our minds and bodies. I like to use the metaphor of thoughts and feelings as clouds in the sky in constant motion. They will eventually clear to reveal their beautiful blue-sky selves that are forever present. Research indicates that regular daily practice of mindfulness meditation can greatly benefit us neurologically, physiologically, psychologically, and socially in school or in our vocations. In fact, people who have been meditating for a long period of time not only have higher levels of positive emotion, optimism, and hope, but have stronger immune systems and are less likely to fall prey to depression, anxiety, self-destructive behaviors, or have difficulties with anger management (Fredrickson, 1999; Hanson, 2013; Hanson & Mendius, 2009; Moffitt, 2012; Pollak et al., 2014; Willard & Saltzman, 2015). Regular meditators tend to be more focused and their problem solving abilities are enhanced. Socially, they are much more present, aware, and attentive, which will help them to strengthen their relationship bonds with family members, close friends, and cultivate new relationships with acquaintances (Fredrickson, 1999). The enhanced ability to be present and have heightened awareness are two good reasons why all therapists should meditate daily. Seven mindfulness mediations and related practices are described below.

THE SOUND MEDITATION

The *sound meditation* is quite popular among adolescents because they regularly access their sound sensory channels several times a day when listening to their favorite tunes. After getting comfortable in a chair or on a sofa, sitting back with open chests with their eyes either opened or closed, whatever feels most comfortable to them, they are simply to pay close attention to all the sounds they hear around them. They are not to try and think about why they hear specific sounds but simply to label the different sounds silently to themselves. For example, they may hear a dog barking outside or people talking in an adjacent room. They are to do this meditation for 10 to 12 minutes.

TAKING A TRIP TO POPCORN LAND

One of the most popular meditations with adolescents is *taking a trip to popcorn land*. After they get comfortable in a chair or on a sofa, we place one piece of popcorn in the palm of the adolescents' left hands. Using all of their senses, we have them take the following steps:

1. Carefully study the piece of popcorn, looking at its shape, rounded edges, indentations, its varying shades of colors, the shadowing around it, and then smell it for 2 to 3 minutes.
2. Next, with their right hands they are to reach over and pick the piece of popcorn up and roll it around on their fingertips with their eyes closed, which accesses their touch sensation. They are to do this for 2 to 3 minutes.
3. The third step of this meditation has the adolescents place their pieces of popcorn into their mouths and roll them around with their teeth and tongues for 2 to 3 minutes. They will begin to salivate while doing this step. They are to focus on what they taste and how the popcorn piece feels in their mouths.
4. The next step involves them slowly and finely chewing the piece of popcorn for 2 to 3 minutes without swallowing it.
5. Finally, they are to swallow their chewed up pieces of popcorn and pay close attention to whatever sensations they experience in their esophaguses and stomachs.

So for 10 to 12 minutes the adolescents are totally immersed in the popcorn eating experience and transported to Popcorn Land!

SIX DEEP BREATHS

This mindfulness meditation can be done in any setting and was inspired by the *acceptance and commitment therapy* approach (Wilson & DuFrene, 2012). Wherever adolescents practice this meditation, they need to sit back with open chests in a chair, on a sofa, or even on a park bench. They can decide whether to do this meditation with their eyes opened or closed. I have added a different twist to this mindfulness practice, which involves having the clients externalize their stressors with each breathing cycle. With each deep inhalation, they are to inhale something or somebody that is stressing them out, and then slowly exhale the source of their stress. This is to be done six times. Often by the sixth inhalation–exhalation cycle they are totally decompressed and cleansed of their stressors. Adolescents often report feeling totally "chilled out."

MINDFUL WALKING

This mindfulness practice also grounds adolescents in the miraculous moment. This can be done as part of a therapy session with the client or done at home with family and/or friends. While walking on a forest preserve path or along a river or lake with lots of trees, bushes, and animals, the adolescents are to pay very close attention to everything they see, hear, and smell. For example, if they see a squirrel they are to describe to themselves the color of its fur, carefully watch its movements on the tree branches, and listen for any sounds it makes. They are to scan up and down looking for interesting-looking and/or pretty birds, other animals, insects, plants, and wildflowers. They are to listen carefully for the chirping of the birds and pay close attention to any distinct smells, such as the greenery, certain flowers, or the mud.

SELF-COMPASSION LETTER WRITING

Adolescents who struggle with internalizing and self-destructive difficulties like depression, anxiety, self-injury, eating disorders, and substance abuse problems often harshly blame and criticize themselves when they fail to achieve their goals, make costly mistakes, experience failure, or when they experience relationship conflicts with and rejection from their peers and intimate others. Unfortunately, we live in a society where young people are unduly pushed to be successful and independent, without conveying that humans are imperfect and unique. We need to educate adolescents about the Buddhist belief that we all possess a vast reservoir of unconditional kindness and compassion that we can tap when we need to comfort ourselves after experiencing emotional distress or life disappointments. Research indicates that people who respond to their own flaws and setbacks in a positive way, rather than beating themselves up about them, will experience greater physical and mental health (Smith, 2015). According to Neff (2010), "Self-compassion is an island of calm, a refuge from the stormy seas of endless negative self-judgment. When we give ourselves compassion, the tight-knot of negative self-judgment starts to dissolve, replaced by a feeling of peaceful, connected acceptance—a sparkling diamond that emerges from the coal" (p. 13).

One powerful and easy self-compassion experiment adolescents can do is *exploring self-compassion through letter writing* (Neff, 2010). There are two parts to this experiment. In the first part of the letter, the adolescents are to write about any issue or difficulty they experienced where they felt inadequate or bad about themselves. After accessing their memories, they are to write about how they felt while reliving these unpleasant issues or life difficulties.

In the second paragraph, they are to write about an imaginary friend who is unconditionally loving, accepting, kind, and compassionate toward them. This friend can see all of their strengths and weaknesses, including the issues and difficulties written about in their first paragraphs. They are to imagine and reflect on how their imaginary friends would embrace, love, and accept them exactly the way they are, no matter what mistakes they make. Their imaginary friends remind them that no matter how hard they try, humans are imperfect, make mistakes, experience disappointments, and suffer at times.

Next, they are to write separate short letters to themselves from the perspectives of their imaginary friends focused on their perceived inadequacies and how they tend to harshly judge themselves. They are to pretend to be in the minds of their imaginary friends while answering the following questions:

"What would this friend say to you about your perceived 'flaw' or tendency to harshly criticize yourself from a perspective of unlimited compassion?"

"How would this friend convey deep compassion he or she feels for you, especially for the emotional discomfort you feel when you judge yourself so harshly?"

"What would this friend write in order to remind you that you are only human, that all people have both strengths and weaknesses?"

"What possible changes would this friend recommend you make?"

In concluding their imaginary friends' perspective letters to them, they are to try to convey in their writing a strong sense of being unconditionally accepted and embraced by them. They are to put down their letters somewhere in their bedrooms for a period of time. Later, when they read them, they are to try to allow the comforting and kind words of their imaginary friends to sink into their minds and bodies and really feel their compassion, as it sooths and comforts them. Finally, they are to remind themselves that they are now one with their imaginary friends and that their love, unconditional kindness, and compassion have become a part of themselves and are forever present to be tapped when needed (Neff, 2010, pp. 16–17).

URGE SURFING

Urge surfing was developed by Alan Marlatt and his colleagues at the University of Washington as an empirically supported mindfulness practice specifically designed to help substance abusers prevent relapses (Bowen et al., 2011). I have found it to be equally effective for adolescents experiencing other self-destructive behaviors like disordered eating, self-injury, sexually risky behavior, and anger management difficulties. My version of urge surfing is slightly different from how it is typically done. After the adolescents get comfortable in chairs or on sofas sitting back with open chests, I begin this mindfulness practice by setting a kitchen timer for 5 minutes. I have them close their eyes and access in their minds internal triggers (mood state or oppressive thought) and/or external triggers (family or peer conflict) that often lead to immediately engaging in their choice self-destructive behaviors. They attempt to sit with the powerful emotions that arise within them without flinching, caving in to the urge to hurt themselves, or losing control and lashing out with anger. They are to pay close attention to physiological changes like rapid breathing, any flushing in their faces, and any other physical discomfort they may experience. We also have them picture themselves on surfboards riding the powerful waves of emotions they are experiencing, trying to keep their balance without wiping out. After they succeed at not flinching or losing control at 5 minutes, they often feel more self-confident and good about not caving in to their old self-destructive behaviors. Next, they can be offered the option of trying the practice for 10 minutes or practicing daily at home for 5 minutes a day for a week until the next scheduled appointment, when we can increase the time. Research indicates that negative emotions begin to decrease on their own after around 28 minutes (Schwartz & Gladding, 2011). So if we can help our adolescent clients get up to 28 to 30 minutes of sitting with their powerful negative emotions without caving in to their former self-destructive behaviors, they will be emotionally tough and resilient enough to take on any major life challenges. This mindfulness practice greatly strengthens adolescents' self-regulation and self-control skills.

Most adolescents are good visualizers, particularly those youth who are passionate about art and photography. One of the most effective visualization distress management tools that we can teach high-risk adolescents is *visualizing movies of success or joy* (Selekman, 2005, 2009). The adolescents pick either something that they accomplished in the past or recently that they were really proud of or a wonderful place they had visited with family or friends that triggered strong senses of joy and exuberance for them. Once they have selected the situation they wish to make into a movie, they are to get comfortable in a chair and picture a blank movie screen in their minds with their eyes closed. I like to have them picture going to their local movie theaters and imagine sitting looking up at one of those screens. Next, they are to do the following steps:

1. Using all of their senses, project on the screen what they see, hear, smell, taste, touch, including color and motion.
2. They are to describe silently to themselves where they are, when this event occurred, their age, who they are with, and what they are doing together.
3. They are to access their thoughts and feelings while in action.

It is helpful to have them do this visualization for 10 to 12 minutes and have them practice daily once or twice per day, even during non-stressful times. Ideally, we want them to get so skilled at accessing their movies that this can become a go-to coping strategy instead of caving in to their old self-destructive habits.

Cognitive Skills Training

Cognitive tools and strategies can help adolescents with internalizing and externalizing difficulties. They become more skilled at challenging what I like to call their "*stinkin' thinkin'* " or their self-defeating irrational thinking patterns. These often are a powerful trigger for falling prey to depression, anxiety, self-destructive, and externalizing difficulties. Once they master the cognitive tools and strategies below for disputing their "stinkin' thinkin'" thoughts and their inner critics' voices, they will be better able to maintain emotional balance, entertain alternative views of disappointing life events, and make more adaptive behavioral choices.

Every adolescent has heard of the famous detective Sherlock Holmes. Have adolescents pretend to be like Sherlock Holmes and search for hard evidence to support their negative and rigid beliefs. After a week of playing super sleuth detectives, they are to bring the hard evidence into the next session to support their negative irrational explanations for disappointing life events. Often, they come in empty handed, which can begin to loosen up fixed beliefs and open their minds to alternative views. When adolescents get stuck clinging to a narrow, self-blaming explanation, I encourage them to ask themselves, "How can I be absolutely certain that it is my fault?" Since we can never be absolutely certain about anything, this question can help open up their minds to other possible explanations.

GAINING A KALEIDOSCOPIC VIEWING OF DISAPPOINTMENTS

Most adolescents know what kaleidoscopes are and that they offer us multiple perspectives when we look through them. Have the adolescents pretend that their minds are like kaleidoscopes when they step back and reflect on disappointing life events they've experienced. This disputation strategy helps adolescents keep their minds open and flexible to be able to entertain the second, third, fourth, and even fifth possible explanation when bad things happen to them.

TRANSFORMING NEGATIVE SELF-TALK AND RUMINATION

Most high-risk adolescents are oppressed by self-defeating and irrational thought patterns and tend to ruminate when things go wrong, which contribute to maintaining their internalizing, self-destructive behaviors. They may be able to identify a critical voice that is the source of their irrational thoughts and unpleasant feelings. This critical voice may be a remnant from what they used to or continue to hear from their parents, caretaking relatives, critical teachers and coaches, or even peers who used to bully and put them down. Andreas (2012, 2014) has developed several highly effective strategies for responding to the critical voice when it is triggered. He recommends the following strategies (Andreas, 2014, pp. 3–7):

1. Change the location from where you hear the voice, such as pretending it is outside of you and in a different location such as in the corner of the room or in an adjacent room.
2. Change the voice's tone, tempo, or pretend you have control over its volume, so frustrate it by lowering and raising back and forth the voice's volume.
3. Add background music to it, such as pretending to hear your favorite tune playing in the background.
4. Adopt the Buddhist mindfulness position of embracing the voice

with loving-kindness and compassion, which simultaneously comforts it and you.

5. View the positive intent of the critical voice as coming from a position of love and concern and desire to protect us from making similar future poor choices with our decisions and whom we choose to associate with.

6. Make use of the critical voice's special abilities by thinking about its wisdom, its unique perceptions, skills, and where and with what specific life situations or challenges you can use this voice to help resolve those difficulties.

According to Kross and his colleagues (2014), how people conduct their inner monologues can greatly contribute to their success in life. These researchers found that instead of addressing yourself with "I," using your first name increases your chances of mastering tasks and quickly rebounding from disappointments and other life challenges. First-name self-talk shifts the focus away from the self and allows us to transcend our innate egocentrism. By gaining psychological distance from ourselves, we have more self-control, gain a new perspective, focus more deeply, and plan better for the future. When faced with a challenging life event, it is helpful for adolescents first to soften it by reminding themselves (using their first names) that they faced similar situations in the past and came out unscathed. The second step is to soothe themselves by remaining calm and taking their time with trying to manage the challenge. The third step is to remind themselves about their strengths and talents and to handle the challenging situation the best they can, knowing that is all they can do (Weintraub, 2015).

Self-Control Management Skills

Self-control management tools and strategies can greatly benefit adolescents in learning how to delay gratification, be less impulsive, and discover what works. According to Kahneman (2010), our brains are primed to pursue the easiest and quickest routes to pleasure and relief from emotional distress. Our willpower is the engine of self-control and helps us to manage our thoughts, feelings, and self-destructive habits and override momentary desires for instant gratification. Like any muscle, our willpower will not operate at its highest potential unless we practice it regularly and get enough sleep. After adolescents succeed in resisting the temptation to cave in to self-destructive habits, it will become easier to resist in the future because they are priming perseverance and self-control over their quick-fix survivalist brain's tendencies (Schoen, 2013). Dweck (2006) also found in her research that when we are faced with a big, stressful challenging situation, we should adopt a realistic mind-set. If we know that it will be a bumpy road, but believe we will make it through, we will be more likely to succeed.

Our adolescent clients need to practice self-control management skills, using them daily in different contexts, even when they are not experiencing triggers or higher levels of stress. This is how they get skilled at implementing them. Discussed below are two self-control management strategies: the three S's and implementation intentions.

THE THREE S's

The three S's is one of the most versatile coping strategies for a wide range of adolescent emotional and behavioral difficulties. They consist of *self-awareness, self-monitoring,* and *self-advocacy*. After defining what each of these important components mean and providing concrete examples, we can have the adolescents apply the three S's to their most pressing difficulties. With the self-awareness and self-monitoring components of the three S's, they can ask themselves the following questions when experiencing their triggers:

"What is happening inside of me physiologically (heart beating faster, rapid breathing, flushing in the face) right now?"
"What am I thinking and feeling in response to this trigger?"
"Are my bodily and psychological responses intensifying?"
"What steps can I take to calm myself down?"
"Whom specifically can I reach out to for support?"

If we can get adolescents to practice the three S's daily or every other day, they will eventually discover that they can confidently take control of stressful situations, better self-regulate, and steer clear of bad choices. They should have two or more people they can reach out to when self-advocating or seeking support at home (a parent, older siblings, or a close extended family member) and at school, including therapists and teachers in classes that they are struggling with. The three S's plus mindfulness practices (increases self-awareness and helps us to stay calm), visualization (triggers positive emotion), and cognitive skills (disputes negative, narrow, and rigid thinking) give teens many effective coping tools and strategies to put into immediate action well before they make contact with their key support people.

IMPLEMENTATION INTENTIONS

According to Brier (2010, 2014), once we have increased adolescents' motivation levels and they can see the benefits of self-restraint, we can involve them in the critical skill of *implementation intentions,* which involves having adolescents identify at least three different pleasurable and healthy actions they can take when faced with powerful triggers or obstacles to self-control. Ideally, the positive actions the adolescents should take are self-generated coping and problem-solving strategies they have successfully used in the past instead caving in to their self-destructive or externalizing difficulties. We can have our adolescent clients respond to the following if–then question: "If situation *X* happens, then I will maintain self-control by pursuing *W, Y,* or *Z.*" It can be most beneficial to give adolescents sheets with this directive written at the top. Below it, they can write what they will commit to doing if they are confronted with powerful internal and external triggers over the next week. Since there will be plenty of white space left on their sheets, they are encouraged to list other creative coping and problem-solving strategies below their first three go-to options. The if–then core component of the implementation intentions coping strategy helps teach adolescents' brains a new and more adaptive way of responding to emotional distress and external stressors.

Brier (2014) recommends that to further enhance positive outcomes with the implementation intentions strategy we can have adolescents picture themselves succeeding in the face of adversity. I like to use my trusty imaginary crystal ball and have adolescents gaze into it, seeing themselves over the next week not allowing triggers and obstacles to derail them. The more detailed their visualization, the more likely they are to pull it off in reality. As part of this crystal ball inquiry, I have them use all of their senses, including color and motion and how they are thinking and feeling, as they are not allowing triggers and obstacles to cause them to lose self-control.

Social Skills Training

Some high-risk adolescents have poor social skills, such as social withdrawal out of fear of being rejected or feelings of inadequacy, personal boundary issues, obnoxiousness, and clowning around too much at the wrong times, and misreading social cues that get them into trouble with the way they interact with others. Two highly effective therapeutic experiments that help strengthen social skills are *observing oneself up high in a bubble* and *perspective taking.*

OBSERVING ONESELF UP HIGH IN A BUBBLE

The *observing-oneself-up-high-in-a-bubble* experiment can help remedy difficulty building and sustaining peer relationships (Selekman, 2006, 2009). On a daily basis, the adolescents pretend that the friendly guardian angel parts of them are in bubbles above them carefully observing every social encounter they have throughout the day. The guardian angels in the bubbles will be paying close attention to everything they say or do that promotes positive communication and meaningful conversation flow. They will also observe what they do that sabotages them, quickly shuts down conversations, or leads to being rejected. It is helpful to give them small notebooks to keep track of their observations and insights about what works and how they self-sabotage and set themselves up for rejection. Most adolescents learn a great deal from this experiment about what works socially and what they need to avoid doing with their peers. The added bonuses of this experiment are that it helps them to develop observing egos and identify what specifically they need to cultivate to become more socially skilled.

PERSPECTIVE TAKING

Perspective taking is one of the most important social skills adolescents need to master. It helps them become more empathic and skilled in establishing strong relationship bonds and resolving conflicts (Hodges, Clark, & Myers, 2011; Myers & Hodges, 2013). Perspective taking is the capacity to put oneself in the shoes and minds of others. It increases motivation to listen generously, validate, and try and help. A nice way to help cultivate in adolescents' perspective-taking skills is to arrange a community service experience helping out homeless people, the elderly, or special-needs children and have teens practice listening generously and validating these others' thoughts and feelings. After they have had their altruistic community experiences, we can process with adolescents what they learned about the individuals' life struggles and emotional suffering. We also can explore whether they learned anything new or view themselves differently after completing their service experiences. They also can practice further honing their perspective-taking abilities while talking with family members and close friends.

Finding Meaning and Purpose in Life

Young people today struggle to find meaning and purpose in life. This can be found through regularly immersing oneself in *flow state* activities (Csikszentmihalyi, 1990, 1997). These are enjoyable and rewarding activities where one loses track of time and becomes totally focused and deeply engaged. People in flow states are capable of producing creative and novel solutions to challenging tasks. Adolescents also can experience meaning and purpose in life by engaging in service work in the community, prevention work at their schools or in their communities, or getting involved in social or political causes. Research indicates that there are many positive physical, psychological, and social functioning health benefits for individuals who regularly engage in altruistic acts, such as enhancing capacities for empathy, loving-kindness, generosity, and compassion for self and others (Post & Neimark, 2007; Ricard, 2015). Below, I discuss two activities adolescents can experiment and increase their involvement with to optimize expanding their horizons by finding more meaning and purpose in their lives.

COMMUNITY SERVICE AND SOCIAL CAUSES EXPERIENCES

We can explore with our adolescent clients whether there is one population they have thought about helping out or that could benefit from their support. This can include the homeless, the elderly, special-needs kids, and deaf, blind, or otherwise physically impaired kids. Some of the adolescents we work with may have strong opinions about certain societal, global, or environmental problems but have never taken any action to advance their views or pursued social change with like-minded others. Once they have picked a community service or social cause they would like to pursue, we can connect them with key people and places in the community that can accommodate their volunteer services. After the clients have committed to their community service or social cause and tried it out for a while, we can ask them the following questions:

> "What have you learned about yourself by doing this important work?"
> "What have you learned about the realities and challenges of being (homeless/elderly/having special needs/being deaf or blind/physically handicapped)?"
> "Did anyone you worked with offer you some valuable words of wisdom that really resonated with you?"
> "Has this work in any way changed your views on life and your future career pursuits?"

ENGAGEMENT IN KEY FLOW STATE ACTIVITIES

We need to have adolescents identify for us their key flow state activities so that we can increase their involvement (Csikszentmihalyi, 1990, 1997). The flow state activities should be things they like to do that are enjoyable and meaningful, such as cooking, baking, playing an instrument, writing lyrics and poetry, rapping, dancing, sewing and making clothes, building things, artwork, and photography. They have to be activities or hobbies where the adolescents find themselves deeply absorbed, losing track of time and feeling. The more we help adolescents with self-destructive tendencies to fill their free time with meaningful flow state activities, the less likely they will be to self-injure, binge and purge, abuse substances, and spend excessive time with video games. If the adolescents cannot readily think of a current flow state activity, we can have them either reinstate a former flow state activity or pursue an area they think would be "cool" to learn more about. Once they identify this area, we can encourage them to cultivate this new knowledge or skill base. We also can help them gain training in this new skill area.

Art and Photography Therapeutic Experiments

Some high-risk adolescents express themselves best through their art and photography and are great candidates for art therapy experiments. Some of these youth may have trouble expressing painful thoughts or feelings, or even identifying what they are feeling. For example, some adolescents who had experienced traumatic life events can develop *alexithymia* and *psychic numbing* (an inability to label and express what they are feeling) (Krystal, 1982; van der Kolk, 2014). They are also ideal candidates for art therapy. Adolescents report it to be fun, relaxing, and nonthreatening to do with their therapists (Selekman, 2009). In this section, I present eight different art therapy experiments: drawing out your oppressive thoughts, feelings, and habits; surrealist art solutions; my family story mural; my imaginary feelings X-ray machine; my strengths collage; my soul collage; my superhero comic strip; and my positive moods photography album and exhibit.

DRAWING OUT OPPRESSIVE THOUGHTS, FEELINGS, AND HABITS

Using crayons and colored pencils on sketchpad paper, approximately 14″ × 17″ in size, the adolescents are to draw what they think their most oppressive thoughts, feelings, habits, or problems look like. Similar to externalization of the problem (White, 2007), this art experiment can help liberate clients from the clutches of their oppressive difficulties by making them external. This gives them more self-control and the freedom to pursue more preferred future realities. Having the power to depict their oppressive difficulties helps to neutralize their grip. After having done this art experiment, some adolescents reported feeling psychologically cleansed.

SURREALIST ART SOLUTIONS

Before providing instructions about how to do this experiment, the adolescents and I talk about what they know about the Surrealist art movement. Most kids have had some exposure to the work of Salvador Dalí and René Magritte. I also find it helpful to bring in my art books of Dalí and Magritte's work to have examples and to get their creative juices going.

On a sheet of sketchpad paper 20″ × 24″, the adolescents are to create a Surrealist illustration that can capture an intriguing dream they have had that is connected to their life story in some way; a scary nightmare connected to some life difficulties they are struggling with; or a picture of their achieving a strongly desired wish, fantasy, or goal. Target areas and outcome goals the adolescents wish to address and achieve often grow out of this art experiment; in some cases these are secrets or concerns that they have never talked about before or resolved. With the help of their Surrealist-informed imagination, they may come up with some novel solutions for their presenting difficulties.

Ann, a 16-year-old depressed and self-injuring white female, made a beautiful Surrealist drawing depicting her present dark and depressed emotional state on the right-hand side of the page and a barbed-wire fence as an obstacle to getting to the brighter "happier" emotional state left-hand side of the paper. Interesting to note on the right-hand side of the page was the black-and-white butterfly she had drawn, which was empty and colorless and represented her (see Figure 5.1). Ann loved butterflies and she would draw and paint them on her arms instead of cutting herself. She also shared that this art exercise is helpful for teens and their therapists alike in that it visually depicts what their desired outcome pictures will look like, including "obstacles that can prevent them from achieving their goals."

In discussing the steps she would need to take to cross the barbed-wire fence to reach the happiness on the left-hand side of her illustration, Ann shared that

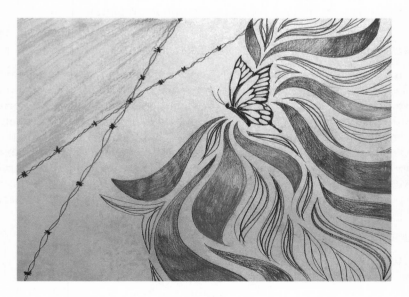

FIGURE 5.1. Ann's *surrealist art solutions* drawing.

she would have to improve her relationships with her parents and make and sustain healthier new friendships.

FAMILY STORY MURAL

At an art supply store, you will need to purchase a large roll of butcher's paper or something similar that does not wrinkle and tear very easily. On a long sheet of paper cut off from the roll, the adolescents are to create murals that best capture how they see their families. Then they are to explain why they depicted their families in certain ways and their rationales for being closer to and more distant from certain family members. They can draw family members in any shape or form they wish. With the help of this art experiment, we can learn a great deal about family conflicts, coalitions, certain roles family members play, key family stressors, and problem-maintaining family interactions. The adolescents become family consultants to us by guiding us in determining what relationships they wish to see changed and what would improve the quality of family life for them. This art experiment can be done in a first session, in the middle phase of family therapy, and around termination to serve as a visual measurement of changes in family relationships. Family members can learn from this how the adolescents perceive the family drama and what their specific concerns are (Selekman, 2005, 2009, 2010).

At times, I have found it to be quite useful to have the adolescents' families join them in constructing the family story mural together. It may be a novel experience for them to do a fun activity together and gain insights in about family members' different perceptions of their relationships and the family politics.

IMAGINARY FEELINGS X-RAY MACHINE

The *imaginary feelings X-ray machine* art experiment can be quite effective with adolescents who have trouble identifying and expressing their thoughts and feelings and/or may have somatic complaints like headaches and stomachaches (Selekman, 2005, 2009, 2010). They may have grown up in invalidating and high-stress family environments.

Adolescents are to imagine a special X-ray machine that could show pictures of what their feelings look like inside of them and where the feelings reside in their bodies. Next, they are to lie down on a long sheet of thicker paper that will not wrinkle and tear easily. After picking the color crayon they wish to have used, a family member of their choosing is to draw the outline of the teen's body on the paper. Once the body outlines are completed, the adolescents are to draw scenes from their lives that capture their major feelings in those areas of their bodies where they reside. This powerful and enlightening art experiment often reveals unresolved conflicts they may have with certain family members and peers, past traumas, secrets, and other major stressors. Observing family members can feel free to share their reactions to and ask questions about the adolescents' X-rays. This process of reflection and dialogue can open up space for possibilities across all family relationships.

STRENGTHS COLLAGE

One fun way we can tap adolescents' strengths is with the *strengths collage*. On a long sheet of paper have a family member draw the outline of their adolescent's body with a crayon. Using magazines and newspapers, adolescents are to cut out words, phrases, and images that capture their major personal strengths. This upbeat and most enjoyable art activity often increases their awareness of their natural gifts, talents, and resiliency, protective factors they can utilize to help to resolve their difficulties and achieve their goals. Discuss in what target areas they wish to deploy their top strengths. Explore whether they have successfully used their strengths in the past and how specifically they achieved mastery at those times through their self-talk and action steps. Parents are often very impressed by their kids' final products and can be asked to share specific examples of where they witnessed their kids shining and achieving at high levels using their top strengths.

SOUL COLLAGE

The *soul collage* art activity not only can raise adolescents' awareness and insight regarding their identities but it also can serve as an excellent vehicle for goal identification and treatment focus. Prior to beginning the activity, we have a conversation about what they think a soul is and where it resides in their bodies. Most kids think their souls comprised their identities and cultural backgrounds; and that they are connected to their life experiences and family stories, their personal values and beliefs, life passions, spiritual selves, and fantasies. The majority of adolescents also believe that their souls reside in their brains. On a sheet of sketchpad paper 14″ × 17″, we first draw the profiles of the adolescents' heads. Next, using magazines and newspapers, they are to cut out words, phrases, and images that they believe would emanate out of their souls if we could take the tops of their heads off and gain access to them. As mentioned earlier, often adolescents gain a great deal of insight after doing this activity and it becomes more clear to them not only what their strengths and talents are, but also specific target areas and patterns of thinking and doing that they would like to change to improve the quality of their lives.

Sixteen-year-old Ann (see her other work in Figure 5.1) made a powerful soul collage, which captured the darkness of her depression and deep sense of hopelessness and despair she was feeling with her life situation (see Figure 5.2). She cut out words, phrases, and images that immediately captures viewers' attention about how shattered and worthless she felt inside, such as "broken windows" and "Will I be remembered?" Ann strongly recommended that therapists use this art exercise early in treatment with teens as an effective way to gain access to their inner "emotional life and core issues" and as a method for establishing short-term goals with them.

SUPERHERO COMIC STRIP

One way we can empower high-risk adolescents is to employ the *superhero comic strip* activity, which utilizes the narrative therapy strategy of externalizing the problem (White, 2007). On a 20″ × 24″ sheet of sketchpad paper, adolescents are to create a comic strip in which they are the superhero with special powers. As superheroes, they are quite clever, and now well equipped to conquer the supervillain oppressive problem that has been objectified into either a human-like form or a monster. We first discuss with the adolescents what their specific powers are, how they picture themselves looking as superheroes, and their strategies for conquering their supervillain problems for good. Next, they are to describe what the supervillain problems will look like, what kind of magical powers they have, how they think, and what their clever tactics are. On their sheets

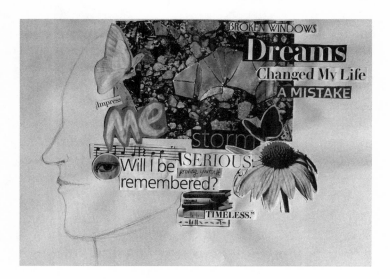

FIGURE 5.2. Ann's *soul collage.*

of paper using markers, crayons, and/or colored pencils they are to create a cartoon strip with large boxes where they can sequentially depict action scenes in which they eventually conquer their problems. Once they complete their drawings, the adolescents often feel liberated from their oppressive problems and more confident. We can explore with them how they would begin using some of the magical powers of their superheroes to improve the quality of their lives, and in what relationships and other contexts. This inquiry can help spark helpful ideas and solutions adolescents can use immediately.

Twelve-year-old Ben was referred to me by his school social worker for attention deficit disorder, depression, anxiety, and fears, as well as his tendency to gravitate toward bullies and other toxic peers. As a young child, he had been exposed to domestic violence, which the social worker felt was still haunting him and contributed to his gravitating toward and being victimized by mean-spirited peers. Since Ben loved art and Marvel comic strip superheroes, I had him create a superhero comic strip in which he was a superhero with magical powers (see Figure 5.3). In the comic strip, he became the Blue Lantern whose super-human abilities included: lightning-fast mixed martial arts fighting moves, quickly putting up his impenetrable invisible force field to shield himself from villains' attacks, and using his large and powerful sledgehammer to knock out and slay any villain. We externalized his "fears" into the super-villain the Green Ghoul, which Ben

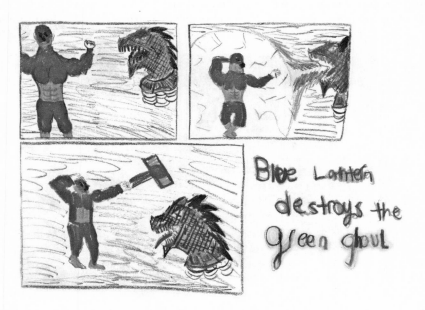

FIGURE 5.3. Ben's *superhero comic strip.*

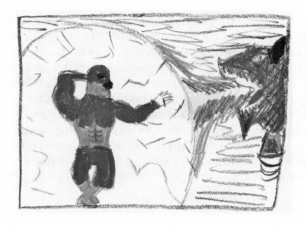

FIGURE 5.4. Blue Lantern's impenetrable invisible force field.

thought would look like a giant "Godzilla head." The Green Ghoul possessed powerful jaws and razor sharp teeth that could tear through any object. It also could blow fire and quickly melt any object to a crisp in less than a minute. In the second frame of Ben's comic strip (see Figure 5.4), the Blue Lantern demonstrates how he uses his invisible force field to both protect himself and repel the Green Ghoul's attempts to burn him to death. When asked about which Blue Lantern abilities he could use in verbally threatening peer interactions, Ben thought pretending to put up his invisible force field would help him to not be afraid and remind himself that he was safe. Additionally, he also felt liberated by the last frame of his comic strip, which captures the Blue Lantern in an action pose after he finally slayed the Green Ghoul. This art activity and other tools Ben put to use helped boost his self-confidence and empowered him to be more assertive with his peers and his parents when necessary.

POSITIVE MOODS PHOTOGRAPHY ALBUM AND EXHIBITION

For adolescents who love photography, we can have them add to their photography portfolio and create a *positive moods photography album*. They can choose to do their photographs in black and white or color or combine the two. They are to use or take photos of beautiful and intriguing nature scenes, beautiful and interesting looking modern and old architecture or monuments, photos of beautiful evening horizons or unusual cloud formations, photos of animals/pets, beautiful photos of family members and close friends, photos of them and their teams or co-performers after achieving great victories or excellent performances. Most important, their photos have to trigger positive emotions for them every time they look at them. After they have taken their photos or picked out old favorite photos, they are to title them, think of short narratives for each one (three or four lines), and determine how they would arrange their photos for an exhibition. They are to come up with catchy titles for their exhibitions. Arrangements can be made at local public libraries and at their schools with their school counseling and art department staffs to have their work exhibited. In addition, there can be scheduled times during the week for the adolescents to present a talk about their photography. Finally, whenever the adolescents are stressed out or experiencing negative emotions they can pull out their beautiful photography albums and leaf through them or look at them online for a strong dose of positive emotion to put them in better moods.

Expressive Writing Experiments

Some high-risk adolescents express themselves best through creative writing and poetry. Therefore, it will be most advantageous to tap into this key strength area of their expertise to spark solutions to their presenting difficulties. I discuss the following eight expressive writing experiments: my favorite author rewrites my story, you at your best story, cut-ups, my humor journal, my habit journal, my gratitude log, my epiphany log, and my serendipitous practices and contexts log.

MY FAVORITE AUTHOR REWRITES MY STORY

When adolescent clients' favorite activities are creative writing and reading books, they are perfect candidates for the *my favorite author rewrites my story* expressive writing experiment (Selekman, 2009). We want to inquire who their favorite authors are, lead characters in these authors' books, and what about these characters really resonates with them. In the session, we can ask them the following questions to get their creative writing juices going:

> "Let's say your favorite author decided to rewrite your individual or family story; what kind of character would you be in this new story?"
> "What special qualities, powers, talents, or interests would your new character have?"
> "How would your favorite author rewrite how your parents, siblings, and close friends are as characters in your new story about your life?"
> "The adolescent then completes the short story of one to three pages or begins it in the session. After the story is finished, ask, 'Are there any aspects of your new character or elements from your

new story that you might want to experiment with in your current life?' "

"How do you think that can make a difference in your relationships with your parents or friends you are having difficulties with?"

"What other advice would your new character give to help you resolve your current difficulty?"

I have had some ambitious clients who enjoyed this writing activity so much that they wrote three or four chapters of their new book. This fun experiment can help generate new views of self and significant others and spark creative solutions for the adolescents' difficulties.

YOU AT YOUR BEST STORY

One way we can empower adolescents with internalizing disorders is through having them do the *you at your best story* writing experiment (Peterson, 2006; Selekman, 2009). This positive psychology expressive writing experiment has shown excellent clinical results with depressed clients. The adolescents are instructed to write approximately three paragraphs about something they are proud of having achieved. They can write about an excellent performance in a sports event, a concert, a play, doing great on a paper or test in a difficult class, doing something very special and kind for somebody, and so forth. After they complete their stories, I like to have them use blue and red pens to underline both their *agency thinking* (blue ink) and their *pathway thinking* (red ink) that had gotten them fired up and helped them to achieve mastery (McDermott & Snyder, 1999). Agency thinking consists of our helpful self-talk or what our best supporters tell us that gets us fired up and highly motivated to achieve. Pathway thinking consists of the specific action steps we took to perform at a high level. We can utilize their agency and pathway thinking to help them to resolve their present difficulties. As the old adage goes, "Nothing succeeds like success." Once they are done writing and editing their stories and write final drafts, they are to read them each night right before they go to bed. Peterson (2006) has found that clients sleep better after reading their stories because of the positive emotions and memories that are triggered for them.

CUT-UPS

William Burroughs, the author of *Naked Lunch,* developed with his friend and colleague Brion Gysin a writing technique called *cut-ups* (Miles, 2015). By cutting through pages of newspapers, magazines, and old books and then randomly juxtaposing the cut-up pages, they produced some very interesting and intriguing text. According to Burroughs:

I would say that my most interesting experience when you make cut-ups is that you do not simply get random juxtapositions of words, that they do mean something, and often these meanings refer to some future event. I've made many cut-ups and later recognized that the cut-up referred to something that I had read later in a newspaper or in a book, or something that happened. (in Miles, 2015, p. 366)

Using Burroughs's cut-up technique, we can have the adolescents cut lines out of pages of old newspapers, magazines, and old books that we were planning to discard or give away and randomly juxtapose the page lines together until some interesting and intriguing text emerges. We can explore with the adolescents if their cut-ups had sparked for them any new meanings for them about their current dilemmas, life stories, or any useful ideas to pursue in resolving their current presenting difficulties. The late David Bowie was greatly inspired by Burroughs's writings and used his cut-up technique to generate lyrics for his new songs (Savage, 2013).

HUMOR JOURNAL

A *humor journal* is an effective way to disrupt negative thoughts and feelings and help prevent self-destructive and externalizing behaviors. When we laugh, our brain chemistry secretes endorphins, which numb bad thoughts and feelings and produce a pleasurable sensation. In journal books or on their iPads or laptops, adolescents are to write down jokes or humorous stories they heard from friends, on TV shows, or in movies. They can also cut and paste funny cartoons, or add their own jokes or funny stories. Whenever they are stressed out or in a bad place emotionally, they can grab their journal or digital devices for a good laugh and as a way to trigger endorphins and positive emotions and put them in a happier and calmer mental state.

HABIT JOURNAL

Self-destructive adolescents have reported that the use of *habit journals* had greatly contributed to their conquering their oppressive habits (Selekman & Beyebach, 2013). As part of their transformative journeys, they are to document the bumps in the road they experienced; any slips they have had; what they learned from these experiences, such as where the structure had broken down; and which specific toxic people and places they needed to avoid. In addition, with each slip we can explore with them what wisdom they gained and how they will manage similar stressful situations in the future. Conversely, clients learn what meaningful and healthy activities they engage in that trigger positive emotions, and details regarding what family members, friends, and adult inspirational others say or do that put them in a good mood and help them to stay emotionally strong and confident. Research indicates that habit journals are effective at empowering obese individuals to lose weight and keep it off (Hollis et al., 2008).

GRATITUDE LOG

Gratitude has been identified as an important ingredient for life satisfaction. It also has many physical, psychological, and social health functioning benefits (Emmons, 2007; Froh & Bono, 2014). I encourage adolescents to start a log either in a journal book or on a digital device where they add new entries three or four times a week of things they are grateful for. The log format has two columns: a *Date* column and a *What I'm Grateful For* column. Whenever they are feeling down or empty, they can look through their gratitude logs for a good dose of positive emotion to elevate their optimism, hope, and happiness.

EPIPHANY LOG

A client extratherapeutic factor that few therapists inquire about with their clients is their *epiphanies*. Epiphanies can occur as flashes of insight sparked by something our clients heard, read, saw, or experienced that was life transforming. It could be a sudden realization that the time was now to quit their alcohol and substance abuse, self-injury, or eating disorder. Unexpected good luck also can be transformative. Miller and C'de Baca (2001) wrote a fascinating book about adults who gave up their alcohol and substance abuse addictions after experiencing epiphanies that had transformed their lives. For their epiphany logs, the adolescents are given sheets with five columns, with these headings: *Date, My Epiphany, Sparked by, Wisdom Gained,* and *Applied to* (see Form 5.1 at the end of the chapter). It also is beneficial to have parents keep track of and write down their epiphanies that have helped them change their negative views of their kids and sparked more positive interactions with them. In our sessions, we can ask adolescents and their parents the following questions to help them to fill out their epiphany logs in the session and at home:

> "Sometimes we read, hear, or see something in a book, out in nature, on a TV show, or in a movie that sparks some new insights about our life or compels us to try something new or daring. Have you had any experiences like that lately or in the past that were really meaningful to you?"
> "After experiencing that epiphany, how have you put that wisdom to use in your life and in your most important relationships?"

"What did you start doing differently as a result?"

"How specifically has your life been transformed by that new realization about your personal capabilities?"

"Are there any other hunches or connections sparked by another epiphany you plan to follow up on?"

We can give clients extra blank epiphany log sheets to fill out between sessions and bring in for discussion. This writing experiment often grounds adolescents in the present moment, and their focusing and concentration abilities are enhanced. Like good detectives, they will be on the lookout for experiences that will spark epiphanies for them.

SERENDIPITOUS PRACTICES AND CONTEXTS LOG

Serendipitous practices and contexts also are client extratherapeutic factors that therapists rarely inquire about. A *serendipitous practice* consists of certain beliefs, positive superstitions, or a positive habit that brings clients good luck. This client strength can serve as a potential building block for solution construction. *Serendipitous contexts* are places our clients go to where they may meet interesting people, get good advice, or gain some insights into their situations. Just visiting this context triggers positive emotion and brings good fortune. I have created a *Serendipitous Practice and Contexts Log* for adolescents to fill out between sessions (see Form 5.2 at the end of the chapter). Similar to the use of the epiphany log, we can use this tool with parents; having them keep track of and write down their serendipitous practices and contexts helps increase their awareness about what works and what to do more of to improve their relationships with their kids. The log has five columns: *Date, Serendipitous Practices and Contexts, Wisdom Gained, Applied to,* and *Positive Outcomes.* We can ask adolescents and their parents the following questions so they can begin filling out their Serendipitous Practices and Contexts Logs in our session and at home:

"Sometimes we discover that certain cherished beliefs we have or practices we engage in seem to lead to positive and surprising things. Do you have any cherished beliefs or practices that seem to bring good fortune or luck to you?"

"What specifically are those beliefs and practices?"

"Do you have any hunches for today—just feelings about actions you should take or things you might do?"

"With your keen sense of openness for possibilities, what pleasant surprises are you anticipating happening over the next week?"

"Can you think of any places you like to visit where it seems like positive surprises or good things seem to happen that benefit you either while you are there or after leaving?"

This writing experiment has the same positive benefits as the epiphany log activity in that it increases adolescents' awareness, grounds them in the present moment, enhances their focusing and concentration, triggers positive emotion, and helps us identify many potential building blocks for solution construction.

Parental Therapeutic Experiments and Rituals

In this section, I present 14 strategies and rituals designed to strengthen parents' bonds with their teens and improve the quality of their relationships, communications, and problem-solving skills with them.

Mindful Parenting: Parental Presence, Loving-Kindness, and Compassion

One of the key characteristics found in research on strong families is *spending enjoyable time together* (De Frain, 2007; Stinnett & O'Donnell, 1996). Therefore, *parental presence* plays a major role in strengthening parents' relational bonds with their adolescents. This involves setting aside some time each day to connect with their kids to find out how their days had been, be empathically attuned to when the teens need comfort, and engage in some pleasurable activity with them. Parental presence also includes consistency with setting limits and enforcing consequences. These are loving acts, in that they help young people develop internal controls and take responsibility for times when they make poor choices. It is important for parents to learn about the Buddhist principles of *loving-kindness* and *compassion* when responding to their kids' emotional distress, meltdowns, or provocative button-pushing behaviors. Rather than becoming emotionally reactive with anxiety or anger, they are instead to remain calm, speak in a soothing tone, offer to listen to them about what is upsetting, offer a hug, or go for a walk and talk about the upsetting situation. When adolescents are suffering and feeling out of control, they need to be supported by a compassionate and empathic parent who is in control. Once the adolescents have mastered a few of the mindfulness meditations described earlier in this chapter, I like to put them in charge of teaching their parents how to do these meditations. They can do them together, or the parents can meditate as a way to decompress after a stressful day at work or as a way to avoid losing control when they are angry with their kids.

Parents Share Their Mistakes, Failures, and How They Bounced Back

Every adolescent or child likes a good story, particularly when it is about their parents' resilience and how they bounced back from life challenges. The storytelling can occur at the dinner table or in some other relaxed setting when their adolescents have some free time. The parents can share stories about mistakes they made with mishandling certain situations, tasks, relationship difficulties, or failures they experienced in school or on the job, the wisdom they gained from these experiences, and the steps they took to bounce back. In many cases, the parents had ventured out of their comfort zones when they made these mistakes or experienced failure. The parents' stories normalize for their kids that mistakes and failures occur in our lives, particularly when we venture outside our comfort zones, and that mistakes can help us become more courageous and resilient. Hearing their parents' stories can increase the adolescents' hope that they too can overcome current difficulties.

Soliciting Regular Feedback on the Quality of Your Parenting

Adolescents are often quite surprised when out of the blue their parents start asking them once or twice a week for feedback on their parenting. We ask parents to share with their kids how important it is to them that they have strong relationships with them and that they are open to making any necessary adjustments to improve the quality of their relationships with their kids. This could include changing the household rules; adding new privileges; revisiting and changing the chore responsibilities; reducing annoying parental behaviors like nagging, lecturing, yelling, and so forth; and learning about old or new activities their adolescents would like to do with them or wish to pursue solo. This major parental shift away from being too authoritarian, rigid, and hands off can dramatically improve parent–adolescent communications, eliminate conflicts in their relationships, and strengthen their relational bonds.

Use of Positive Consequences

Parents can experiment with *positive consequences* as a great alternative to groundings and taking away privileges and valuables from their adolescents. Positive consequences consist of having adolescents do a good deed in the community for a designated period of time instead of being grounded or losing privileges. Positive consequences can include working with homeless, elderly, special-needs children, or handicapped people, or getting involved in some social cause to better their communities. Although the adolescents may initially balk at the parents' carefully selected consequences, afterward kids often feel good about what they did. It helps build character, compassion, empathy, and may even spark a potential career path for them. Some kids like their consequences so much that they voice a strong desire to continue to volunteer for the organization that hosted them or request working part-time over the summer.

Institute a Compliment Box

The *compliment box* can help spark more positive family interactions. The parents are to get an old shoebox and cut a slit in the top. Each day, family members are to write down on signed slips of paper things that they really appreciate about one another and what other family members have done and continue to do for them that has positively resonated. After dinner, family members are to pass the shoebox around and take turns reading what is written on the slips of paper. Often, family members hear things that they never knew the others appreciated. This triggers positive emotion and infuses more warmth in their relationships. Destructive family interactions are replaced with more positive family communications and mutual respect.

Becoming Super Sleuth Solution-Oriented Parenting Detectives

Parents of high-risk adolescents are often anticipating problems to occur with their kids, which sets negative self-fulfilling prophecies in motion. We need to coach these parents to step back, and pull out their imaginary magnifying glasses, and on a daily basis carefully look for those sparkling moments when their adolescents are respectful toward them—doing their chores, not tormenting their siblings, and not acting up. Like good detectives, they need to find hard evidence of their kids' positive behaviors and pay close attention to what they are doing differently during those times that is helping. They may discover that they had changed their tone of voice, refrained from nagging or yelling, avoided power struggles, and had been good listeners. Once parents find what they do that brings out the best in their kids, we need to encourage them to do more of it!

Taking Charge of Technology Use: Helping Kids Find Balance in Their Lives

One of the major problems that parents struggle with today is providing firm guidelines for their kids' daily technology use and being aware of what websites and specific activities they are involved with online. On the average, adolescents are spending 7 to 8 hours on their technology devices per day (Sales, 2016; Turkle, 2015). James and Jenkins (2015) contend that youth today are blind to moral and ethical dimensions of their conduct while they are online. For example, many adolescents in their study indicated that someone else's property online is "free for all" and that spreading rumors or being hostile toward their peers online was "just a joke." They believe that parents need to become much more knowledgeable about what their kids are doing online, become more digital savvy, and help them to cultivate ethical thinking skills and moral citizenship while online, which they refer to as *conscientious connectivity*. One way we can empower parents to become more savvy is to put their kids in charge of mentoring them and teach them their knowledge and skills about social media, what kids are into, and help them to improve their technical skills with digital devices.

A second reason why parents need to provide firm guidelines for screen usage is that it is driving a wedge in family relationships, lessening quality time spent together to connect with one another. Screens do not teach valuable social skills like empathy, compassion, conflict resolution, and assertiveness (Turkle, 2011, 2015). They are learned best in the offline world. To help make room for one-on-one high-quality parent or family time, the parents can institute a *digital-free day*, where all of the kids' interactions are in the offline world one day a week.

A third important reason parents need to help their kids balance daily online and offline time is the epidemic of adolescents with sleep disorders. Research finds that adolescents' excessive technology use greatly contributes to sleeping difficulties, such as shorter deep REM sleeping durations, difficulties falling and staying asleep, and 5 or fewer hours of nightly sleep. Most adolescents need on the average 8 to 9 hours of sleep in order to wake up alert and well rested the next day (Hysing et al., 2015). In addition, when adolescents fail to get enough sleep they tend to be more irritable, more likely to argue with their parents or others who cross them, and have less willpower. This can lead to lower of impulse control and an increase in their self-destructive and externalizing behaviors (Baumesister & Tierney, 2011).

Do Something Different

For parents that are entrenched in the authoritarian position ("My way or the highway!" or "I'm the parent and you're the kid, so you need to listen to me!") or the hyper-responsible position (the more responsibility the parent takes on, the more irresponsible the adolescent behaves), the *do something different* experiment is highly effective (de Shazer, 1985, 1988; Selekman & Beyebach, 2013). The parents are given the following directive:

> "It is obvious to me that your kid has gotten your number. He or she can tell what's going to come next by the looks on your faces and the way you are standing there. So over the next week, whenever your teen does anything to push your buttons, I want you to do something different than your usual course of action, something really off the wall or surprising that he or she has never experienced before from you. Good luck and have lots of fun with this!"

Parents often come up with some pretty creative responses that can shock their adolescents into accommodating their changes and changing their challenging behaviors. This experiment also helps improve parental self-reflection, that is, to step back and think about their options rather than engaging in their former unproductive behaviors of yelling, threatening, or rescuing and overindulging their kids. The case example below illustrates how powerful the *do something different* experiment can be at dramatically turning around a severely acting-out 15-year-old Orthodox Jewish girl named Yael with highly conservative parents at their wits' end after exhausting all of their attempted solutions.

For the past year, Yael had been doing drugs, skipping school, sleeping with older adolescents and young adults, and not following the parents' rules. There were no reports of physical or sexual abuse. The only major change that the parents reported was that Yael was now "running around with a negative group of girls" who were "corrupting" their daughter and "taking her to all-night rave parties." Yael had reluctantly come to our first family therapy session, stayed for half of it, told me to "fuck off" when I supported the parents' need for her cooperation, and walked out of the session saying she would never return. I gave the parents the *do something different* experiment to try, which they enthusiastically embraced. One week later, the parents came in all smiles. They tried two extremely off-the-wall responses when their daughter started to push their buttons. The first outrageous thing they tried was to buy large water guns, fill them up, and from Yael's bed fired away at her when she returned one night from a party by crawling through her bedroom window. Another time, the mother earned an Academy Award for walking around with her head down acting deeply depressed. She had baked Yael her favorite chocolate cake but had not told her was that she had put too much salt in the cake batter because she was "not myself anymore." When Yael had happily dug into the big wedge of cake, she nearly spit it out because it was too salty. After yelling at her mother, the mother responded with, "I'm sorry dear, I'm just not myself anymore." Three days later, not only did Yael get up early in the morning but also she approached her mother, asking, "I'm really worried about you, is there anything I can do to help you out?" The mother glanced at her and said, "Well, it would be nice if you could go to school, but you probably won't." She then shuffled off with her head down into the living room. Not only did Yael go to school that day but she also showed up at our next family session requesting my professional services in helping her to help her mother "be less crazy." We explored a variety of things Yael thought she could do to help her to be less crazy. From this point on, Yael would regularly attend our family sessions so that together we could help prevent relapses from occurring with her mother.

Be Mysterious and Arbitrary

The *be mysterious and arbitrary* experiment can remedy cases in which the adolescent wields all of the power and controls the family mood. The experiment puts the parents back in charge. The parents are given the following directive:

> "It is clear to me that you are like your son's/daughter's hostages or prisoners in that you two don't have a life anymore and he/she calls the shots! It is not fair, nor right that he/she robs you of having lives outside of your home. So I would like to propose we try an experiment over the next week. When either one of you wishes to go back to your jobs, feel like going shopping, or like getting together with close friends to have some fun, I want you to just take off through the door and do it! Don't tell your son/daughter where you are going and when you will be back—just go! When you eventually do come back and your son/daughter asks, 'Where were you?', respond with, 'Oh, I just felt like going out.' No further conversations are necessary; just move on to something you need to do in the house. It may take a week or two for this to start working, so be patient and do expect some backlash or testy behaviors from your son/daughter."

After about a week or two of the parents being mysterious and arbitrary, the adolescent's power and hold over them is neutralized because the parents are now calling the shots. As a result of this powerful parenting experiment, the adolescent is backed into the corner, where he/she can either start taking responsibility like going to school, staying out of trouble with drugs, stop self-injuring, and so forth or dig in more. However, even the most difficult adolescents have difficulty coping with the fact that they no longer have any control over their parents, which leads them to shaping up.

Parents Pretend the Miracle Happened

In clinical situations where the parents cannot identify any past successes that curtailed or resolved their adolescents' problematic behaviors or any pretreatment changes, the *pretend the miracle happened* experiment is a great therapeutic option (de Shazer 1988, 1991; Selelekman & Beyebach, 2013). After we have asked the miracle question earlier in the session, we will have gained access to the specific parental changes the adolescents greatly desire from their parents after the miracle occurs. It is these behaviors that the parents are going to pretend to engage in. The parents are given the following directive:

> "Over the next week, I would like you to pick two days to pretend like the miracle really happened in your interactions with your son/daughter and engage in the miracle-like behaviors that he/she would like to see from you. While you are pretending, I want you both to pay very

close attention to how your son/daughter responds to you. Keep track of which miracle-like behaviors he/she responds the best to in terms of his/her interacting with you in a more respectful and positive way, including any surprises like being more responsible with doing his/her chores or homework without reminders. Please write down what you thought worked the best and the positive responses you got from your son/daughter and bring your list to the next session. Give it your best shot as actors and go for those Academy Awards!"

What is great about this therapeutic experiment is its effectiveness at producing meaningful exceptions to the adolescents' former challenging behaviors that the parents are often quite pleased about. It also injects positive emotion into their relationships with their kids and elevates their hope that they have the power and control to resolve their adolescents' difficulties.

Externalizing Oppressive Parenting Patterns and Practices

Many burned-out, frustrated parents of high-risk adolescents get stuck engaging in negative problem-maintaining interactions with them. It is as if these destructive interactions have a life of their own. These family patterns can be intergenerational. In these clinical situations, I like to externalize their parenting patterns and practices (White, 2007). These parents can be asked the following questions:

> "Tell me, when you were growing up, did 'yelling' get the best of your relationships with your parents?"
> "What effect did that have on you?"
> "Sometimes these parenting practices and patterns take on a life of their own and become intergenerational. Do you think 'yelling' is trying to ruin your relationship with your daughter?"
> "Have there been any times lately where you started to get upset but you refrained from 'yelling' at your daughter?"
> "What did you tell yourself or do instead to pull that off?"
> "Now that you see who the real culprit is in this family, are you going to rewrite history and put an end to the intergenerational reign 'yelling' has had over family relationships, or are you going to allow it to destroy your relationship with your daughter?"

The case below of Juanita and Yolanda illustrates the effectiveness of externalizing a destructive intergenerational family pattern.

I once worked with a Mexican American family that was being pushed around by an "I'm right, you're wrong" intergenerational family pattern. Juanita was seeking family therapy for her 18-year-old daughter, Yolanda, for parent–adolescent conflicts, her daughter's lack of communications about her whereabouts, and verbal abuse toward her. It turned out that what was intensifying their conflicts and communication breakdown was the "I'm right, you're wrong" intergenerational pattern, which both of them described as being quite skilled at pushing each other's buttons. Once I externalized this oppressive intergenerational family pattern, I discovered that this pattern used to get the best of Juanita's relationship with her mother, her parents' relationship, presently in Juanita's relationship with her husband, Hector, and in Yolanda's relationship with her boyfriend, Josh. I got Juanita and Yolanda emotionally fired up as a team to put an end to the "I'm right, you're wrong" pattern's intergenerational reign over their family. I first asked them what they wanted to call their team. Juanita and Yolanda agreed to call their team the "A-Team." Next, I set up a ritual where on a daily basis they were to keep track of what they told themselves and did to stand up to the "I'm right, you're wrong" pattern and not allow it to get the best of them. They also had to keep track of the "I'm right, you're wrong" pattern's victories over them, where they needed to tighten up the structure and try to figure out how to outsmart it. When asked what percentage of the time they were in charge of the pattern prior to seeking family therapy, they indicated they were in charge of it 50% of the time. After three sessions, the A-Team was not only in charge of the pattern 90% of the time, but feeling like they had conquered it! I awarded Juanita and Yolanda with an achievement award (see Figure 5.5) for their excellent teamwork and for conquering the "I'm right, you're wrong" family pattern.

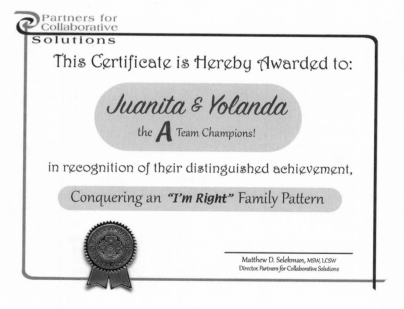

FIGURE 5.5. Juanita and Yolanda's achievement award.

Creating Intensity

Creating intensity with parents can be an effective strategy in clinical situations where the parents are burned out, too permissive, highly inconsistent with setting limits, and skilled at getting helping professionals to take over and try to prevent dire consequences from happening with their adolescents (Alexander et al., 2013; Fishman & Minuchin, 1981; Henggeler et al., 2009; Liddle, 2010; Szapocznik et al., 2003). As hypnotist Milton H. Erickson once said, "It is the patient who does the therapy. The therapist only furnishes the climate, the weather. That's all. The patient has to do all of the work" (in Zeig, 1980, p. 148). We should never be working harder than our clients. We work from behind them as consultants, empowering to utilize their strengths and resources to resolve their adolescents' difficulties. To help parents to step up and take charge, asking the following pessimistic sequence questions (Selekman, 2009; Selekman & Beyebach, 2013) can spur them to action:

> "Let's say a police officer rings your doorbell this Saturday morning at 3 A.M. and tells you that your son had died. What affect would his loss have on you individually?"
> "What affect would his loss have on your marital relationship?"
> "What will you miss the most not having your son around anymore?"
> "Who will attend your son's funeral?"
> "What will the eulogies be?"

After responding to these questions even the most burned-out or laissez-faire of parents are not going to allow something dire to happen to their kids. They will begin to step up and collaborate in the change effort with us.

Parental Unity and Teamwork

Often in families with seriously acting-out adolescents with chronic behavioral difficulties, there is a lack of parental unity and teamwork, which is contributing to the maintenance of the presenting problems (Alexander et al., 2013; Donohue & Azrin, 2012; Henggeler et al., 2009; Liddle, 2010; Selekman & Beyebach, 2013; Szapocznik et al., 2012). In cases with delinquent and substance-abusing adolescents, the parents often disagree about how best to resolve their kids' difficulties. They don't back each other up, and the adolescent may be sitting on the shoulders of one of their parents in a coalition against the other parent. This leads to the parents' disqualifying each other and neutralizes their power and authority over their adolescents. Like inspirational coaches, we have to create intensity to get them emotionally fired up to be a dynamic duo in charge of their adolescents. I like to use superhero and sports metaphors as examples of successful teamwork. Finally, it also is beneficial to explore with the parents about their past successes of effective teamwork in managing their kids' problematic behaviors. We can then experiment with having them try out their past successful problem-solving strategies with their kids' current difficulties.

Nonviolent Passive Resistance Tactics

Omer (2004) was the first to research the use of nonviolent passive resistance tactics like sit-ins and letters to disarm severely acting-out children and adolescents and successfully put parents back in charge of the family. It is very difficult for even the most aggressive adolescent to continue to act out without a sparring partner. Two of the nonviolent passive resistance tactics he and his colleagues like to use are *sit-ins* and the *announcement letter*. In order for these tactics to work, both parents need to be willing to sit cross-legged inside their son's or daughter's bedroom door without losing control for as many hours as it takes for him or her to come up with solutions to their problematic behaviors. Omer (2004) has found that for explosive and violent adolescents it is best for the parents to have someone else in the house (a relative or close friend of the family) when they stage a sit-in in their bedrooms. This keeps the adolescents in check and makes it very difficult for them to try to hurt their parents.

Parents are to type up their announcement letter and present it to their son or daughter as a unified team. It should read as follows:

Dear _____,

Your mother and I and probably you have not liked the ways things have been in our family. As the leaders of our family, we would like to take our family in a much better direction. So your mother and I have agreed to stop yelling, nagging, threatening, giving you lengthy consequences, and lecturing at you as a positive step in that new direction. If we are willing to commit to making those changes that we know in the long run you will really appreciate, we need you to make the following changes:

- *No more smoking weed.*
- *No more swearing at and being disrespectful toward us.*
- *You will do your daily homework and chores without reminders.*
- *You will go to school daily.*
- *You will respect your curfew time.*

The other changes we plan to make are letting relatives know what has been happening in our family and no longer keep it under wraps. On the positive side, your mother and I are going to work on consistently praising you for your efforts to turn your behaviors around and the positive steps you are taking to be responsible and respectful. When these positive things happen, one of us will make ourselves available to do something fun and pleasurable you would like to do. It is very important to us that we can enjoy spending high-quality time together with no tension or fighting. We will only spend this high-quality time together when you are upholding and honoring all of our above requests of you.

Love,

Mother: _____

Father: _____

Most high-risk adolescents like the fact that their parents are willing to put forth the effort to change their "annoying" behaviors to improve their relationships with them. Since they have been wielding the power in the family so long, they initially don't like to hear that their parents are going to let relatives or others know about their "bad" behaviors. Predict for the parents that, even after they dramatically change the way they interact with their adolescents, there will be some backlash and limit testing. Parents have to be patient and maintain their composure. Eventually, the adolescents will get the message that provocative, threatening, and aggressive behaviors no longer can control and neutralize their parents' power. Once this clicks for the adolescents, their negative behaviors will begin to dramatically decrease.

Systemic Therapeutic Experiments and Connection-Building Rituals

In this section, I present a wide range of systemic therapeutic experiments and connection-building rituals. These are designed to alter outmoded family beliefs, disrupt long-standing problem-maintaining interactions, and strengthen parent–adolescent relational bonds. Some of these playful and upbeat systemic interventions tap family members' imagination and inventiveness to generate their own high-quality solutions to presenting difficulties. I discuss the following six therapeutic experiments and connection-building rituals below: imaginary time machine, adolescent mentoring his or her parents, invisible family inventions, the secret surprise, solution-oriented enactments, and pattern intervention strategies.

Imaginary Time Machine: Five Major Uses

The *imaginary time machine* is one of the most versatile family interventions that can be used at any stage of treatment (Selekman, 2005, 2009; Selekman & Beyebach, 2013). When adolescents or their parents are time traveling, it is important to have them use all of their senses, including color and motion, to bring their experiences to life as much as possible. I also like them to describe what they are thinking and feeling while in action in their choice destinations. I like to use the imaginary time machine in five different ways: to bring back the best from the past; to experience future selves to establish new parent–adolescent relationships in the now; to say "hello" in order to say "good-bye" to lost parents, siblings, and close relatives and friends; and to take the time machine anywhere in time. Below, I describe in what clinical situations each of these uses of the time machine can produce good results.

Bringing Back the Best from the Past

When there appears to be an emotional and physical disconnection between the adolescent and one or both parents, we can have the adolescents hop into the imaginary time machine. They are to take it back in time to a place where they felt very emotionally close with one or both parents and engaged in a fun or meaningful activity. Have them close their eyes and try to transport themselves back in time to relive these special and wonderful experiences with one or both parents. Most adolescents long to reconnect with the most disengaged parent; they used to be close, but after the parents separated or divorced he or she may have checked out of their son or daughter's life. Once adolescents have arrived at their choice destinations, they are to use all of their senses, including color, motion, to describe how they are thinking and feeling while with this disengaged parent. If the parents are present in the session, they usually start smiling and chiming in about how much they had enjoyed those experiences as well. Together with their adolescents, they can determine what pieces of this past positive experience they would like to reinstate in their relationship now. They might make plans to do this activity again in the near future. The use of the imaginary time machine often leads disengaged parents to agree to participate in future family sessions and be more present in their adolescents' lives.

When we are working with burned-out, frustrated parents, we can have them hop into the time machine and take it back to a place in the past where they felt a strong emotional connection with their adolescents. Whatever worked in the past that infused more warmth and emotional closeness in their relationships with their teens can be restored in their present relationships.

Taking the Time Machine Back to an Exuberant Life Experience

This use of the time machine can be done in both individual and family therapy sessions. Using all of their senses, the adolescents are to go back in time to a place they had been to that was magical, incredibly special, and emotionally uplifting to them. For the family members listening to the adolescents' marvelous time-traveling experiences, it serves as an injection of positivity and warmth in their relationships. If family members participated in the adolescents' exuberant life experiences, they can chime in their positive feelings and memories. It is a reminder of what works in their relationships and what they can reinstate in the here and now.

Experiencing Future Selves to Establish New Parent–Adolescent Relationships in the Now

When working with highly demoralized parents, the future can serve as fertile ground for all kinds of possibilities for them and their kids. In the family session, we can have the adolescents hop into the imaginary time machine. When they step out of it they are 24 or 25 years old, have completed their community or regular college education, are working, and have their own apartment alone or with friends. They have come over for Sunday night dinner with their parents. We can ask the parents and adolescents the following questions:

"Which one of you parents will faint first when this happens?"
"What will you be the most eager to share with your parents that is going well for you in your life?"
"Which one of you parents will be the most surprised to hear that?"
"When your parents ask you how you pulled that off, what steps will you tell them you took?"
"What else will you share with them that is helping you be so successful in your life?"
"Dad, is there anything that you had wanted to do with your son in the past that you now are more likely to do with him?"
"If you were to walk us back in time spelling out the steps that you took to achieve each one of those great accomplishments [completing college, getting a job, being financially self-sufficient], what will you tell us? What did you tell yourself and what were the specific steps you took to make it happen?"

For the parents, this future conversation of success can trigger positive emotion and greatly elevate their hope. This also will change their negative and pessimistic view of their son or daughter, which will improve their communications. The added bonus is that using the future this way can be helpful for goal setting, particularly if this had not happened due to the parents' feelings of hopelessness and despair.

Saying "Hello" in Order to Say "Good-Bye" to Lost Parents, Siblings, and Close Relatives and Friends

Adolescents who have experienced the painful loss of a parent, sibling, close relative, or friend may struggle with the grief process and get stuck at the point of the loss. This may be due to the fact that they had never had a chance to say good-bye to their departed loved one or close friend. More straightforward therapeutic attempts to facilitate the mourning process may not work. Here is where the trusty imaginary time machine can be most useful. If the adolescent is not suicidal or emotionally vulnerable, we can invite him or her to hop into the time machine and take it back to a place where he or she had done something special with the departed person. Using all of their senses, including color, motion, and how they were thinking and feeling at the time, they are to relive this meaningful and special experience. They are to say whatever they wished they could have said to the one they lost, to hug and kiss them, and think about the positive qualities they would like to carry on in honor of their special loved ones. Typically, when they return from their time traveling they start crying and so do the other family members. This opens up space for the adolescents and their families to begin mourning and reminiscing about their lost ones.

Taking the Imaginary Time Machine Anywhere in Time

A final way we can use the imaginary time machine is to have adolescents take it anywhere in time they wish. Some adolescents go back in time and meet famous historic figures from many different professional disciplines, such as people like Steve Jobs, Malcolm X, Martin Luther King, Jr., Eleanor Roosevelt, Mother Teresa, Pablo Picasso, Ben Franklin, Thomas Edison, Gandhi, and so forth. Other adolescents take the imaginary time machine into the future, where they have landed on Jupiter and met up with some aliens who taught them some interesting scientific and technologically advanced ideas and exposed them to their inventions. At the end of their time in their chosen destinations, they can invite their historic figures or new alien friends to join our family sessions to serve as consultants and offer advice for improving the adolescents' relationships with their parents and for other important areas of their lives.

Adolescent Mentoring His or Her Parent(s)

Another way that we can facilitate connection building and strengthen the parent–adolescent bonds is through the use of the *adolescent mentoring his or her parent(s)*. This ritual empowers adolescents to shine in their key competency areas and dramatically alters their parents' unhelpful and negative views of their kids. Adolescents can pick the parent they feel the most disconnected from for this ritual. They are first to identify their top skill areas, such as specific sports skills, cooking, dancing, playing an instrument, creative writing, acting, building and fixing things, and so forth. I avoid having them do activities on the computer or video gaming because it detracts from their staying connected with one another. The adolescents and their parents are to come up with a schedule of 45 minutes to an hour of dedicated time daily or every other day when the adolescents are in charge of teaching their parents their top skills and helping parents to achieve mastery in these areas. The adolescents are the teachers and their parents are the respectful students. They can ask questions for clarification but they cannot challenge or criticize their adolescent teachers. Often after a week of lessons with their kids, the parents discover how special and competent they are, which alters their former negative views and injects a big dose of positivity in their relationships. The parents often shower their adolescents with compliments, and in some cases request ongoing lessons with their kids. The adolescents are often all smiles and quite proud of being so patient with their parents.

Invisible Family Inventions

High-risk adolescents who are great with technology, sciences, and tinkering with and building things are excellent candidates for the *invisible family inventions* experiment (Selekman, 2005, 2009; Selekman & Beyebach, 2013). Some of these kids have already launched their careers as inventors by making things or have hot ideas for future products they would like to get on the market. In the family session, they have the option of doing this experiment alone with their therapists or in the company of their families. To launch the experiment and get their creative juices going, they are asked the following questions:

> "If you were to invent a machine or a gadget that would benefit other kids and families like yours, what would it do?"
> "What would it look like?"
> "How would it work and benefit you and your relationships with your family members?"

Like all inventors, they are to make a prototype sketch of their new machine or gadget. Next they are to come up with a name for it. I encourage them to present their sketches to their family and explain how it will work. Many adolescents get so excited about their new inventions that they will enlist their family members and try to build their new contraptions at home. Over the years, I have been so amazed, and so have their parents, about the high level of creativity they bring to their inventions. Some examples of these wonderful inventions include the Family Helper Machine, designed to alter your brain cells—you go in it when feeling down or stressed out and when you exit you are happy; the Anti-Annoying Parent App that parents can have on their digital devices which tracks their blood pressure, breathing, and heart rates prior to being annoying with their kids, such as nagging and yelling, and flashes a red warning sign on their screens indicating that they need to "chill out" and regain their composure before approaching their kids; or the deamplifiermagatizerrenatorrenator 2007, which was a large reverse megaphone designed for noise control in the household. It would suck up and trap the noise in it like a vacuum cleaner. Two warring adolescent brothers came up with this great invention to help reduce all of the yelling. Their 8-year-old autistic brother got up almost daily at 3 A.M. running around the house making sound effects, so nobody ever had peaceful uninterrupted sleep in this family. Not only were the boys' parents pleased to see that they could work together peacefully, but they loved their creativity and their wonderful infomercial. They also went home and built it with their father using plywood and cardboard, and added a bent light to it with a cord so it could be plugged into the wall and light up.

Secret Surprise

The *secret surprise* is a fun and upbeat therapeutic experiment to use as a way to inject more positivity into adolescents' relationships with their parents (O'Hanlon & Weiner-Davis, 1989; Selekman, 2005, 2009). During the family session, we meet alone with the adolescents and ask them, "How would you really like to blow your parents' minds?" This gets them intrigued and on the edge of their seats wanting to hear more about what their therapists have in mind for them. They are given the following directive:

> "Over the next week, I would like you to pull two secret surprises that will really shock your parents in a positive way. They need to be surprises that they will notice, really appreciate, and not expect from you. The important thing is that you are not allowed to tell them what the surprises were; your parents are going to be asked to play detectives and try to figure out what they were. In our next session, we will see what great detectives they were and we can talk about the surprises at that time. I can't wait to hear how you really blew their minds and they nearly fainted because of your great surprises!"

It is helpful while presenting the secret surprise experiment to have the adolescents come up with some surprise possibilities and write them down, so that they leave with some concrete ideas. When we reconvene with the parents, we let them know that there are going to some surprises happening over the next week that will shock them in a positive way. They are instructed to be like detectives, pull out their imaginary magnifying glasses, and try to figure out what the surprises were. We will compare notes in the next session.

Sometimes I will reverse who will be pulling the surprises and have the parents be the ones to surprise their kids. Their adolescents are the detectives trying to figure out what they were. This reverse strategy is particularly useful in clinical situations where the adolescents complain a great deal about how rigid and negative their parents are. Finally, in situations where the adolescents are having conflicts with particular teachers, we can have the adolescents perform the secret surprise in their classes and have their teachers try to identify what the surprises were.

Solution-Oriented Enactments

Originally, Minuchin (1974; Minuchin & Fishman, 1981) developed the family therapy technique of *enactments* as a great way to disrupt problem-maintaining patterns of interaction in family sessions. In his family sessions, he would have the family reenact a recent destructive interaction that may have led to the adolescent severely acting out or to some other crisis. The traditional use of enactments can be quite effective when the family therapy has become much more problem-focused and the family is deeply entrenched in rigid and destructive ways of interacting.

What I call *solution-oriented enactments* are useful early in treatment if family members are reporting noteworthy solution-building interactions and we want to get all of the details about what they are all doing differently during those times. We can have them practice the most useful and effective solution-building interactions both in and out of our sessions. In fact, when old destructive or unproductive interactions occur at home, a family member can make a time-out hand signal indicating that the family needs to freeze, shift gears, and engage in one of their most effective solution-building interactions with one another. With regular daily family practice time, eventually the solution-building patterns of interactions will become more natural, easier to engage in, and replace old unproductive family interactions.

Changing the Family Dance: Pattern Intervention Strategies

When the family therapy has become much more problem focused we can track problem-maintaining family interactions and disrupt them with *pattern intervention strategies* (Cade & O'Hanlon, 1993; Haley, 1983;

Havens, 2003; O'Hanlon, 1987; O'Hanlon & Weiner-Davis, 1989; Short et al., 2005). The first step is to invite one of the parents or another family member to provide a detailed motion picture description of the problem-maintaining interaction that triggers the adolescent to act up and what happens after that. This picture can be mapped out on a flipchart, which provides us with several locus points in which to intervene and break up the pattern. We can change the following:

- Change the order of family members' involvement.
- Add something new to the context in which the problem occurs.
- Schedule and prescribe for the adolescent to pretend to engage in a problematic behavior; the parents have to figure out if he or she is pretending or not.
- Change the time, duration, frequency, and location of the problem's occurrence.
- Make it an ordeal for the adolescent to engage in his or her problematic behavior.
- Predict that certain family members may struggle with the discomfort and consequences of change and then intervene to maintain the status quo, which can lead the family members to rebel against the therapist to prove him or her wrong.
- Have a crisis-prone family forecast what the next crisis is going to be, where it will happen, when, and who will be involved with it.

All of the above pattern intervention strategies can break up the problem life support systems in which the high-risk adolescents' challenging behaviors are embedded. Paradoxical pattern interventions are particularly effective with highly psychologically reactive adolescents who have not responded to more straightforward interventions (Rohrbaugh, Tennen, Press, & White, 1981; Weeks & L'Abate, 1982). On a cautionary note, paradoxical interventions should not be used with suicidal, violent, or psychotic clients. We should never prescribe self-destructive or destructive behaviors that could potentially harm the client and family members.

FORM 5.1

Epiphany Log

Directions: Every day, write down epiphanies that occurred to you, what sparked them, any wisdom gained from them, and how you applied them to resolving your difficulties or coping with them better.

Date	My Epiphany	Sparked by	Wisdom Gained	Applied to

Serendipitous Practices and Contexts Log

Directions: Every day, monitor and document any serendipitous practices and contexts that have brought you good luck or benefits. Specify what wisdom you have gained from these practices and resources, how you applied them to resolving or coping better with your difficulties, and the positive outcomes you experienced.

Date	Serendipitous Practices and Contexts	Wisdom Gained	Applied to	Positive Outcomes

CHAPTER 6

Family–Social Network Relapse Prevention Tools and Strategies

One small crack does not mean that you are broken; it means
that you were put to the test and you didn't fall apart.
—LINDA POINDEXTER

It is my contention that the relapse prevention process should begin at
the start of family therapy, whether or not the clients have elected to push
for total abstinence. We need to normalize for families that slips go with
the territory of change. They should be expected and seen as an indication that the family has already made good headway. By normalizing slips
in this way, families are less likely to perceive them as meaning they are
back to square one. Instead, they are valuable opportunities to learn, gain
wisdom, and discover together where they need to tighten up. The more
key resource people we have involved from our adolescent clients' social
networks providing support, the less likely slips will occur.

In this chapter, I present several major relapse prevention tools and
strategies that we can teach adolescents, their families, and key concerned
resource people from their social networks. I discuss what to do when the
adolescents' main peer group is highly toxic and the resources in their
social networks are limited. Finally, I address what strategies to pursue
with high-risk adolescents and their families who are constantly having
slips or prolonged relapsing setbacks, in spite of our team's best efforts.

Goal Maintenance and Relapse Prevention Is a Family–Social Network Affair

Often, therapists provide relapse prevention training with the adolescents
alone or in a group therapy setting. The parents are educated about their

kids' diseases if substance abuse is the main presenting problem or are educated about how their enabling behaviors contribute to their kids' substance abuse and other problematic behavior. They also learn alternative communication skills. Other actively involved key members from their social networks are typically excluded from the relapse prevention planning and strategizing process. If we are to adopt a true systemic relapse prevention approach and greatly optimize for adolescents' treatment success well beyond the completion of family therapy, we need to actively involve all of the key resource people from their social ecologies. When beginning the relapse prevention planning and strategizing process, I always invite the adolescent and his or her family to share with me what key people from their immediate and extended family and from their social network we need to invite who can help them to conquer their difficulties. Once engaged, the families and key resource people from their social networks are walked through the following four steps of the relapse prevention planning and strategizing process:

1. Consolidating gains and amplifying changes: The use of consolidating and future-vision questions.
2. Know thy triggers: Positive and negative.
3. Worst-case scenarios and action steps planning.
4. Solution-oriented behavioral rehearsing and practicing positive slip prevention management skills and strategies at home.

Below, I discuss each of these important therapeutic operations.

Consolidating Gains and Amplifying Changes: The Use of Consolidating and Future-Vision Questions

Although some of the recruited key resource people from clients' social networks may already have been involved earlier in their treatment process, we want to continue to tap their expertise. They can help consolidate client gains and share their powerful and positive future visions of success. After making great progress and achieving their goals, a questioning process will be used with the adolescents, their families, and key resource people. I provide below examples of both categories of these questions.

Consolidating Questions

"What would you have to do to go backwards at this point?"
"What are you now doing instead to not cave in to cutting?"
"Are you aware of how you're able to pull that off?"

"What are you telling yourself that is really helping?"

"What will you need to do to continue to make that happen for you?"

"How about with your parents, what are they doing differently that's helping you do so great and continue to stay on track?"

"How about with your grandmother, what is she doing differently that really helps?"

"How about with Mr. Sperry [the adult inspirational other], what specifically has he been sharing with or recommending to you that you think has contributed to your turnaround?"

"Mr. Sperry, what are you hearing from and seeing with Rosalind that you think has contributed to her incredible progress?"

"What about with Jackie [the adolescent's best friend], how has she contributed to your great success at quitting weed?"

"Tell me, Rosalind [the adolescent client], how are you viewing yourself differently now as a person versus how you used to view yourself when we first started working together?"

"How about the two of you [mother and father], how have your view and perceptions of Rosalind changed since she conquered her cutting problem?"

"Let's say I were to invite you in as guest consultants to help me with a family just like yours. What advice would you give them to help turn their situation around?"

"How specifically will that change make a big difference for them?"

"What else would you highly recommend to that family that you think will really work?"

Future-Vision Questions

"Let's say that we mutually decided to meet again in 4 weeks due to your tremendous progress. Now, if I had a crystal ball and we all gazed into it and we are watching all of you taking positive steps to further improve your relationships, what specifically are you doing that is really working?"

"How are you thinking and feeling different when your parents are treating you that way?"

"Mom and Dad, what are we watching Stan do differently in relation to you that is helping you get along even better together?"

"Let's say we have a 1-year anniversary party in my office after we had successfully completed our counseling together. What will be the number one change each of you will be eager to share with me?"

"How have those changes made a big difference in your relationships with one another?"

"What else is much better?"

"If your grandmother attends the anniversary party, what family change will she be the most delighted to share with me?"

"What will your best friend, Della, share with me at the party that she really noticed that changed with you Elisa [the adolescent client]?"

"Let's say we were to run into each other at your favorite shopping mall 6 months down the road, after we had completed counseling together. And Candy, you see me at a distance and come running up to me excited to tell me what further progress you had made. Which change will you share with me first that will really blow my mind?"

"Now that you are getting along much better with your father, what will you tell me you are doing together that is making a big difference in your relationship?"

"What else will you tell me about that is going great in your life?"

"Wow! Mr. Parker, your former school social worker, must have noticed us from a distance as well and is heading over here. What will he be the most surprised to hear that changed with you and your family situation?"

"Mrs. Davenport [Candy's mother], what will you share with me that you're happiest about that either further improved or changed in your relationship with Candy?"

Know Thy Triggers: Positive and Negative

When it comes to self-destructive behaviors, most therapists tend to only ask their adolescent clients and their parents about their negative triggers, and not what they and others do during good times that triggers positive emotion for them and helps them to resist slips. We also want to find out in detail from the adolescents what their parents, siblings, and key resource people from their social networks do that triggers positive emotions and interactions with them. One highly effective relapse prevention tool that I like to give adolescents to fill out weekly is *my positive trigger log* (see Form 6.1 at the end of the chapter). Between sessions and on a daily basis, the adolescents can keep track of what they, their parents and siblings, their closest friends, and other involved professionals do that triggers positive emotions and thoughts and keeps them from caving in to their internalizing or externalizing behaviors. It also is most advantageous to have them circle what they and others do that helps the most, so that these coping strategies can be the first to turn to during high-stress times. After a week of experimenting with their my positive trigger logs, they bring them in and we can learn what works the best for them. We can make copies of their positive trigger logs and they can fold up the originals to keep with them. They can be pulled out in emergency situations, offering many positive options to pursue. I like to give the adolescents a stack of positive trigger logs to take with them and continue to fill out as new creative coping strategies come from them and others.

For negative triggers, we need highly detailed and comprehensive inquiry with the adolescents, their families, and involved key resource people from their social networks. Adolescents' negative triggers can be:

- Certain toxic people
- Certain toxic places
- Certain objects
- Certain musical tunes
- Certain images, memories, and mood states
- Certain thoughts and feelings
- Certain websites and/or online games
- Certain video games
- Certain parental tones of voices and nonverbal facial or bodily postures
- Being triangulated into taking sides against one parent
- Being set up by a sibling or peer to get into trouble
- Being rejected by peers or a romantic love interest
- Being publicly humiliated or having rumors spread about the adolescent by peers on popular social media sites
- Failing a test or doing poorly in school
- Not getting enough sleep

By no means are these all of the triggers that adolescents typically report, but they are some of the most common ones I have heard in my office. The family members and involved key resource people from their social networks also may be able to identify unmentioned triggers that they have observed over the years for the adolescent as well. It is important for the adolescents to let all members of their relapse prevention teams know what specifically each can do to help when they encounter triggers. It is critical to educate parents about the same coping tools and strategies we have taught their adolescents, so as to create a bridge from our offices to their homes. For example, if an adolescent client experiences one or two triggers the parent can ask her, "What do you think can help you best right now, doing the *visualizing your movie of success* or doing the *six deep breaths*?" Once my adolescent clients get more skilled at using their tools, I will put them in charge of teaching them to their parents. Many parents greatly appreciate learning coping tools and strategies, particularly mindfulness meditations in order to decompress after stressful days at work.

Worst-Case Scenarios and Action Steps Planning

One of the biggest mistakes therapists make after their clients have made considerable progress is failing to prepare clients to constructively manage worst-case scenarios that could trigger a prolonged relapse. Therefore, a critical component to a solid relapse prevention plan is doing *worst-case scenarios and action steps planning* with the families and their involved key resource people from their social networks. I have developed a special form that clients can fill out with their relapse prevention support teams so that everyone is clear what specific steps they need to take if the adolescent's identified worst-case scenarios should occur (see Form 6.2 at the end of the chapter). These steps are to be written down on the form, and all members of the relapse prevention team receive a copy of it. It will be mailed to absent involved people from the clients' social networks. What is most important is that the adolescents take the lead in sharing with their family members and concerned key members of their social networks what specifically they could do to help them constructively manage worst-case scenarios. It also is important to have parents identify potential crisis situations that they might have faced with their kids in the past and have them identify both which key resource people from their social networks they would like to call upon for support and what specifically these others could do to help stabilize the situation. Finally, the faster the members of the relapse prevention support team can intervene when worst-case scenario situations occur, the more likely they will be able to prevent slips.

Solution-Oriented Behavioral Rehearsing and Practicing Positive Slip Prevention Management Skills and Strategies at Home

Once the adolescents identify what specific types of positive and supportive interactions their parents and key resource people from their social networks engage in that prevent them from having slips, we can have them practice their solution-maintaining interactions in sessions. This underscores what works and what to increase doing, reduces the likelihood of their returning back to destructive interactions, increases their positive emotion levels, and reinforces the benefits of good teamwork. At home, even during low-stress times, it can be beneficial to have the family and members from social networks practice their solution-maintaining patterns of interaction a few days a week. The adolescents can pretend that two or more triggers are pushing them around or they experience an unexpected worst-case scenario. The family members and key resource people from their social networks can rapidly respond in the adolescents' identified best ways to help slips from occurring.

Other Goal Maintenance and Relapse Prevention Tools and Strategies

In this section, I discuss six other goal maintenance and relapse prevention tools and strategies: daily engagement in positive virtuous habits; externalizing solutions to thwart problem comebacks and sneak attacks; using former client alumni as expert guest consultants; using weak-link peers and untapped adult inspirational others; imagining yourself as _____ to stay on track; and the 10–10–10 risk management strategy.

Daily Engagement in Positive Virtuous Habits

There are three major contributing factors to why high-risk adolescents often experience slips: lack of skills to cope with unpleasant negative emotions, high stress, and a lack of healthy activities during their leisure time or at school (Donohue & Azrin, 2012; Marlatt & Donovan, 2005; Peele, 2014). This is why, as early as possible in the treatment process, we need to expose the adolescents to a wide range of *positive virtuous habits* derived from their key strengths and interest areas that they can build into their daily schedules (Selekman & Beyebach, 2013). First we need to find out from the adolescents what types of positive flow state activities they could either reinstate from the past, such as playing an instrument again, or new flow state activities they can increase their involvement with. We also need to find out from them if they can identify any unexplored areas of curiosity that might be worth exploring and/or pursuing at school or during their leisure time, such as rock climbing or taking a martial arts, yoga, or hip-hop dance class. Once we have a good sense what our adolescent clients' key strengths, talents, life passions, and possible career interest areas are, we can share our ideas and build into our therapeutic work the mastery of positive virtuous habits, which can include the following:

- Learning and daily practicing mindfulness meditations and visualization.
- Learning and practicing wise mind dialectical behavior therapy distress management tools and strategies (Miller, Rathus, & Linehan, 2007; Rathus & Miller, 2015).
- Engaging in some form of daily exercise: running, biking, walking, swimming, and/or weight training.
- Trying out for a school sport's team.
- Adopting a healthier diet and getting enough sleep.
- Reducing one's daily involvement in the use of technology and striving to find the balance of offline and online interactions with others.

- Getting involved in a school club.
- Once a week, strive for some form of prevention work at school or service work in the community, involvement in a social cause, or do a good deed for a family member, friend, or neighbor.
- Keep a gratitude log and regularly acknowledge and thank those in one's life for their kindness and generosity.
- Challenge oneself to learn about and master something new, like learning how to play an instrument, a new dance, a new sport, or acting.

Adolescents' participation in such daily habits should decrease their negative emotions, help reduce stress, and increase meaning and purpose in their lives. Over time, this should ultimately help stabilize their internalizing and externalizing behaviors. After we collaboratively determine with the adolescents which positive virtuous habits they wish to cultivate, let them know that initially their new habits will feel unnatural. They should expect bumps in the road while practicing, and it will take discipline and hard work to master them.

Externalizing Solutions to Thwart Problem Comebacks and Sneak Attacks

Long-standing adolescent problems that seemingly have had a life all of their own don't die easily even after lengthy periods of calm, and regular use of their coping tools. Just as certain bacteria become resistant to antibiotics, problems can become resistant to certain coping tools and strategies. They can lose their strength, particularly after family crises that trigger high levels of negative emotion and stress, making them vulnerable for problem comebacks and sneak attacks. In the spirit of narrative therapy, I like to externalize the adolescents' and families' top solutions as a way to see how they may need to be strengthened to help thwart their problems' comeback efforts and sneak attacks. Some examples of *externalizing solutions questions* to ask clients include:

> "In what ways can you call upon and use your trusty self-talk strategy, 'Stephanie, stay calm and remind yourself that you are a kind, caring, and compassionate person' instead of caving in to 'cutting's wishes that you will cut yourself in the girls' bathroom,' after Courtney rolls her eyes and makes some nasty comments to you in front of her friends when she passes you in the school hallway?"
> "Are there any other positive qualities or words you would like to add to your self-talk strategy that you think would make it even more potent and resistant to 'cutting's brainwashing efforts to get you to brutalize your body'?"

"In addition to telling yourself, 'Stephanie stay calm and remind yourself that you are a kind, caring, and compassionate person,' what other helpful coping tools and strategies can you come to school armed with that could serve as good backups to immediately use if your self-talk strategy appears to be neutralized by 'cutting's wishes for you to punish yourself'?"

Externalizing solution questions tap the expertise of the adolescents to see how they can further strengthen the potency of their choice coping tools. Invite them to be mindful about the importance of having good backup coping tools and strategies to immediately put in place if their first choices are ineffectual and are being neutralized by the powerful resurrected problems. These types of questions also remind them to be flexible, stay on their toes, and be open to further honing their coping skills, particularly during high-stress times or following crisis events.

Using Former Client Alumni as Expert Guest Consultants

For years, I have maintained an alumni association of adolescents and parents I formerly worked with. They have agreed to serve as expert consultants in the future to help me with more challenging families that could benefit from hearing their solution-determined success stories, specifically what worked and has continued to work for them. With adolescents deeply rooted in gang life, heavily into drugs, bullying other kids, and engaging in other high-risk behaviors, it can be of great benefit to bring in alumni who conquered these difficulties, particularly if they are fairly close in age. The alumni can help clients find legitimate jobs, do better in school, help them to safeguard themselves from experiencing slips and making poor choices, and expose them to healthy leisure activities like joining a basketball league at the local recreation center, practicing yoga, service work, mindfulness meditation, and so forth. In some cases, the clients may become good friends outside of therapy sessions, which can be another plus. Before carefully matching and recruiting alumni for my family sessions with the adolescents, I first secure written consents from both the parents of the clients and the alumni, the adolescents, and the alumni adolescents/young adults giving me permission to invite these resourceful others to participate in our sessions. I explain to everyone the importance of respecting client confidentiality.

Bringing in alumni parents can be quite uplifting for these challenging parents who hear that their adolescents' difficulties can be overcome. What is most beneficial for these stuck parents to learn about is how the alumni turned their situations dramatically around.

Using Weak-Link Peers and Untapped Potential Adult Inspirational Others

When high-risk adolescents' main peer groups are highly toxic, goal maintenance is on shaky ground. We can engage two potential resource people and tap into their expertise with the relapse prevention process and ask for additional support between sessions and well after treatment completion: *weak-link peers* and *untapped potential adult inspirational others.* Weak-link individuals can be acquaintances or people our clients have met in different contexts who they may have liked or been intrigued by because of their interesting work, talents, or their shared interests, but for whatever reason did not take the extra steps to try building relationships with them (Koch & Lockwood, 2010). For high-risk adolescents and their parents or legal guardians, these weak-link others also can be strangers they have heard about in the community or at school because of their knowledge and expertise, or they have observed or overheard them talking to others in social contexts. The adolescents may have thought them to be "nice, friendly, clever, and interesting" people and worth getting to know (Gregerman, 2013). Other important weak-link individuals are *positive deviants* or outliers who used to have similar difficulties but came up with creative, high-quality solutions for resolving their problems (Pascale, Sternin, & Sternin, 2010). We can learn about these resourceful positive deviants from school social workers, specialized adolescent treatment programs, community-based self-help groups, through various forms of the social media, and so forth.

Over the years, I have had a great deal of success with having my high-risk adolescent clients venture out of their comfort zones and attempt to establish relationships with their weak-link acquaintances and strangers in their social ecologies. More often than not, these weak-link peers are quite receptive to getting to know them and building relationships with them. Prior to embarking on their risky social missions, we discuss in sessions the necessity of expanding their social horizons and the dangers and risks of continuing to run with the same crew of peers who have cost them big time. Once the clients have cultivated relationships with these weak-link peers and friendships are solidifying, they can be recruited to join us in our family sessions to share their creative ideas about helping the clients stay on track and serve as a relapse prevention support system for them outside of sessions.

For high-risk adolescents who do not have adult inspirational others present in their lives, we can explore whether they can think of anyone in their social ecologies who could serve in this role. If so, I will encourage them to step outside of their comfort zones and attempt to connect with these potential adult inspirational others to help provide them with added support. In clinical situations where the adolescents cannot identify an adult for this role, I have recruited experienced adult inspirational others who I knew from work with former clients. They are often delighted to serve in this capacity. However, if they are to see the clients outside of school or you would like them to participate in family sessions, it is important to have the adolescent's parents or legal guardians sign a consent form.

Imagine Yourself as _____ to Stay on Track

Since most adolescents have a great sense of imagination and are quite curious, the *imagine yourself as* _____ *to stay on track* experiment can be an intriguing and fun relapse prevention tool they can add to their repertoire. We need to talk adolescents through the following five steps:

1. Have them identify a famous person they are inspired by.
2. Have a brief conversation with them about what personal qualities, strengths, and talents made them so successful in their professions and lives.
3. Have them close their eyes and see themselves having a conversation with their selected famous person, telling him or her about their personal situations and concerns about staying on track and preventing slips.
4. With their eyes closed they are to share with you the advice or words of wisdom their famous person is sharing with them, particularly what steps the person would take to successfully manage their problem situations if he or she was in their shoes.
5. Next, have the adolescents imagine seeing themselves shake hands with or hugging their famous person, imagine merging with them. The person is now a friendly and caring part of them that will influence their thinking and action to help them to successfully cope with negative triggers and crisis situations. Finally, have the adolescent practice by imagining a crisis and using the internalized famous person to help them to manage it.

With the last implementation step, it is important for the adolescents to remain as calm as possible when faced with triggering negative emotions. They are to access the image and the words of their selected famous people who will direct them on how best to handle the crisis situation. Like all coping tools and strategies, we need to have the adolescents practice using this coping tool even during nonstressful times.

The 10–10–10 Risk Management Strategy

The 10–10–10 risk management strategy is helpful with collaborative risk management and is effective at preventing adolescent slips from happening (Steiner, 2014; Welch, 2009). Whenever the adolescents are experiencing any of their powerful triggers and feeling vulnerable for a slip, they are to say to themselves, "If I cave in to the urge to [cut myself, get stoned, binge and purge, etc.], I need to ask myself, 'What will be the advantage of my doing this in 10 minutes?'; 'In 10 hours?'; 'In 10 weeks?' "

Adolescents can do this exercise any time they are tempted to engage in former self-destructive or externalizing behaviors. This allows them time to stop and reflect, which can help prevent poor decisions.

It is also critical to teach high-risk adolescents how to use the mindfulness mediations, visualization, and cognitive and self-control tools and strategies discussed in great detail in Chapter 5, which I include as part of the relapse prevention arsenal. We need to encourage our adolescent clients to practice using them daily, even during nonstressful times, so that they can be confidently and easily used when they are experiencing negative emotions and high stress.

Being Mindful for Impending Slips

Throughout the course of family therapy with high-risk adolescents and their families, we need to carefully listen to and observe the following in and out of sessions from our clients:

- The structure is breaking down during leisure time.
- Picking up on adolescent and parental indications that they are slipping back into former negative family interactions, experiencing increased stress and negative emotions.
- The adolescents' testing their willpower by putting themselves back in the company of toxic people and places, and in risky situations.
- The adolescents' becoming increasingly more secretive and ducking under the radar of family and involved caring others from their social network.
- Decreasing or stopped practice of their coping tools and strategies and engaging in healthy activities.

All of these situations can set the stage for adolescents to have slips. As therapists, it is important not only to amplify and consolidate our clients' gains session-by-session but also to make room for exploring any recent worries, crisis events, losses, newly diagnosed serious family illnesses, or other stressors. They may be contributing to the above actions. This includes any family members' worries or concerns outside our goal maintenance and relapse prevention plan areas. We can ask the families the following questions to find out this important information:

"Is there anything we have not talked about up to this point or happened recently that could lead to a major setback or relapse situation occurring unless we address it soon?"

"Is there anything else going on outside of our goal or relapse prevention plan areas that any of you are concerned about that could come back to haunt us or derail your progress unless we address or resolve it now?"

Once the adolescents' and their families' concerns are identified in close collaboration with their involved members from their social networks, we can put our heads together to strategize about how best to resolve their concerns. In some cases, families are so shaken by a loss or crisis event that they stop doing what had been keeping them solidly on track and they inadvertently fall back into old habits and problem-maintaining family interactions.

Managing High Slip Rate and Prolonged Relapsing Adolescents and Families

One of the most challenging clinical dilemmas we will face are those clients who have high slip rates and prolonged relapsing periods. Some of these families may be grappling with frequent crises and family disruptions; multiple symptom-bearing family members with serious DSM disorders; acclimatization to the presence of the original adolescent presenting problems that makes change feel like a threat to status quo; and difficulty with maintaining the necessary structure and teamwork among family members and concerned others in their social networks for reducing the frequency of slips and likelihood of prolonged relapsing situations. Below, I present seven strategies we can pursue both with the key resource people from their social networks and in our family therapy sessions to try and reduce the clients' high slip rates and prevent prolonged relapsing crisis situations from occurring: can–if mapping and strategizing; using a reflecting team; using a therapeutic debate team; the negative consequences of change; the compression technique; declaring impotence and firing oneself from the case; and risk management (periodic detoxes, hospitalizations, and temporary alternative living arrangement respites).

Can-If Mapping and Strategizing

In Chapter 4, I introduced the creative and idea-generating *can–if map* strategy for both coming up with high-quality solutions and for determining missing important areas to cover that can help empower our clients to resolve their difficulties (Morgan & Barden, 2015; see Chapter 4 and Form 4.2). Include in the can–if mapping and strategizing meetings as many of the key people as possible from our clients' social network and involved helping professionals from larger systems. The more brainpower and creativity we have around the circle, the more likely we will be able to co-generate multiple novel high-quality solutions that can be immediately implemented. The solid backup support can help reduce the frequency of slips and prevent prolonged relapsing crises from occurring.

Using a Reflecting Team

The *reflecting team* consultation method can be quite helpful with stuck cases and family situations where we are picking up on innuendos of family secrets that could be responsible for why the high-risk adolescents are constantly having slips or prolonged relapsing episodes (Andersen, 1991, 1995; Lax, 1995; Selekman, 2005, 2006). The reflecting team consultation format consists of three or four team members who will have a 6- to 7-minute conversation in front of the family around 40 minutes into the hour-long session. They dialogue and pose questions from a position of curiosity about what the clients may have left unsaid or what they speculate may be the family's current dilemma or difficulties. Team members can take big risks with their probing. It is important that they (1) present their ideas and questions in a tentative way, with qualifiers like "I wonder if . . . ?," "Could it be . . . ?,"; "I was struck by . . ."; (2) avoid at all costs placing blame on any one family member; (3) use possible logical and intriguing explanations versus negative explanations when framing reflections; and (4) try not to bombard the family with too many ideas (limit the team conversation to two to three possible ideas or themes). After the team completes their dialogue, the family is invited to reflect on what the team had to say, which can open up space for the revelation of the unsaid. It may be a family secret or some other concern that has never been talked about before.

In practice settings equipped with one-way mirrors and adjacent observation rooms, the family and team can switch rooms when the team reflects and listen attentively and quietly to their conversation for ideas, themes, and questions that resonate with them. When the team's reflection is over, they switch rooms and the therapist invites the family to reflect on what they had to say. If your practice setting does not have one-way mirrors or observation rooms, the team can sit in the therapy room positioned back behind the family and therapist. At the 40-minute point of the session, the family and therapist can turn their chairs to observe and carefully listen to the team's dialogue. The case below with Tricia, a 16-year-old white girl, and her parents illustrates the therapeutic benefits of the reflecting team consultation method with a difficult case. I was asked to serve as one of the reflecting team members for a colleague who was feeling stuck after four unproductive family sessions.

Tricia had a 2-year history of severe bulimia, self-injury, and anxiety. She was having difficulty remaining abstinent from bingeing and purging and self-injuring. The reflecting team members posed the following questions during their dialogue: "Could it be that Tricia's bulimia and cutting are metaphors for her possibly feeling cut in two with her family loyalties and experiencing indigestion from that?" "I wonder what's not being talked about in this family that might need to be addressed?" I posed my question in response to the first team member's question, "I wonder if there is something that happened in the past or recently that might be difficult for Tricia to swallow or digest?" For a few more minutes, as a team, we played around with the metaphors of split loyalties and some possible family event that has been difficult to digest. After Tricia heard the team's questions and dialogue, she grew anxious and asked if she could talk to her father alone. The therapist honored her request to talk alone with her father without the mother present. For the first time, Tricia disclosed to the father that she had seen on his laptop some email exchanges with what appeared to be a woman she suspected he was having an affair with. The father reacted with, "Oh my God!" Tricia confronted him with, "Is it true?" He admitted that he had been having an affair for the past 2 years, which coincided with the onset of Tricia's bulimia, self-injuring, and anxiety difficulties. Tricia went on to say that she had been keeping a lid on this information for the past 2 years and protecting both the father and her mother. The father apologized to Tricia for putting her through such an "emotional ordeal." Tricia started crying when her father hugged her, and she shared with him, "You've got to tell mom." The therapist explored with the father how he wished to handle the situation, and he requested that his wife join them and for Tricia to wait in the lobby. What transpired next in the session was the father's telling the mother about his extramarital affair. Although she was quite furious and hurt by this painful information, she was open to trying to save the marriage. Apparently, she had noticed that her husband had been emotionally and intimately withdrawing from her over the past 2 years. The couple ended up contracting with my colleague for marital therapy. Tricia started doing much better as her parents committed to improving their relationship.

Using a Therapeutic Debate Team

The *therapeutic debate team* strategy is quite effective when family members are deeply entrenched in rigid role behaviors and adolescents are experiencing high rates of slips and prolonged relapses (Papp, 1983; Selekman, 2006, 2009; Selekman & Beyebach, 2013; Sheinberg, 1985; Sheinberg & Frankael, 2001). Since they have become so acclimatized to having problems and moving from one crisis to the next, these therapeutic veteran families may view any changes to their situation as a threat. Throughout my career, I have worked with a number of therapy-veteran families whose adolescents were using the threat of violence and suicide to control and hold their parents hostage. Needless to say, these powerful and tyrannical adolescents were not quick to give up the secondary gains they got from ruling the roost in their homes.

With the therapeutic debate team format, two to three of your colleagues serve as the debate team. Around 40 minutes into the hour, the team members join the family and therapist and launch into a debate in their company. The team members represent different family members' positions, such as the adolescent, the parents or legal guardians, including one team member pretending to be a personified version of the problem. Similar to the reflecting team dialogue, they can be provocative and take risks with what they debate about, such as speculating about inequities in power and control dynamics in specific family relationships, unexpressed family secrets, the dilemmas and costs of change, and so forth. Family members often will chime in agreement with or challenge what debate team members are saying. In some cases, family members will share secrets, concerns, or topics with one another that had never been expressed before. The high-risk adolescent may rebel against the debate team member who is taking the side of his or her parents and predicting that he or she will dig in more and continue to rule the roost at home and refuse to change, despite the rapidly mounting life consequences he or she is experiencing. The debate team member taking the side of the adolescent may lead the teen to sharing for the first time with his or her parents or legal guardians the unresolved conflicts he or she is still harboring with them or what specifically has been missing in his or her relationships with them that could make things better. The debate dialogue should not exceed 10 minutes. Following the team's debate, family members can share what they had heard that resonated with them, any new ways of viewing their family situation, their relationships, or the problem, and new directions they wish to explore as a family.

The Negative Consequences of Change

When goal maintenance tools and relapse prevention strategies are failing to stave off slips or prevent prolonged relapse situations, we can use the MRI brief strategic major intervention of the *negative consequences of change* (Fisch & Schlanger, 1999; Fisch et al., 1982). Therapy-veteran families in particular are often highly entrenched in unproductive patterns of interaction and cling to very rigid views of their difficulties. Therapists get into trouble with these types of families in their zeal to push for change using straightforward therapeutic tools and strategies. Families will resist and not implement their proposed interventions. Rather than continuing to do *more of the same,* therapists instead need to slow the change process down and be curious with these families about the dangers and potential costs of their changing. We can wonder aloud with them and pose the following provocative questions:

"I wonder, if Sidney stops smoking weed, whether your younger teenage son will start experimenting with drugs to keep you [the parents] on your toes?"

"I wonder when you [the parents] no longer have to worry about Mary's anorexia whether the two of you will start arguing more?"

"Johnny, I wonder if you step down from your throne in your family whether your dad will have to fight his own battles with your mother?"

"Do you think he can handle it, or will he need your help?"

"Mary, if you stop carving deeply into your arms do you think you will become an invisible person in your family?"

"Steve, do you think if you conquer OCD and stop its reign over you and your family that there will be an emptiness in your life and your family life in general will become really boring?"

The hope here is that the family will be pried out of their nochange position and rebel against the therapist's provocative predictions. When they start to dismiss these predictions and offer alternative outcomes, not only do I write down their responses but I like to respond to them with the following *restraint from immediate change* questions:

"How can you be absolutely certain _____ will happen instead?"

"What makes you think that?"

"Don't you think that will be really hard for you to pull off?"

"Wouldn't that be like stepping into no-man's land for you, going outside your comfort zone in that way?"

What often happens is that family members begin to take steps in the direction of change to prove their skeptical therapists wrong. Conversely, when we prove to be accurate fortune-tellers with our provocative predictions we can be confused and curious with the family about how what they claimed could not possibly happen came to pass.

The Compression Technique

The *compression technique* (Stanton, 1984) can be in order with therapy-veteran and other parents who have long histories of being hyperresponsible or overprotective, robbing their adolescents of being more self-sufficient and taking responsibility for their actions. Typically, straightforward rational attempts at convincing these parents to discontinue their unproductive enabling and controlling behaviors are met with an onslaught of "Yes, but . . ." responses. Therefore, we need to pursue a counter-illogical direction with them. You can share with them that you have been all wrong with your approach to the situation and that you are now switching gears. Next, we want to encourage them to increase their hyperresponsible, loving and caring behaviors with their adolescents, by doing the following: waiting on, checking in on, and texting their adolescents more often when they are at home or out with friends; if they are home sick, check their temperature every hour and keep regularly replenishing their fluids; and if they have papers that are due and need to be written immediately, write them for them. When the teens are out with friends, play detective and follow them in your cars and stage stakeouts outside of their friends' houses to make sure they are safe and where they say they are supposed to be. The compression strategy may not change the parents' behaviors for a week or two, but eventually, a neon sign will light up in their minds flashing: THIS IS CRAZY! WHAT HAVE I BEEN DOING! I'VE GOT TO STOP THIS MADNESS! Once this happens and the parents abandon their unproductive solutions, their adolescents' problematic behaviors begin changing. The parents become open to learning more effective parenting tools and strategies.

Declaring Impotence and Firing Oneself Off the Case

When teens escalate their high-risk behaviors despite their parents' efforts to help them, *declaring impotence* may be worthwhile (Andolfi, Angelo, Menghi, & Nicolo-Corigliano, 1983). The parents or legal guardians declare to their adolescents that they have finally discovered that there is nothing more that they can do to help them. They have decided to stop having any expectations for them or even attempting to parent them. This declaration can include discontinuing washing and drying their clothes, waking them up in the mornings to go to school, being their chauffeurs, cooking their favorite dishes, and so forth. When approached by their perplexed adolescents about what is wrong with them or why the sudden change in their behaviors, they are to respond arbitrarily with: "I am/We are emotionally and physically exhausted," "I am/We are tired of battling with you," "It is my/our turn to take care of myself/ourselves," or "You win, we surrender." After giving these arbitrary responses, they are to avoid further elaborating on their new positions vis-à-vis their adolescents and move on to something they wish to do or take care of. This dramatic parental move away from former power struggles, threats, lectures, withholding highly prized possessions and privileges, and bribery can lead to their adolescents' beginning to cooperate more with their rules and expectations and improvement in their problematic behaviors.

Another variation of this strategic intervention is for the *therapist* to declare impotence and fire him- or herself off their case. This should be a last resort intervention after we have exhausted both straightforward and other indirect strategic interventions. In addition, there should already have been conversations between the frustrated therapist and his or her supervisor about referring the family to another therapist who uses a different approach. To add further drama to this unexpected therapeutic move, the therapist can bring in a letter written by his or her supervisor to read to the family which states that he or she is being removed from the case because his or her involvement was not improving their situation and indeed it appeared to be getting much worse. The supervisor can also indicate in his or her letter that in situations like theirs it can be quite beneficial to have a new therapist with a fresh approach. Often after hearing the supervisor's letter, the family will not only disagree with his or her skeptical supervisor but fight to keep their therapist on the case. Families typically respond in the following ways: "We like you, we don't want to start over with a new therapist!" "That is mean of your supervisor to do that!" "Can we meet with your supervisor and tell her we want to keep you as our therapist?" In some cases, families will go the extra mile to fight for their therapists by talking to their supervisors and advocating for us. What I have observed with this strategic intervention that often families not only are more ready to establish cooperative partnerships with their therapists but they start to talk about issues or difficulties they had never brought up before in earlier sessions, which had been keeping the treatment process at a standstill.

Risk Management: Periodic Detoxes, Hospitalizations, and Temporary Alternative Living Arrangement Respites

With high-risk adolescents heavily abusing substances and exhibiting clear signs of physiological dependency, periodic detoxes may be necessary so that they can be closely medically monitored. Some aftercare days or a week in a partial day hospital or an intensive outpatient program may be in order if they are still in a vulnerable state after detox. The same is true for teens with anorexia who are physically in jeopardy and formerly suicidal adolescents who could greatly benefit from short stays in the hospital to make sure they are safe and medically stabilized. Some follow-up aftercare in either partial day or intensive outpatient programs may also be appropriate for further support.

When the conflict is extremely high in the home or there is the potential for violence and a no-violence safety plan is in place, it can be of great benefit to all parties for the adolescents to live temporarily with an older sibling or close relative until they are in better places emotionally to deal with their difficulties. Once a decision is made to reintegrate the adolescents back into their homes, we can have the older sibling or relative they lived with join us in family therapy to help ease the transition process.

FORM 6.1

My Positive Trigger Log

Directions: Every day, carefully keep track of what you, family members, and resource people from your social network say or do to trigger positive emotions for you and help you steer clear of slips. In the last column, write down what specific thoughts and feelings are triggered for you by your personal steps, as well as the actions of others who care about you.

Date	What I Did	My Parents/Siblings	Friends	Other Involved Helpers	Positive Thoughts and Feelings Triggered

Worst-Case Scenarios and Action Steps

Directions: As a team, collaborate to list four or five worst-case scenarios that could occur. In the second column, the teen is to write the steps he or she will take to constructively manage each of the situations. In the last column, write down the steps you would like family members and key resource people from your social network to take to help you to stay on track.

Worst-Case Scenario	Individual Steps I Will Take	The Steps We Will Take (Partner, Family Members, Key Resource People from Social Network)

CHAPTER 7

"The Atomic Bomb Kid"
Working with a Violent Adolescent

Character cannot be developed in ease and quiet. Only through experience of trial and suffering can the soul be strengthened, ambition inspired, and success achieved.

—HELEN KELLER

In this chapter, I present a full-length case example of my work with a violent gang-involved Mexican American 17-year-old boy named Alejandro, his mother, and key resource people from his social network, which included his school social worker, probation officer, and the family's priest.

Referral Process and Intake Information

Alejandro was referred to me by his high school social worker, Ms. Danner, after being expelled from school for beating up a rival gang member so badly on school grounds that the latter ended up being hospitalized. Apparently, the rival gang member had punched and robbed Alejandro's 15-year-old brother, Eduardo, and this was considered a retaliatory act. Prior to his being expelled, he was about to be placed in a highly structured therapeutic day school due to his "fighting with peers, self-injuring by smashing his fists into walls when angry, alcohol and marijuana abuse, and school truancy problems." Alejandro's violent and aggressive behaviors dated back to fifth grade, when he was constantly getting into fights and bullying his peers. In fact, the same school district psychologist who had conducted two case study evaluations with him, one in sixth grade and one in tenth grade, had described him as "The Atomic Bomb Kid" because of his very short fuse, poor impulse control, explosiveness, and punching walls when angry. According to Ms. Danner, Alejandro had been a member of one of the oldest and toughest Latino street gangs in the city since he was 12 years old. While serving as a loyal street fighter, drug dealer, and thief for his gang, Alejandro had been stabbed and shot a few times, witnessed some of his best friends being killed and severely maimed on the streets, and had had multiple incarcerations in the juvenile detention center. Ms. Danner had been seeing Alejandro weekly since he was a high school freshman. When asked about his past treatment experiences, Ms. Danner reported that he had had two inpatient psychiatric treatment experiences for his aggressive and explosive behaviors and for not following the parents' rules. He had also had seven outpatient treatment experiences dating back to when he was in fifth grade.

When asked about his relationships with his parents, Ms. Danner shared that he has a good relationship with his mother who prays daily for him with their priest that Alejandro will not be killed on the streets. Ms. Danner pointed out to me that Alejandro hates his stepfather, Pedro, who used to harshly discipline him and would never go to any of his past family counseling sessions. Neither Alejandro nor Eduardo had ever met their biological father because he had abandoned the family when they were toddlers. She also shared with me that although he had bullied his brother in the past, Alejandro did care about him, as evidenced by his going after the rival gang member who had hurt and robbed him. Finally, she stressed that Alejandro had many strengths: he was very bright, had a great sense of humor, and was incredibly talented with auto mechanic work and computers. Apparently, he was the top student in his high school autos class.

I called Alejandro's mother, Sylvia, to set up an appointment. We had a nice conversation and she expressed her fears of losing Alejandro on the streets if he kept running with the gang. I provided empathy and support. Prior to ending our conversation, I gave her the pretreatment experiment of daily carefully watching for any responsible and respectful steps she observed Alejandro taking, writing her observations down. In addition, I had her keep track of what she had been doing during those times that may be contributing to Alejandro's positive behaviors occurring. Finally, I explained to her that this experiment would teach me more about her and Alejandro's strengths, resourcefulness, and self-generated coping and problem-solving strategies.

The First Family Therapy Session

In attendance at our first family session were Alejandro and Sylvia. When asked about why Pedro had not joined them, Sylvia and Alejandro shared with me that they had never invited him and that he probably would not have come anyway. After hearing their perspectives on the reason for their being referred to me, and my gathering some additional background information, I moved into finding out the results of the pretreatment changes experiment I had given them in the initial phone conversation. Sylvia reported that Alejandro had been like "an angel" lately, helping her out around the house, coming home in the early evenings, and not running with the gang. Alejandro shared that he was "chilling and hanging by the crib (home) more since being expelled" to stay out of further trouble. Apparently, after having assaulted the rival gang member and being expelled from his high school, his probation officer had put him in the juvenile detention center for 5 days as punishment for violating his probation contract. I amplified and consolidated everything they had been doing to keep Alejandro out of further trouble. Alejandro disclosed that he was quite worried about his probation officer' s looming threat of long-term incarceration if he were to get into any further trouble.

Next, I began the goal-setting phase of the session by asking them both the best hopes and miracle questions (de Shazer, 1988; Ratner et al., 2012). There was dead silence in the room for a few minutes and then Sylvia started to cry. She shared how she feared Alejandro would die if he continued to run the streets with his gang. Alejandro attempted to console and comfort his mother, saying that he will not let that happen. Sylvia went on to share with me how she had been meeting with and praying daily with Father Rodriguez, their priest, so that Alejandro would not be killed. She added that she could not take any more visits to the hospital after Alejandro had been shot or stabbed. After providing empathy and support to Sylvia, I gently asked her to describe for me what she will be the most surprised about the day after the miracle happened. She said Alejandro would no longer be running with his street gang, he would be back in school somewhere, not shoplifting, and not abusing drugs anymore. Alejandro said in his ideal miracle picture that he would be out of his house because he takes "too much shit from my stepfather." I asked him how his stepfather would change after the miracle happened and he said angrily, "That would be impossible! He's a fucking asshole that can't change!" Sylvia chimed in with, "Watch your mouth!" Alejandro started to get visibly agitated and looked like he was ready to explode. I had flashes in my mind of the psychologist's "atomic bomb kid" description and an image of volcanoes erupting as Alejandro was losing control. After comforting him, I decided to abandon the goal-setting process, separate them, and meet alone with Alejandro first.

During my individual session time with Alejandro, I provided plenty of empathy and support until he cooled down. Once he was more relaxed, I asked him how I could be most helpful to him with his situation at this time. Alejandro shared that the reason he came for counseling was "not to get the pain away because it was unavoidable" but "for later in life, when I have kids I don't treat them like shit!" He shared that sometimes his use of weed and alcohol helped calm him down and block out "bad thoughts and moods." He went on to share with me several abusive incidents inflicted by his stepfather toward him dating back to when he was 5 years old. Alejandro disclosed that he had always "dreamed to have a father that cared about" him and "wanted to do things" with him. At this point, Alejandro started to cry while sharing these painful stories. I listened generously and validated his thoughts and feelings. Next, he shared with me that his stepfather told him the day he was expelled from his high school, "If your mother and I get divorced, it's your fault!" Alejandro started to get angry again and mimicked his stepfather taunting him and saying, "Come on, you think you are a man!" Alejandro said, "If he ever lays a hand on me again, I will kick his ass!" In a highly insightful way, Alejandro alluded to the cycle of intergenerational abuse, by sharing with me that he has found himself hitting his brother out of the blue when in a bad mood and then feeling badly that he was treating Eduardo the same way his stepfather had been beating up on him. He said, "He ain't no little animal, he doesn't deserve to be treated that way. I just did to him what my stepfather does to me! It's not right!" Finally, he said, "I hate my stepfather! If it was up to me, he would die today and I will not go to his funeral!" This was the emotionally heaviest part of our session, but I could tell that Alejandro's having the opportunity to vent his strong emotions, be listened to, and embraced empathically had provided some relief for him. I sensed that a working alliance was starting to develop. To end our individual session time, I circled back to my original question to Alejandro. He was able to express a strong desire to learn how to better manage his "hot temper" and help with how to get his GED, so that he could go to the community college auto mechanic school program. Alejandro declared to me that he wanted to avoid at all costs going to "long-term juvie jail" and planned to "stay away from his gang homies." I shared with him that I would be right by his side helping him to accomplish all of these great and responsible goals he had for himself. I pointed out that it would be hard work with bumps in the road, but if we worked together as a team, we would succeed. I praised and thanked Alejandro for courageously sharing his painful story with me and that I looked forward to working with him. Alejandro thanked me and smiled.

With only 15 minutes left in the session, I met alone with Sylvia and shared with her how impressed I was with her son. I noted that underneath his tough façade is a young man with a big heart, sensitive, caring, and bright. She started to cry and thanked me for being there for them. She acknowledged that he was a "fine young man" and the teachers have told her a lot how smart he is. I asked her how I could be helpful to her. Sylvia wanted me to see Alejandro individually and also wanted me to help her with parenting skills. Sylvia said that it would be counterproductive to involve Pedro and that he apparently had been having an affair and might be moving out soon. She acknowledged that she and Alejandro had a very close relationship, but that she felt that his street gang had become his family and she had lost her parental hold on him. I stressed that the best way to help Alejandro break free from his gang and turn his life around is with a lot of structure and a team approach. I asked Sylvia who we should have serve as Alejandro's solution-determined collaborative support team and she recommended that we invite Mr. Gomez, the probation officer, Father Rodriguez, and Ms. Danner. Sylvia also shared that she really liked Alejandro's probation officer and that her son had a good relationship with Father Rodriguez. She also raved about how wonderful Ms. Danner was and how much she cared about Alejandro. Since there were only a few minutes left with our session time, I had Alejandro join us and asked him how he felt about having a team of the above concerned individuals working with us. He completely supported the idea.

Next, I wanted to make sure we had a double safety plan in place in case the threat of violence was imminent between the stepfather and Alejandro, and what he should do if the rival gang in the neighborhood should come after him. First, I had them identify some concrete steps each of them could take if the stepfather was coming after Alejandro or Sylvia, which had never occurred. Alejandro came up with the following three options if his stepfather provoked him: lock himself up in his bedroom, go to his non-gang-involved friend's house, or go for a walk to "chill out." I added as another option for Alejandro to pursue the *six deep breaths* coping strategy (Wilson & DuFrene, 2012). I walked him through and wrote down the steps so he would know how to use this coping strategy. After trying it, he reported feeling really "chilled out." Sylvia recommended that he call Ms. Danner, Father Rodriguez, or me for support. I gave them the name, address, and phone number of a shelter in their community as another option if Sylvia or Alejandro were concerned that the stepfather might hurt them. When asked about what steps Alejandro would take if the rival gang members came after him on the streets, he responded with the following three options: duck into a store, call his mother to pick him up, and run and hide until it is safe to head home. I wrote down the concrete steps of their safety plans that they could take with them as reminders about what to do when the threat of violence was imminent.

I ended the session by complimenting Sylvia and Alejandro on their resilience and perseverance in spite of all of the crises they had been through together. I told them that I could tell there was a lot of love in their relationship. I commended Alejandro on taking the huge responsible step of showing up for our session, in spite of being expelled. I pointed out that it was clear that he was at a crossroads with his choice making after being expelled from school; he could have said to himself, "Fuck it! I'm just going to run with my gang and not make something out of my life!" Instead, in those closing minutes of our first session, he said with confidence, "I want to get a GED and go to the community college and attend the auto mechanic program there." I responded, "Wow! That is so mature and responsible! What do you think of that Sylvia?!" Sylvia smiled and told Alejandro how happy she was to hear this. I also complimented Alejandro on his tremendous courage and self-control sharing a lot of painful things with me without exploding in the session and storming out of the office. I said, "Another huge growth step on your part!" Alejandro smiled and his mother shared with him how proud she was of him. I had them sign consent forms so I could talk to and invite the other professionals to our next family session.

Prior to closing out the session, I asked Sylvia and Alejandro what our first family session was like for them. Sylvia smiled and said it was "really nice" and she was proud of Alejandro and his willingness to talk to me. Sylvia also shared that she had "new hope" and that "Jesus's light was now shining brightly on Alejandro." Alejandro disclosed that he too felt "hopeful" that "I want to turn my life around." He also thanked me for "listening and not judging." I asked him what he meant by that and Alejandro pointed out that many of his past therapists had "lectured at and blamed" him for the family problems without giving him any session time to talk about his "concerns and what I want." Finally, I asked them if there was anything they were surprised I had not asked them about their situation, and they both felt like we had covered everything that was necessary to talk about. We scheduled our next family meeting for the next week. Alejandro gave me both a firm handshake and a big smile. Sylvia thanked me again for being there for them.

Postsession Reflections

My first session with Alejandro and his mother was emotionally intense with all of Sylvia's crying and Alejandro's rage and tears as well. I felt that through the generous use of empathy, validation, and support, I had successfully set in motion working alliances with both of them. Although there had been some important pretreatment changes, which I had underscored with them, these changes were overshadowed by a lot of strong affect and fears about the future for both of them. I would have done both Sylvia and Alejandro a terrible disservice if I had continued to push with the miracle inquiry and with the goal-setting process in the early part of the session. They both had long and painful stories to share with me, which required generous and respectful listening on my behalf. Later in the session, once they were safely able to tell their stories and verbalize their painful feelings, they both were able to identify some individual target goal areas they wanted help with. Sylvia wanted help with parenting skills and Alejandro wanted assistance with learning how to better manage his anger and how to get his GED in order to get his high school diploma.

It was clear to me that the best way to help Sylvia and Alejandro achieve their goals was by implementing more structure in Alejandro's life and a team approach composed of caring and concerned significant others. With these tough case situations, it is helpful to mobilize these key concerned others to assist us between sessions to help optimize for these high-risk youth to steer clear from their gangs, help prevent further incarceration, and turn their lives around. Finally, I wanted to make sure we had a double safety plan in place so that the family could take constructive steps to be safe when the threat of violence was imminent between the stepfather and family members and the Vice Lord gang members and Alejandro. Since there had not been any physical abuse incidents in 3 years between Alejandro and the stepfather, I did not see the need to call child protective services. Instead, I gave them the name, address, and telephone number of a shelter in their community they could go to for safety.

Having worked with many adolescent gang members in the past, Alejandro's presentation and background shared a lot of similar characteristics, such as loss and rage issues; a cognitive bias toward hostile intent; the gang had become their primary family where they felt a strong sense of belonging, respect, love, had older male role models, and power and control; abusing substances to anesthetize painful thoughts and feelings; repeated past abuse inflicted by parental figures or key caretakers; and a chaotic and unpredictable family environment in which the parents lacked any leverage or authority over managing their adolescents' behaviors due to a lack of parental unity and the strong influence of the gangs.

Hardy and Laszloffy (2006) have researched extensively gang youth and their families and have identified the loss/rage common thread. The loss dimension represents either the physical or emotional absence of a parent following parental separation, divorce, or family abandonment. Loss also takes the form of shattered dreams, that is, always hoping to have loving and emotionally present father figures who valued their relationships with their kids. This was the case for Alejandro, who wished his relationship with his stepfather had been different. His biological father also had abandoned him. The rage has a twofold purpose: (1) It serves as protective armor to cover up their vulnerabilities and emotional wounds from past traumas and repeated invalidation and (2) it is a powerful and intimidating way to distance others.

According to Dodge (2006), adolescents grappling with explosive and aggressive behaviors may have a *cognitive bias toward hostile intent,* which fuels their verbally threatening and physically aggressive behaviors toward others. They assume that the target of their rage poses a threat to them, so they lash out first as a form of self-protection. What contributes to this cognitive distortion is growing up in chaotic and unpredictable family environments. The young person does not know when he or she will be yelled at or hit next.

The First Family Solution-Determined Collaborative Team Meeting

Present at our first solution-determined collaborative team meeting and seated in a circle were: Sylvia, Alejandro, Father Rodriguez, Mr. Gomez, and Ms. Danner. I thanked everyone for coming and established rapport with new members of the team. I invited each professional to share their stories of involvement with the family. Father Rodriguez said that he had known Alejandro since he was 5 years old and he thought he had "unlimited potential." He went on to say that Alejandro is "bright and has a good-hearted side to him." Looking directly into Alejandro's eyes he said, "I'm here for you my son, you can be saved from the horrors of the streets." Alejandro thanked Father Rodriguez for his support. Ms. Danner chimed in, saying she wanted to add to Father Rodriguez's identifying Alejandro's strengths. She pointed out to all of us that she had known Alejandro since he was a freshman at the high school and had come to discover that he has "loads of strengths." I asked her to share with us what she thought his "loads of strengths" were. She responded, "He is super bright, he has natural leadership abilities, he is a talented basketball player, he is incredibly talented with his hands, particularly when it comes to auto mechanic work and building things in his wood-shop class, and he is very skilled with technology." I turned to Alejandro and asked him if Ms. Danner was a charter member of his fan club. Everyone laughed, including Alejandro who said, "Ms. Danner is cool."

Mr. Gomez said that he thought "Alejandro is capable of being a good kid but that he keeps making bad choices, like getting himself kicked out of high school and going after a rival gang member." He also shared his concerns about Judge Braddock possibly deciding to send Alejandro to the department of corrections for long-term incarceration due to his repeated violation of his probation contract. Alejandro looked visibly scared about this possibility and wanted to know what he could do to prevent this from happening. Mr. Gomez shared that he would either have to attend a therapeutic day school that he had arranged for him or getting his GED, staying alcohol and drug free, and that he must get a job. He also was going to have random hair follicle drug analyses done to make sure Alejandro was staying alcohol and drug free. Mr. Gomez firmly stated that there could not be one more violation of his probation or any other police involvement. Finally, he also wanted him to follow his parents' rules and steer clear from his gang.

I asked Sylvia and Alejandro to share with Father Rodriguez, Ms. Danner, and Mr. Gomez how they could be most helpful to them at this time. Sylvia requested that if she was having a hard time managing Alejandro or getting him to comply with her rules that she would like to know that she could count on Father Rodriguez and Mr. Gomez to come by the house and back her up. She made it clear to us that she could not count on her husband to support her and that he was planning to go live at his girlfriend's house soon anyway. "See what an asshole he is!" shouted Alejandro. "I hate the way he treats my mom!" The two men agreed to be there for Sylvia. Alejandro asked Ms. Danner to find out where he could take a GED class and the test. He told us that he thought it would best for him to get his GED and try to get into the auto mechanic associate's degree program at the local community college instead of going to the therapeutic day school. Alejandro also asked for help to get a work permit so he could try to get a job. Ms. Danner offered to both assist him with finding a GED study guide and class in the community and help him with the work permit situation.

Much to our surprise, it turned out that Mr. Gomez's brother, Ricardo, owned an automobile shop and he had already talked to him about taking on Alejandro as a part-time worker and apprentice once he secured a work permit. Alejandro was thrilled about this prospect. The rest of the team thought this would be a terrific opportunity for Alejandro.

We revisited Sylvia and Alejandro's treatment goals with the team. In family therapy, Sylvia wanted to learn parent management skills and improve her communication with Alejandro. Since Alejandro wanted to work on his difficulties with anger management and self-control, I offered to teach him mindfulness, visualization, and cognitive skills to help cool the inner flames that ignite inside of him when he is angry and frustrated. He also welcomed seeing Ms. Danner once a week pro bono for a while to help keep him on track. Ms. Danner offered to provide added support for Alejandro with home visits when he wanted to talk, with emergency situations, or when in a bad place and tempted to "get stoned or hang with his gang homies." Finally, I presented to the team our double safety plan in case the potential for violence in the home or on the streets was seemed imminent for Alejandro and his mother. I asked the team if they could think of other ways to keep Alejandro and his mother safe. Mr. Gomez said that he would not only field emergency calls from Alejandro but also that he would talk to the police patrolling in his neighborhood to make them aware that there may be some gang activity and retaliation occurring at or near his house. Father Rodriguez and Ms. Danner also offered to make themselves available with support or impromptu meetings in emergency situations.

In wrapping up the team-meeting portion of our session, the following goals and action steps were put in place:

1. Family therapy would teach Sylvia parent management skills, improve family communications, and increase Alejandro's compliance with following household rules.
2. Individual session time with Alejandro will be devoted to teach him mindfulness meditation, visualization, the three S's, and cognitive skills to help to better manage his anger, improve his self-regulation capacities, and maintain self-control.

3. Father Rodriguez and Mr. Gomez will back up Sylvia with parental rule and consequence enforcement and also be available to provide additional support to Alejandro for impromptu phones calls and meetings if emergencies occur.
4. Ms. Danner will help Alejandro secure a work permit, find a GED study guide and class for him to attend, provide individual counseling in the home once a week, and make herself available for emergency impromptu meetings when necessary.
5. Mr. Gomez will arrange work at his brother's automobile mechanic shop once Alejandro secures a work permit.
6. Mr. Gomez will institute random hair follicle drug analysis to ensure that Alejandro is remaining alcohol and drug free and enforce his probation contract.

We all agreed to stay in contact until our next scheduled meeting in 2 weeks. What was really beautiful to bear witness to in the team-meeting portion of our family session was how incredibly supportive, caring, and resourceful the team members were toward Sylvia and Alejandro. They all could see how motivated and passionate Alejandro was about doing auto mechanic work and turning his situation around.

Since there was only 20 minutes left in the session, I chose to meet alone with Alejandro to begin teaching him some mindfulness meditations and visualizing movies of success. Out of all of the meditations I had time to expose him to he really liked *six deep breaths* and *taking a trip to popcorn land* because he really loved popcorn. I also taught him *visualizing movies of success.* He selected the movie of him scoring 30 points for his eighth-grade basketball team to help them to win their league championship. In fact, while accessing this movie with his eyes closed he was smiling. Alejandro reported really enjoying the visualization exercise. I asked him to practice daily, even during nonstressful times, the two meditations and the visualization exercise. I also gave him a three-page handout of mindfulness meditations and cognitive tools and strategies with detailed descriptions about how to implement each one, including the ones we practiced in the session. He was to read through the pages to see if there was any additional tools and strategies he wished to experiment with and we would discuss them in the next session.

Prior to ending our session, I complimented Alejandro on what a fine job he had done in the collaborative meeting portion of our session and had shared that it was clear to me that he was truly committed to pioneering a new and more positive direction with his life. Sylvia also reiterated how proud she was of Alejandro in voicing his needs and career goals. I assured Sylvia that in our next family session we will have plenty of time to work together

The Second Family Therapy Session

Alejandro and his mother came to our second family session smiling and in great spirits. Alejandro not only had gotten his work permit but he had started to work at Gomez's Auto Mechanic Repair Shop 20 hours a week. He loved it! Ricardo, Mr. Gomez's brother and the owner of the shop, reportedly was "a great guy" and had already taught him some new skills. In fact, Ricardo had complimented Alejandro on the knowledge and skills he already possessed. I responded with, "Wow!" I gave him a big high-five for already making his mark at his new job. Sylvia chimed in how proud she was of Alejandro. She also shared some other great news. Ms. Danner had secured a GED study guidebook for Alejandro and she had paid for his GED class that was to begin in a month. Sylvia also reported that Alejandro was pleased that he was following her rules, steering clear from his gang and the stepfather, and has already had two clean hair follicle drug analyses. Alejandro smiled and said that, "as an auto mechanic," he saw "no place for alcohol and drug use," and that "it is important to be able to concentrate and focus on what you are doing." He further added that ultimately he wanted to increase his hours at Ricardo's repair shop and possibly land a full-time job there once he completed the auto mechanic associate's degree program and got certified. I gave another "Wow!" I asked him, "Are you aware of how you came to those realizations about cutting out the alcohol and weed and the job goal?" In a mature way, Alejandro said, "It is time to grow up, man; I need to further myself and get a good-paying job, and my own crib." I turned to Sylvia and said, "You must be so proud of your son the way he is really growing up and already taking big steps to turn his life around." I asked the two of them to rate their current situation on a scale from 1 to 10, with 10 being total confidence that he can kick the gang lifestyle and succeed with achieving his career goal and 1 not at all. Alejandro rated himself presently at a 6. Sylvia also went with a 6. When asked what each of them are going to do to get up to a lucky 7, Alejandro answered first by saying, "Getting to my job on time and doing a great job there, not drinking or smoking weed, and staying away from my King homies." After going over all the details with him about how he would pull all of those steps off, Sylvia said, "He will get to his job on time, stay alcohol and drug free, study his GED guidebook daily, avoid confrontations with his stepfather, and continue to follow my rules." Finally, I taught Alejandro the three S's (self-awareness, self-monitoring, self-advocacy) and how to use this coping strategy when he starts to feel angry or tempted to use substances. He identified adults he could turn to both at home and at school for support when necessary.

At this point in the session, I shifted gears and met alone with Sylvia. She told me that her husband had already started "spending a few nights and some weekends at his girlfriend's apartment." In addition, she had met with a lawyer about pursuing a divorce because of his long history of cheating on her. I commended her on taking a stand with him. Sylvia felt that she could handle raising her sons alone and that she was already used to it. When I asked her what was working for her in bringing out the best in Alejandro's behavior now, she pointed out that she is "tougher and also more protective of him." She is daily having him set aside time to study the GED guidebook and making sure that he gets up in the mornings or leaves the house early enough to get to his job on time. I acknowledged that this kind of structure and parental consistency is needed to help him succeed. She also reported feeling empowered by randomly deciding when to administer drug tests and appreciated having Mr. Gomez stop by weekly to monitor the situation. Finally, Sylvia had done a great job of breaking up a confrontation between Alejandro and his stepfather by sending her son to his bedroom until Pedro left the house. In addition to complimenting Sylvia on the great job she was doing at taking charge and providing more structure and parental toughness with Alejandro, I asked her if I could feel her right bicep to see if she had been lifting weights to see what was increasing her confidence and toughness as a parent. Sylvia said, "Go ahead!" While laughing Sylvia shared that she knows that "Alejandro needs this type of parenting style" and she really wants to "prevent him from dying on the streets." I asked her if there were any parenting skills that she felt she needed more help with. Sylvia pointed out that the only consequences she could enforce with him were "the threat of calling Mr. Gomez" if he planned to violate her rules. This seemed to be an effective cue for getting Alejandro to think twice about breaking her rules. I encouraged her to keep using this strategy with him. She also can have Father Rodriguez, Ms. Danner, or myself come by if Alejandro is losing control and she needs backup. Apparently, sometimes Alejandro would go out at night after she had warned him not to because of the dangers of being possibly jumped by the Vice Lords or the risk of getting involved again with his King friends. However, she did share that this was occurring less frequently since he had started working and was more tired. Another positive thing that Sylvia had done for Alejandro was getting him a membership at the YMCA so he could work out and play basketball there. I praised her for coming up with that great idea. Finally, I sought Sylvia's permission to have Alejandro sit in and co-facilitate an "alternatives to violence" group session with me for eight junior high boys who had been referred by their school instead of being suspended for aggressive behaviors and fighting. Sylvia thought this would be a great idea and nice way for Alejandro to help himself.

I met alone with Alejandro and commended him on the great, responsible job he was doing at turning his life around. I went on to tell him about my wish for him to co-facilitate my next "alternatives to violence" group session with junior high boys. Without hesitation he said, "That would be sweet, man!" I explained that most of the boys had problems with bullying; fighting, swearing a lot, and all of these boys had thought it would be cool to join a gang. I said to Alejandro that he knew best what it was like to feel tough and powerful with thrills at times on the streets. It is not cool to be nearly killed or witness your friends get killed or physically maimed for life or doing "juvie" time. Alejandro shared with me that he would be happy to tell the truth about the gang reality to these young men.

Next, I explored with him how the mindfulness meditations and visualizing his best basketball game movie was working for him. Alejandro reported that daily he had been doing this visualization and the six deep breaths mindfulness practice. Both of these coping strategies had come in handy after he had the confrontation with his stepfather. While he was in his bedroom he used both of these coping tools to "chill out." He only did the taking a trip to popcorn land mindfulness practice once and did not like it as much as the other coping tools. He also mentioned to me that his mother got a membership for him at the YMCA and that he has been "working out and shooting hoops" there. I amplified and consolidated all of Alejandro's gains.

Finally, I did worst case scenario planning with Alejandro to come up with concrete steps he could take if the Vice Lords came after him or his King friends came by to try involving him in some risky activity. With the Vice Lords situation, he said he could call any member of the collaborative team for support or duck into a store and hide. If the gang came by his home, he would just tell them that he has to lay low for a while because he had potential long-term prison time hanging over his head.

Since we were out of time, I reconvened with Sylvia so we could wrap up the session. I complimented Sylvia on all of her loving, consistent, and tough parenting with Alejandro. With Alejandro, I complimented him on all of the responsible steps he was taking to better manage his anger, break free from the gang, and turn his life around. I asked the two of them to keep daily track of the steps they will take to get up to the lucky 7 on their scales.

Postsession Reflections

It was quite clear that some significant individual and family changes were occurring. Sylvia was becoming the confident and tougher parent she needed to become to help pave the way for Alejandro's success at staying out of further legal trouble, working, and keeping him alive. She was being much more consistent with setting limits and enforcing her rules and expectations with Alejandro and at the same time striving to keep the lines of communication open and regularly punctuating the positive and responsible steps he was taking. Alejandro was highly motivated to work, get his GED, and go on to complete the associate's degree auto mechanic program at the local community college. He also was not going out as much in the evenings, was practicing his mindfulness and visualization coping tools, playing basketball at the local YMCA, and trying to add more hours at work to steer clear from the temptation to run with his gang friends. This structure building process that he and his mother had put in place was making a big difference in keeping him out of further trouble. Finally, I thought giving Alejandro a taste of altruism in helping young teenagers not fall prey to the gangs could be therapeutic for him and worth trying.

Alejandro as Guest Co-Facilitator of the "Alternatives to Violence Group"

After securing signed consent forms from the group participants' parents giving me permission to expose their kids to Alejandro's wisdom about the dark side of violent behavior and street gangs, I had the green light to invite him to join me as my co-facilitator. The junior high school principal and social worker supported my idea as well. It was clear to me that Alejandro had excellent leadership skills; he quickly established rapport with and grabbed the attention of all eight boys in the group. By the way they were relating to him, it seemed like they thought that he was really cool. Alejandro opened up by sharing his long, painful story, which some of the boys in the group could relate to, especially about their emotionally distant or "mean fathers." Some of the boys had wide eyes and grimaces when he showed them his scars from being shot and stabbed multiple times and the stories behind each of the scars. He also told them how he had been expelled from high school and the horrors of having to fight to survive in the juvenile detention center. On the upside of Alejandro's storytelling was how he was presently pursuing turning his life around, which included staying out of the gang, working, getting a high school diploma and eventual college degree, and remaining alcohol and drug free. By the end of the group session, each participant had thanked Alejandro for coming and shared how they were inspired by him to think twice about joining a gang. The group even requested that he come back again and talk with them. Once the boys left the room, I gave Alejandro a lot of praise for the stellar job he had done at inspiring the group participants to turn their lives around by steering clear from gang life. I treated him to his favorite meal at McDonald's.

Emergency Phone Call from Sylvia
Regarding Alejandro's Being Gunned Down in a Drive-By Shooting

One week after running the group together and prior to our second solution-determined collaborative team meeting, Sylvia called me crying and said, "Members of his rival gang gunned down Alejandro in a drive-by when he was on his way home from his job." She said he had been "saved by Jesus" because he had gotten "shot in the leg, arm, and the third bullet lodged in his ribs had missed major organs." I comforted Sylvia on the phone and got her permission to see Alejandro at the hospital. Although he was in a lot of physical pain, Alejandro was in good spirits and thanked me for coming by. I told him how grateful I was that he was alive and how much I cared about him. Apparently, I was the first member of the team to visit him. Surprisingly, Mr. Gomez knew about the shooting incident but had not notified me. The good news was that the rival gang members in the car, including the kid Alejandro had beaten up, were all apprehended and were being charged with attempted murder. They had been pulled over for speeding in a school zone and the arresting officer saw that the car matched the description of the one involved in the shooting. Apparently, there were multiple witnesses who had taken down the car license plate and description information. One witness even had a cellphone photo of the car. I found out from Alejandro that he had called Mr. Gomez, Father Rodriguez, Ms. Danner, and Ricardo to let them know what was going on with him, and they all were planning to visit him and bring some great Mexican food for him later. The discharge plans were for him to get out of the hospital in a few days. We postponed our next solution-determined collaborative team meeting for early the next week.

The Second Family Solution-Determined
Collaborative Team Meeting

Sylvia, Alejandro, Mr. Gomez, Father Rodriguez, Ms. Danner, and Ricardo attended the second team meeting. Alejandro began by sharing how much he had appreciated all of the support they had provided for him while he was in the hospital. Everyone around the circle shared how grateful they were that he was not killed and that he did not experience long-term injuries. I invited the team members to share with the group all of the great strides Alejandro had made since our first meeting. Sylvia shared that Alejandro had been a "real angel" with following her rules, staying alcohol and drug free, steering clear from his former gang friends, not provoking or getting into arguments with his stepfather, working hard at his job, and regularly studying for his GED class and upcoming test without any reminders. I asked Alejandro to tell us what his mother has been doing differently that had helped him turn his situation around. He said, "She stopped nagging and bitching at me, she has been very loving and caring, and has been tougher with me." I chimed in that clearly Sylvia had evolved into the leader of the family and become an excellent authoritative parent, balancing nurturance and consistent limit setting. Father Rodriguez also had picked up on Sylvia's important changes. Ms. Danner asked Alejandro if she could share with the team what he had told her about his mother, and he nodded his head in approval. She said he had told her, "I am so blessed to have my mom as my mother." Sylvia was touched, and with tears coming down walked over to hug and kiss Alejandro. Everyone in the room appeared moved by Alejandro's loving words and their loving embrace. Mr. Gomez and Ms. Danner commended Alejandro on his great work and all of the responsible steps he was taking. Ricardo chimed in and told Alejandro that he had "done a super job" for him and that his "position is waiting for him when he is physically ready to return to work." He turned to Sylvia and said, "You have one fine son there." Sylvia and Alejandro both smiled.

Next, we revisited our goals and action plans. The family felt that it would best to keep collaborating and doing what was working. Alejandro recommended that his brother come to the next family meeting so that he could formally "apologize to him after all the years of bullying him." Sylvia and all the team members thought this would be a great idea. We agreed to meet in 1 month to discuss Alejandro's further progress and any team planning changes.

The Third Family Therapy Session

For our third family session, Eduardo came with Sylvia and Alejandro. I welcomed Eduardo and established rapport with him. I asked Alejandro and Sylvia to tell me whether they had both made it up to the lucky 7. They both thought the situation was at an 8. Alejandro was delighted to report that he was really enjoying his GED class and was scoring high grades on quizzes and tests. Sylvia shared that she was very happy about Alejandro's doing well in the GED class and that physically he was doing much better. He was receiving physical therapy for his left leg where he had been shot. Both his doctor and physical therapist said he should be ready to work again in another week. For his upper body, Alejandro's wounds were healing nicely. Also, Sylvia reported that Alejandro was respecting her rules and remaining alcohol and drug free. Finally, she shared that Pedro had moved in with his girlfriend with all of his belongings and the divorce process was under way. Alejandro was happy about this and Eduardo had mixed feelings. Although Eduardo did not like the way his stepfather had treated Alejandro, they got along really well because he was a star soccer player on the high school team and got good grades. I learned from Eduardo that his stepfather used to play professional soccer in Mexico and helped him to improve passing and shooting skills. Apparently, they were still seeing each other since Pedro had moved out.

At this point in the session, I decided to meet alone with Eduardo and Alejandro. I put Alejandro in charge of seeking Eduardo's forgiveness for all of the years he had bullied him. Alejandro said, "I never told you this before but I am sorry for all of the times I sucker punched you and put you down in the past; you did not deserve it. I can be better than that and besides, I am your big bro, you should be able to count on me to be there for you, not be scared of me." Alejandro got out of his chair and hobbled over to Eduardo to hug him. Eduardo accepted his apology and thanked him for being his brother. It was really beautiful to watch these two young men convey their brotherly love for each other. In fact, although Eduardo did not want his brother to get expelled and go into the juvenile center, he did appreciate that he had stood up for and tried to protect him from the Vice Lord who had assaulted and robbed him. I asked the two of them whether there were any activities they either used to do together or would like to do together in the future, now that they had reconciled. Alejandro shared that they used to "play the soccer Xbox game: *FIFA 15 X Box One* together a lot." Eduardo chimed in that he had enjoyed doing that with him. They also used to play *NBA Live 14-Xbox One* and both "shoot hoops and kick the soccer ball around" together. We also discussed how they pictured their ideal relationship to look like in the future. Although Eduardo did have a girlfriend, he pictured that once "Alejandro got hitched with a girl," they would go out as couples. I asked Eduardo whether he had been scoping out any older girls who might be a good fit for Alejandro. He said that there was a girl named Raquel who was quite popular and attractive and also a junior at their high school. Alejandro pointed out that she was "real hot" but "hard to get." I asked Eduardo if his girlfriend had an older sister. He shared that her older sister was 24 years old and finishing up college. Jokingly, I turned to Alejandro and said, "She's not too old for you, is she?" They both laughed and Alejandro said, "Drop the idea, Matthew!" Alejandro did share with us that he had met "a cute girl" named Lucinda at the hospital who was also having physical therapy and was also 17 and went to a private Catholic girls' high school. He went on to say that "I had a great rap going and I think she liked me." Eduardo asked, "Did you get her number so you could text her?" Alejandro responded, "Yeah, and we have been texting a lot, man." Eduardo said, "That's great, bro!" Alejandro said that he had hoped in a few weeks he could take her out. We both acknowledged that would be great for him. I said that maybe they would have their couples' night out in the not too distant future. I complimented them on their great work together and told them that I needed to meet with their mother.

Sylvia told me that she had gotten a big raise at the dental practice where she was working as a technician. The dentist who owned the practice had been extremely supportive and understanding with all of the problems she was having with Pedro and Alejandro. Sylvia's dream one day was to go to dental school and eventually become a dentist. I told her I hoped that, once things settled down with the divorce going through and Alejandro's life being back on track, she may be able to pursue her dream.

Next, I complimented her on doing such a fine parenting job with her two boys. I pointed out how they were able to reconcile with one another and make plans for taking their relationship to a higher and better place. Sylvia was delighted to hear this and did point out to me that Pedro had helped a great deal with Eduardo since they shared a love for soccer. When asked if she had any concerns, Sylvia felt that everything was under control.

I reconvened the family and complimented each of them. To start, I asked the boys to give their mother a high-five for doing such a great job as a parent. I asked them to each share with her one thing that they really appreciated about her. Instead, they both shared the same two compliments like a chorus: "We know she really loves us and she is an awesome cook!" Sylvia smiled and laughed. I complimented the boys on how mature they were in the positive way they were able to reconcile their differences and bring peace and love to their relationship. I pointed out how I have worked with some adult siblings who were not capable of accomplishing what they had pulled off together in one session! Sylvia chimed in that she was proud of them. I complimented Eduardo on being so understanding and open to accepting Alejandro's apologies and wanting to have a better relationship with him.

I did want to let the family know that although their situation was going great, unexpected slips do happen as part of the change process. I asked them whether they anticipated anything that might crop up that could derail them. Alejandro did have in the back of his mind fears of the rival gang trying to take him out again, and of his gang putting pressure on him to get back into action with them. We discussed as a group how to deal with these concerns, and I conducted worst-case scenario planning with them again to see whether they had any new ideas. We all felt that Alejandro needed to be vigilant when out in the streets and to make emergency calls to any members of our collaborative team when he felt at risk. We also discussed the importance of steering clear from certain people and places that were considered Vice Lord and King territory inside and outside of their neighborhood. I pointed out that once he started working full time and taking evening classes at the community college he would be off the streets more, which would greatly benefit him. Our next meeting would be with the collaborative team.

Postsession Reflections

What was most beautiful to experience in this session was to witness Alejandro and his brother reconciling and giving each other a lengthy brotherly loving hug. Alejandro had even shed some tears after his brother had accepted his forgiveness and while hugging him. They also took the relationship to the next level, planning future activities to make their bond even stronger.

With minimal parent management training on my behalf, Sylvia really stepped up with her leadership and toughness, which also greatly contributed to Alejandro's growth. She now was much more confident and competent as a parent. I also was impressed with how she stood up to Pedro and decided she had had enough of his cheating and pursued a divorce with him.

Finally, since I had done minimal relapse prevention nor asked about any other concerns family members had, I wanted to make room for discussing these matters. This is where Alejandro disclosed his concerns about safety issues regarding the rival gang and his former gang and I conducted worst-case scenario planning with them. Past experience has taught me that even when clients have made huge changes, it is critical to cover the back door because unexpected crises or slips can happen. Unless we normalize and prepare them for this inevitability, they will interpret slips as disastrous and feel like they are back to square one. By the end of the session, Alejandro appeared to be much less anxious about these concerns. I told him if these worries should enter his mind at home, he could turn to his meditation and visualization coping tools to help calm him.

Alejandro's Surprise Visit
to the Last "Alternatives to Violence" Group Meeting

Alejandro asked if he could sit on our last "alternatives to violence" group to check in on his "young homie gang wannabes," tell them about the recent drive-by shooting, and to see what progress the group members had made. I had no problem with this and I thought it would be great for Alejandro to share his recent life-threatening ordeal and he steps he had been taking to turn his life around. Alejandro also told the group that he was going to church again and that his faith in God had given him the inner strength and confidence to heal and change his life. Spirituality has been found to be a resiliency protective factor (De Frain, 2007; Miller, 2015). In addition, I felt it would be therapeutic for both Alejandro and the group members to have him sit in with us. For the second time, Alejandro did a stellar job capturing the hearts and the minds of these young men. The participants all thanked Alejandro for inspiring them and helping them choose different life paths. After the group, I thanked Alejandro for being such a positive and inspiring influence on the group members.

The Third Family Solution-Determined Collaborative Team Meeting

Present at our third solution-determined collaborative meeting were Sylvia, Alejandro, Eduardo, Father Rodriguez, Mr. Gomez, Ricardo, and Ms. Danner. The team members were delighted to meet Eduardo and glad that he had come to the meeting. Alejandro opened up the meeting by sharing his great news about acing the GED exam and working close to 40 hours a week at Ricardo's automobile repair shop. Everyone around the circle congratulated Alejandro on his great accomplishments. Ricardo chimed in and reported that "Alejandro is doing a terrific job and becoming much more skilled as a mechanic." He turned to his brother, Mr. Gomez, and thanked him for sending Alejandro his way. Mr. Gomez said that his intuition had told him that Alejandro would work out great. Father Rodriguez told us that Alejandro had paid him a visit one day at the church after he had been sitting in the chapel praying that he would not lose his life on the streets. He was pleased that Alejandro had "sought solace and strength in the house of God" and shared his concerns with him. Father Rodriguez turned to Alejandro and said that he would love to see more of him at church and that he was glad he now was joining his mother and Eduardo for Sunday morning services. Eduardo also told Alejandro that he was glad that he was joining them Sunday mornings.

Ms. Danner reported that she had been working with Alejandro to reduce his anxieties and fears about losing his life, which she felt was connected to his experiencing posttraumatic stress disorder after being gunned down by the Vice Lords. He let her know that he was regularly using his mindfulness and visualization tools. Ms. Danner was also teaching him some other closely related dialectical behavior therapy skills to help stabilize his anxiety and catastrophic thoughts (Linehan, 1993). All members of the team reiterated that they would make themselves available to field emergency calls from Alejandro and meet with him on the streets when he truly was in danger. Alejandro said that he appreciated everyone's willingness to help and really felt like he was "doing much better with his worries" and that the combination of family therapy, individual sessions with Ms. Danner, and now meeting with Father Rodriguez once a week was helping a lot. Alejandro also told us that he was really glad that he and Eduardo were getting "much tighter" in their relationship. Eduardo said he was glad about this too.

Mr. Gomez reported that Alejandro officially had four more months on probation and that he had talked to Judge Braddock about how great he was doing and that the long-term incarceration placement idea at the department of corrections had been dropped due to his progress. Alejandro jumped out of his chair and shouted, "That's awesome!" As a group, we decided to meet one more time in 2 months. We all agreed that if within the 2-month interval period any team member had other great news to share about Alejandro or they had any concerns, we would communicate with one another.

The Fourth Family Therapy Session

I kicked off our fourth family session by asking the family what further progress they had made. Sylvia rated the situation at a 10. I fell out of my chair out of amazement. All family members laughed at my surprise move. I asked Sylvia, "Wow! Are you aware of how you got your family situation up to a 10?!" She reeled off the following: "I have been asserting myself with Pedro and not backing down with him when he comes by the house to see Eduardo and drop off some money for us; I stopped Alejandro from going out with an old gang friend, even though I liked him out of all the crew that he hung out with; I came up with regular chores for the boys and make sure that they do them daily; Alejandro registered for the community college auto mechanic program; Alejandro has not been using alcohol or drugs; and he now gets up on his own daily to go to his job." I reached over to feel Sylvia's bicep and said to her, "Are you now lifting weights! That is one firm bicep!" The boys and Sylvia started laughing. I told the boys, "You better avoid at all costs pushing your mother's buttons or she will do 10 reps of military overhead presses with the two of you apiece!" They laughed again. I complimented Sylvia on how she had evolved into a model authoritative parent, balancing nurturance and limits when necessary. I asked her, "What is your consultation fee if I need you to come into a family session and serve as a guest consultant for those parents?" She said, "I would do it for free."

Next, I asked both Alejandro and Eduardo what they would rate the family situation at now, and they both agreed with their mother that they were at a 10. I asked them to share specifics of how they got up to the 10. Alejandro shared that he was "living my dream." When asked what he meant by that, he said, "I got my GED; I love my job; I got into the auto mechanic program at the community college; Ricardo offered to pay for part of my education with the understanding that I would continue to work for him full time; my bro Eduardo and I are getting along great; I love my great team behind me; and finally, the best news of all, Lucinda and I have been seeing each other for the past 2 weeks!" I responded, "Wow! That's really great! I know you really liked her." Sylvia had Lucinda over for dinner one night and really liked her too. Even Eduardo said he thought she was very special. In fact, they had "double-dated one night."

Alejandro wanted us to wrap up the session earlier so he could go see Lucinda. I asked Sylvia if this was OK with her, and she let him go. As he was walking out the door, I said to him, "Have a great time and remember to be a gentleman!" He said back, "I know, man!" I turned to Sylvia and asked her how blown away she must be by his tremendous growth. Sylvia acknowledged that she was very proud of him. When asked if there was anything else to work on since she now was like the captain of the ship, she shared that she was quite content with where things were. We decided to have a check-up session in 2 months.

The Last Family Solution-Determined Collaborative Team Meeting

Present at our last collaborative team meeting were Sylvia, Alejandro, Eduardo, Father Rodriguez, Mr. Gomez, Ricardo, and Ms. Danner. Across the board, all team members had nothing but praise for Sylvia and Alejandro. Everyone had glorious things to say about Alejandro's growth and his acting like a responsible adult. Alejandro and Sylvia thanked everyone around the circle for all that they had done to support them with their unconditional love and compassion. They both shed tears as they complimented each member of the team and cited specific words of wisdom and encouragement and things they had done that had made a big difference for them. I had Alejandro give a brief speech about where he was at the beginning of his journey and where he was now. It was a beautiful speech and Sylvia hugged and kissed him and he got a hug from Eduardo as well. I initiated my trademark high-five ritual with Alejandro and all the other members followed my lead. The other team members offered great speeches about Alejandro's transformation as well that were quite uplifting. The good news was that Mr. Gomez was able to negotiate with Judge Braddock to end Alejandro's probation after this last team meeting. Alejandro shouted, "That's really sweet! Thanks, Mr. Gomez!" I had brought a big sheet cake, which had written on it, "Great Work Team!" Beverages were also provided for the team so we could toast Alejandro and his family for a job well done. I really wanted to honor the family and team for their efforts in coauthoring with Alejandro and his family a solution-determined family success story.

The Fifth and Last Family Therapy Session

Two weeks after our last collaborative team meeting, we had a short check-up family meeting to find out what further progress they made. We had a surprise guest—Lucinda, Alejandro's girlfriend. It was clear immediately how bright, articulate, sweet, and special she was as a person.

Since she and Alejandro were so serious about their relationship, Lucinda decided to go to a university in the city so that they could continue to see each other. Alejandro was very happy about this. Sylvia, looking over at Lucinda, shared, "I'm so glad you are in Alejandro's life, you are good for him." Lucinda smiled and thanked Sylvia. Alejandro hugged Lucinda. I asked Alejandro and his mother if they had broken the scale with a 15! Both Sylvia and Alejandro said they were at a 16! I amplified and consolidated all of their gains. Alejandro and I met alone for a short time. I praised him for all of his great work and told him that Lucinda was very special and to take good care of her. We shook hands and hugged. I asked him whether he would be willing to serve as a guest consultant to help me in the future with other young men trying to get out of gangs or co-facilitate other "alternatives to violence" groups, and he said, "Count me in!" I thanked him.

I reconvened the family and wished them the best of luck. I also mentioned that I routinely check in with families I had worked with at 6 months, 1 year, and 2 years later to hear what further progress they made. They thanked me for my help and we ended the session.

Final Reflections and Case Follow-Up

In looking back at all of the risk factors and challenges I was up against with Alejandro and his family, I truly believe without having used a collaborative team approach we would not have had such a positive treatment outcome. With a high level of compassion and commitment, the professional members of the team gave 110% throughout the course of treatment to be there with support and advocacy for Alejandro. Ms. Danner, an incredibly caring and committed school social worker, was like my co-therapist providing support and taking over with cognitive skills training with Alejandro. Having Father Rodriguez, an arm of God in our collaborative meetings, had paid off on multiple levels for Alejandro. He had another caring adult to talk to and pray with, which eventually led to his joining the family for Sunday morning church services. The spiritual side of me believed that Jesus's light and strength also helped empower and heal Alejandro to be resilient enough to overcome the big challenges that he faced. He could have died in the drive-by shooting incident. Finally, it was like a miracle, not just a coincidence, that Mr. Gomez's brother owned an auto repair shop, which perfectly played into Alejandro's number one work strength area and life passion.

One of the key contributing factors I believe that paved the way for Alejandro's transformation was Sylvia's becoming an authoritative parent and assuming a consistent and solid leadership role in the family.

Alejandro clearly needed lots of limits and structure in his life so he could develop better impulse control and capacity to self-regulate his moods, make better choices, and be accountable for his actions. Not only did she get tough with him in a loving and caring way but she also stood up to Pedro and initiated the divorce process, which took tremendous courage and self-confidence.

Another important contributing factor to Alejandro's changes, commitment to family therapy, and attending our collaborative meetings was the empathic bond and emotional resonance between us that was established in our first family session. He felt respectfully listened to, empathically embraced by me, and enough safety to lower his psychological armor, cry, and share his painful story, which I believe set in motion our working alliance. This was a novel experience for him because he was used to not only regularly being emotionally invalidated and verbally and physically abused by Pedro, but some of his former therapists had taken his mother's side against him, and his needs and voice were lost in the treatment process. In my work with Sylvia, I really did minimal parent management skill training with her once I impressed upon her the importance of providing structure and consistent limit setting with Alejandro.

Alejandro's anger management, substance abuse, and gang involvement became nonissues for him once he regularly started using mindfulness, visualization, the three S's, cognitive coping skills, and regular physical exercise. He also had a strong calling and personal mission to secure his GED, complete the auto mechanic program at the community college, get certified, and work at an auto repair shop as his career. Once all of these pieces fell into place, there was no stopping Alejandro with his drive and determination to succeed. Finally, the last great thing that happened for Alejandro was meeting Lucinda, the love of his life.

I followed up with Sylvia and Alejandro at 6 months, 1 year, and 2 years later. At 6 months, I was able to talk with Sylvia and Alejandro. They both indicated that there was no longer any gang involvement, no substance abuse, and Alejandro was working full time at Ricardo's and making good grades in his auto mechanic program at the community college. One year later, I received the same report from both of them. Prior to my next follow-up telephone conversation with the family, Alejandro had helped me twice with two adolescent clients of mine who were struggling to get out of their gangs. At 2 years, Alejandro had completed the community college program, got certified as a auto mechanic, was financially self-sufficient, and was living with Lucinda in a two-bedroom apartment. In fact, they were now engaged and they planned to get married once she was done with her undergraduate university schooling.

CHAPTER 8

From "Numbing Out Bad Thoughts and Feelings" to "Welcoming Death"

Working with a High-Risk Suicidal Adolescent

> When you're following your inner voice, doors tend to eventually open for you, even if they mostly slam at first.
>
> —KELLY CUTRONE

One of the most intimidating and challenging clinical situations therapists face is an adolescent with a long career of self-injury, substance abuse, and suicide attempts. In this chapter, I present a biracial 17-year-old named Amara, who had been cutting herself since age 12, began abusing marijuana and alcohol at 13, had difficulties on and off with bulimia, and had made two serious suicide attempts at ages 15 and 16.

Referral Process and Intake Information

Amara was referred to me by her high school social worker, Ms. Carson, for self-injury, substance abuse, and being at high risk for a suicide attempt (due to her extensive history of these self-destructive behaviors and serious family problems). Ms. Carson told me that Amara had come out to her about being lesbian and that she had a girlfriend. Recently, her parents caught her and her partner "making out on the couch" in the living room when they had come home from the theater earlier than expected. Apparently, they "ordered her partner out of the house, took away all of Amara's technology, and grounded her for a month." According to Ms. Carson, when Amara had come out to her she disclosed that ever since she was 12 she found herself physically attracted to and fantasizing about being intimately involved with girls. Ms. Carson pointed out to me the huge challenge Amara was up against, which was "her mother was a staunch Catholic from Puerto Rico and her father was a Muslim from Iran." Amara's sexual orientation was unacceptable to them and they demanded that she not see her partner anymore and change her behavior immediately. This intense pressure to change led to an increase in her cutting and substance abuse behaviors behind the scenes. She also was sneaking out of her bedroom window some nights to rendezvous with her girlfriend.

According to Ms. Carson, the family had hospitalized Amara in psychiatric wards three times in the past. The first time was after a drug overdose when she was 15 following a confrontation with her parents. The second time she was hospitalized after running away from home. More recently, she was hospitalized after slicing her wrists following another major confrontation with her parents over her sexual orientation. Following all of these hospitalizations, Amara had numerous individual and family treatment experiences, which failed to stabilize her self-injuring, substance abuse, and resolve the sexual orientation impasse with the parents. In fact, they had kicked Amara out of the house on two occasions after she had snuck her partner back into house and the parents caught them making out again. On both occasions, Amara ended up living temporarily at her best friend Cindy's house. Cindy's parents knew about Amara's family problems and completely supported her.

The last area Amara was struggling with was her grades. According to Ms. Carson, Amara was "failing three major subject areas, had a D, and the rest C grades." Ms. Carson suspected that all of the emotional turmoil that Amara was experiencing was greatly contributing to her poor grades. Amara's poor grades further fueled the conflicts and arguments with her parents. Ms. Carson gave my name and telephone number to Carmen, Amara's mother. Carmen called me the same day to schedule an appointment for Amara. Prior to ending my pleasant telephone conversation with Carmen, I asked her to try out my pretreatment change experiment and bring in her written observations to our first family therapy session.

The First Family Therapy Session

In attendance for our first family therapy session was Amara, Hassan, the father, and Carmen. After coming to know everyone by their work and key interest areas, I opened up the session by exploring with the family what their best hopes were for our work together. Hassan began the conversation by sharing how he and his wife had "a big problem," which was "Amara's not respecting our religious beliefs about homosexuality being wrong." According to Hassan, such behavior in his culture is "unacceptable." Carmen also chimed in that she was a "devout Catholic and raised that homosexuality is not right or supported in the Bible." Amara got angry with her parents and shouted, "You guys will never understand me!" Hassan responded with, "You're the one that needs to change here, not us!" At this point, I intervened to break up this destructive interaction and asked if there had been any noteworthy pretreatment changes prior to our session. Neither Hassan nor Carmen could identify anything that was going well with Amara's behavior. Amara could not think of anything positive happening either. I shifted gears and asked the miracle question, and neither parent could even play around with the idea of a miracle ever happening with Amara. I was tempted to ask the parents the coping question regarding how they had prevented the situation from getting much worse, but I wanted first to see how Amara was going to respond to the miracle question. Amara had a number of miracle wishes: "Mom and Dad would accept me for who I am, which includes my sexual orientation; I would be happier and probably do better in school; and my partner, Cassie, could come over to the house and my parents would accept her." I asked her what effect all of those changes would have on her. Amara responded, "I would be much happier, my parents and I would get along better, and I probably would stop cutting myself and partying with weed and alcohol." I asked the parents which one of them would faint first when those changes occur. In a negative and invalidating manner, both parents responded by telling me that "she should not be hurting herself and doing drugs anyway, and in order to stay in their home in the future she has to be heterosexual and change her ways." Amara stormed out of my office at this point. I asked the parents if they would let me meet alone with Amara and had them go out to the lobby. When I went out to collect Amara, I discovered that she had stepped outside to smoke a cigarette and "chill."

I felt it was critical to meet alone with Amara to try to build an alliance with her and prevent her from dropping out after her parents had invalidated her. Amara told me with tears in her eyes how hard it is to live at home. She pointed out that all of the past therapists they had been to had failed to change her parents and she was not at all hopeful that my work with them would make a difference either. I asked her how I could be helpful to her at this time. Amara was not sure where to live if she moved or got kicked out of the house again. One option was to live with her married 27-year-old sister, Maria, who she did get along with, but the major problem was that she would have to go to another school and leave all of her friends, which would be very difficult for her. The other option, if it would be OK with her parents, was to live at her friend Cindy's house since she got along well with her parents. I asked her whether she thought her parents would approve of this and she was not sure. I made a mental note to explore this possibility with the parents as a future option to pursue if we failed to change the toxic family interactions.

I first empathized with Amara about how hard it must be that her parents did not accept her sexual orientation. I thanked her for coming back and being open to talking with me. Next, I wanted to be transparent and thorough in assessing Amara's risk potential for another suicide attempt, since she did have a history of trying to take her life and the home situation was so volatile. I told her that Ms. Carson had told me she had been cutting, using alcohol and weed, and had made some past suicide attempts. I pointed out that her safety was my top priority while we were working together and that I needed a commitment from her that she would let me know if she ever felt so down and out of control that she was in jeopardy of wanting to end all. Operating from a position of curiosity, I wanted to learn how self-harming fit into her life story and whether there was ever a time when she and her parents had a closer and more positive relationship. Amara said that she cut, drank, and smoked weed for "numbing out bad thoughts and feelings." Using a harm reduction and a risk management approach with her, I strongly recommended that she try to schedule her daily cutting and substance abusing habits at separate times if she felt still compelled to engage in both of them. I said, "I have been working with self-harming kids for 30-plus years and never lost anyone who was cutting and abusing substances, and I don't want you to be the first one." I added, "When a person is stoned or drunk, she may not be paying close enough attention to where she is inflicting her wounds and accidentally sever a major blood vessel." Amara acknowledged that she understood where I was coming from and that she would strive to separate the two habits. Amara also pointed out to me that because all of the stress at home she did not think she could abstain from the cutting and substances because they were like "good friends" helping her to cope and because she had engaged in these habits for so long.

Since Amara loved music and wanted to give her one go-to relapse prevention tool and harm reduction strategy, I offered her my *sound meditation*. After trying the sound meditation for 12 minutes, Amara really liked it because it helped calm her. I encouraged her to experiment with the sound meditation daily over the next week and keep track of the times when she used it instead of cutting herself, getting stoned, or drinking and how it worked for her.

When we discussed the nature of her relationship with Maria, she reported that they had an ambivalent relationship. Apparently, Maria was always her parents' "perfect child." She was an A student, graduated from college, got married to a great guy, they have children, and a nice home because her husband was a doctor. Although Maria was "always kind and caring" toward her and recently had been trying to broker peace between Amara and their parents, she always felt like she lived "in the shadow of Maria's greatness" and was "never good enough" in her parents' minds. For Amara, this feeling of "never being good enough" and "feeling deeply depressed hit hard" when she was 12. She felt jealous and envious of her sister's closeness with their parents. Amara also started having strong feelings for and being physically attracted to girls, which she felt she could not talk about with anyone. Amara then shared with me that she started cutting herself as a way "to quickly get rid of feeling bad" and as a way "to punish myself for not being good enough." As the years passed, Amara became increasingly depressed and anxious about her future. She had "poor grades," her "parents were constantly yelling at" her, and she "relied on cutting, alcohol, drugs, and running away to cope." At times, she felt such a strong sense of "hopelessness and despair" and being "a burden and a mistake" to her parents that she tried to kill herself. This happened on three occasions. With the last suicide attempt, she truly wanted to die and she said, "I was welcoming death to claim my life and saw it as a beautiful and peaceful thing." I asked Amara how her parents had responded to her suicide attempts. She said that for a short time they would be concerned and then "once I got home from the hospital, they would start yelling at me about my grades, alcohol and drug use, and my sexual orientation. They also would wave in my face, 'Why can't you be like Maria!'" She turned to me with a sad and frustrated look on her face and said, "You see what I have to live with, and it really sucks!" I provided empathy and support.

At this point in the session, I shifted gears and wanted to find out from Amara what former therapists did with her and her family that was a real drag for her or made the home situation much worse. She shared with me that most of the former therapists took her parents' side against her. According to Amara, three of her past therapists were homophobic and tried to talk her out of being lesbian. Other therapists appeared to be quite anxious and intimidated by her cutting and scars. This made her feel frustrated unwilling to open up to them about her problems and wanting to "blow off" future appointments with them. I asked her, "If you were to work with the most perfect therapist, what would he or she be like as a person and make happen with your family?" Amara took time to reflect and responded, "Well most important, the therapist would accept me for who I am, you know, my sexual orientation. The therapist would be stronger then all of the others in standing up to my parents and trying to help them be less negative, listen to me, and show me that they love me no matter what my sexual orientation is." I said to Amara these were great and ideal long-term outcomes we could work hard to try to make happen with her parents. I asked her in the short-term, "What would be one thing you would like to achieve either with your parents or individually at this time?" Amara shared that "if we could simply talk together and they would listen to me without them yelling or lecturing at me, that would be huge!" Finally, before meeting with her parents I asked Amara if she had any adult inspirational others outside the home that she has turned to for advice and support. Amara said that she could always count on Ms. Carson and Mr. Slive, her biology teacher, for support and advice. Apparently, he had a long ponytail and was a hip-looking teacher. Amara said, "He's a cool dude." I asked Amara if she would feel comfortable having them join us in her family meetings if her parents were OK with that, and she really liked the idea. I also wanted to know if it would be helpful to involve her sister in our sessions and she was OK with my inviting her to participate as well. I thanked her for courageously opening up to me and helping me better understand her story.

Next, I met with the parents alone for the remainder of the session. Immediately, both parents began asking me if I could miraculously change Amara and "stop her from living a life in sin as a lesbian." I first acknowledged how her sexual orientation conflicts with their traditional cultural values, practices, and religious beliefs, and how difficult it must be for them to cope with and manage this dilemma with Amara. However, I felt that, with our limited time, we needed to shift gears and address safety issues, particularly what steps they would take to prevent a future suicide completion from happening with Amara. As a way to *create intensity* (Fishman & Minuchin, 1981) with them and get the parents more involved in helping their daughter in a different way and inject more warmth and positivity into their relationship with Amara, I asked them the following tough questions:

> "Let's say it is 3 o'clock Saturday morning and a police officer rings your front doorbell. When you open the door he says, 'I feel badly about having to tell you this, but your daughter has killed herself.' What effect would her loss have on each of you individually?"
> "How about as a couple?"
> "What would you miss the most not having her around anymore?"
> "Who will attend her funeral?"
> "What will the eulogies be?"

In response to my questions, Carmen said, "We can't let that happen! It would really devastate me." Hassan responded with, "I, too, would be devastated by such a painful loss." I asked the couple, "What would happen to your relationship after this devastating event had occurred?" Carmen shared, "Well, I would feel emotionally numb and not have much left to give to Hassan." Hassan thought, "We would not have much to talk about if my Amara were not here. You know I named her." I said, "So, in a sense, Amara provides your daily agenda for conversational topics and your entertainment." Both parents agreed and admitted that there would be "an emptiness" in their relationship without Amara being present. I was tempted to cross the bridge to address their marital issues but I felt it may be too premature and could revisit this topic later. Instead, I pushed on by asking what the eulogies would be at Amara's funeral. Carmen said that her eulogy would be, "Amara was a big help" to her with "preparing meals and baking." Hassan's eulogy would be that "Amara a great babysitter, especially with Maria's kids."

Since my line of questioning dramatically changed the climate and appeared to raise their anxiety about what the loss of Amara would mean for them individually and as a couple, I wanted to tap their expertise about what steps they could take to help prevent them from losing her permanently. In exploring specific steps both parents could take, Hassan came up with the idea of their discontinuing their incessant lectures and yelling at her about how she should live her life. Carmen agreed, and felt that they needed to show her that they cared about and loved her. One of her theories about why Amara was so self-destructive and lesbian was because they "did not show her enough love." I took a big risk and told them that, after working for over 30 years with kids like Amara with long careers of self-harming behaviors, these kids often have felt emotionally invalidated, unlovable, and, in extreme cases, truly believe that they are a burden to their loved ones who would be a lot happier if they were no longer around. The parents looked troubled. Suddenly, Carmen asked, "Do you think Amara feels this way?" I suggested that I bring in Amara so they could ask her that question. Before bringing Amara in the room, I double-checked with the parents whether they were OK about having this heavy and important conversation. Once Amara sat down and got comfortable, I had Carmen look at her daughter directly and tell her what we had been talking about and pose her important question. In response, Amara courageously, while shedding tears, told her parents that she has "felt for years" that they "loved Maria more" than her, that she was "never good enough," and that sometimes she "felt like dying" so they "would not have to deal with" her anymore. Both Carmen and Hassan looked troubled by what Amara had said. Carmen responded, "I'm sad that you feel that way, honey, but we love both of you equally." Amara chimed in, "I really don't believe you. You and Dad are always comparing me to Maria and saying, 'Why can't you be like your sister, you are so difficult.'" Hassan admitted that they said that a lot and that they had to stop doing it. I asked Amara what she needed from her parents at this moment. She said, "Well, you guys have not hugged me for a long time. Also, I wish we could just talk about anything and you would listen, without either of you lecturing at me or getting angry at me."

Prior to ending the session, I complimented the family on being resilient and persistent in their efforts to seek solutions for their difficulties and not giving up. I praised the parents for their willingness to see the goodness and strengths that Amara possesses. I let them know that they did a fine job of listening to Amara and taking to heart her unique needs and recognizing that she and Maria are two different people and require two styles of parenting. I pointed out to the parents how badly Amara needs to be validated, listened to, and feel loved and appreciated by them, which would make her feel happier, less likely to engage in self-harming behaviors, and more likely to do better in school. Finally, I showered Amara with compliments about her courage to rejoin the session after storming out and, unlike many teenagers, her incredible ability to clearly articulate her thoughts, feelings, and needs to her parents and me. I encouraged the family to go home and set aside one-on-one time for the parents and Amara where they could practice just talking, listening, and responding. The only ground rule was to keep the conversation light and avoid all loaded hot topics for now. I predicted that this might be a struggle for them, since it could feel very unnatural for them to talk without conflict. Rather than allowing defensiveness and personal discomfort to undermine their conversations, I recommended that when necessary one or both of the parties could flash a time-out sign and take a short break from talking until he or she is feeling more relaxed. I asked them to keep track of what works in terms of keeping the conversations flowing in a positive way. I also asked the parents if it would be OK for Maria, Ms. Carson, and Mr. Slive to come to our next family meeting and they agreed.

When I asked how the session was for each of them, both parents said it was helpful in that they had never heard before how Amara was feeling about herself and their relationships with her. Hassan shared that he thought Amara did a great job of opening up to them. Carmen felt the session was enlightening because she could see the need for her and Hassan to change the way they were interacting with Amara, so that she could feel better about herself and count on them more. Amara said that she thought the session was more productive than any other family session she had had before. When asked to elaborate, Amara said that I listened to her and respected her, and she thought I had done a good job with her parents, in that they were able to listen to her and acknowledge that they had to make changes as well. I asked them if there was anything they were surprised I had not asked them about their family situation and they all felt that we had covered a lot of territory and the session had been productive. Finally, because of the long history of destructive interactions and conflicts in this family and not totally trusting the staying power of the positivity that had occurred toward the end of the session, something in my gut told me to predict that over the next week some kind of argument or conflict might erupt to derail the new direction they were beginning to pursue as a family. I told them that predicting is like forecasting the weather—we can never be certain of anything but I hoped they would prove me wrong. We scheduled our next appointment in 1 week.

Postsession Reflections

I was exhausted and ready for a shower after this tough session. I felt like I had been like a traffic police officer in a very busy intersection between Amara and her parents. The parents initially were so focused on the "evils" of Amara being lesbian and trying to get me to fix her that I did not think I could get them to shift gears and discuss more critical issues like preventing their daughter from killing herself. The dramatic turn occurred during my private session time with the parents when I had surpassed their pessimistic, negative, and rigid views of Amara by asking pessimistic sequence questions (de Shazer et al., 2007; Selekman & Beyebach, 2013), which presented a dark and dire future scenario of their daughter's suicide completion and its painful emotional aftershocks. Following the parents' responses to my questions, I was able to get them to have a heart-to-heart and meaningful conversation with Amara about what had been fueling her self-harming behaviors and what she needed from them now.

Earlier in the session, when Amara had stormed out of my office, I was quite concerned that she would leave the premises and drop out of therapy. Through the use of empathy, validation, and support, I was able to create an emotionally safe climate for Amara to share her long self-harming story with me. This was quite informative and insightful and revealed to me the family dynamics and what was fueling Amara's self-harming behaviors. I felt like we established a good working alliance.

Having worked with self-harming youth and with gay, lesbian, bisexual, and transgender adolescents and their families for more than 30 years, I could see that this family possessed many dynamics I had seen before, such as emotionally invalidating interactions, emotional disconnection, using self-injury and substances to get quick relief from emotional distress, and the self-harming adolescent being constantly compared to more successful siblings (Selekman, 2009; Selekman & Beyebach, 2013). We also know from research that adolescents with long histories of self-injury are at high risk for suicide attempts due to conquering their fears of death, perceiving it as being a beautiful outcome, and perceiving themselves as a burden to others (Joiner, 2005; Joiner et al., 2002). Prior to her past suicide attempts, Amara had had these very same thoughts. Finally, Hawton and Rodham (2006) and D'Angelli, Grossman, and Salter (2005) have found in their research that it is quite common for adolescents to engage in self-harming behaviors, including attempting suicide, when struggling with sexual orientation issues prior to "coming out," or after doing so and fearing or experiencing rejection from family or peers. In fact, Hawton and Rodham (2006) found that adolescent females struggling with sexual orientation issues are four times more likely to self-harm than boys and girls who do not have these concerns.

Because Amara was at such a high risk for another suicide attempt, I felt it would be most advantageous to organize a team of concerned and caring others from her social network to help support her. I was delighted that the parents were in favor of having Maria, Ms. Carson, and Mr. Slive join us in our next family session.

The First Family Solution-Determined Collaborative Team Meeting

Present in our first solution-determined collaborative team meeting were Amara, Hassan, Carmen, Maria, Ms. Carson, and Mr. Slive. After establishing rapport with the new members of the team, I invited them to share their stories of involvement and we discussed the purpose of meeting as a group. Maria opened up the conversation by saying how much she loved and cared about Amara and had repeatedly invited her to live with her and her family. Apparently, over the years when Amara and her parents were embroiled in intense conflicts and arguments, it was decided that it would be best for her to live with Maria so they could have time away from one another. I was curious whether Maria had ever gone through tough times with her parents as a teen. According to Maria, she was a very serious student, was involved in a lot of school clubs, and worked hard so she could try and get a scholarship to Stanford, which she eventually landed. Hassan chimed in how proud he and Carmen were of Maria and thought she would go on to law school. I looked over at Amara's face and I could tell that she did not like all of the praise Maria was getting from her parents. Carmen added, "Well, she decided to become a mother instead. We really love her husband, Trevor, and their two beautiful children, Eloise and Sean." Maria reiterated, "If it would help not tearing our family apart, I would gratefully have Amara live with us." Amara chimed in, "I appreciate it, Maria, but I would have to start over at a new school and be too far away from my friends." I turned to the parents and asked, "If Amara changes her mind about living with Maria, is that a viable option in the future?" Both parents acknowledged that things were presently going better between them and this option would only be pursued if things dramatically deteriorated. I wanted to seize this opportunity and find out from the parents and Amara what was going better between them since our last family session. According to Amara, "They both were really listening to me, we didn't get into anything heavy, and we went to my favorite Italian restaurant." Carmen added, "It was less stressful at home and nice to get along."

At this point in the meeting I shifted gears and wanted to hear Ms. Carson and Mr. Slive's involvement with Amara and how they saw her and their thoughts about what was going on in the family. Ms. Carson shared that she had a 3-year history of working with Amara and had had many telephone and face-to-face conversations with Carmen. She pointed out, "Amara is a very assertive young woman and stands up for her convictions." I jokingly interjected, "Maybe Amara will be the future lawyer in this family!" Everyone laughed, including the parents. Ms. Carson had told Amara if she could pick up her grades and took her history class more seriously, she would be great on the debate team. Ms. Carson was a former college debater and helped out the high school team. Hassan chimed in, "She could probably be one of the top debaters! The words 'cooperation' and 'I give up' are not in her vocabulary." Amara pointed out that most of the debaters she knew were "nerdy geniuses" and not part of her "crew of friends." Hassan began to lecture Amara about not having "an attitude about smart students." Something told me in my gut that this could digress into a negative exchange between the parents and Amara, so I shifted gears and invited Mr. Slive into the conversation.

Mr. Slive had had two biology classes with Amara at the high school. He reported that he really liked Amara a lot and she contributed a great deal in his current class with her. Apparently, her downfall was not completing and turning in her lab and homework assignments. However, he contended that she had a great memory and often scored high on quizzes and tests. This was why she was getting a B in his class. He described her as "having the mind of a scientist" because of her "high level of curiosity and openness to all possibilities." I chimed in and said to Amara, "Maybe this could be your mantra: 'openness to all possibilities.'" This kind of true Buddhist mind can be used in any conversation with any person. All parties around the circle agreed about these valuable words of wisdom. Mr. Slive shared with all of us that he was a Buddhist and he practiced mindfulness meditation daily. I wanted to seize this wonderful opportunity and see whether he would be willing to set aside a little after-school time to teach Amara some mindfulness meditations that he thought could benefit her. Mr. Slive welcomed the opportunity to teach Amara if she were game and the parents supported it. Amara shouted, "That would be sweet!" The parents were OK with it as well.

I caught the new team members up with how we were trying to improve the family communications and I wondered whether they had any suggestions that might aid them in this area. Ms. Carson put herself on the line and said that Amara has been wanting for some time "to feel loved and appreciated by her parents unconditionally, without being judged and criticized because her values and choices are different from theirs." Maria chimed in before the parents spoke and said, "Yes, I have said this to my parents a lot that just because Amara has different values and may be making some radical choices, they need to love her unconditionally." Hassan responded, "I hear what you are saying but it is unacceptable to us for her to do poorly in school and live in sin as a lesbian!" Amara abruptly responded, "I thought you guys were trying to change, but I guess I was wrong." Carmen chimed in, "We will not accept your choices here." Maria intervened with, "Stop it! Stop it! You can't treat Amara like this! I don't want this to tear our family apart!" Maria convinced her parents that Amara should spend the night at her place. Amara thought this would be a good idea so she could "chill."

Since we were running out of time, I decided to move the group conversation in a different direction. I wanted to find out from the team members what their goals and action steps were going to be. I list them below:

1. Ms. Carson will continue to provide weekly individual sessions, emergency sessions when needed, and monitor her schoolwork and put support resources in place to help increase Amara's academic performance.
2. Mr. Slive will set aside after-school time on Tuesdays and Thursdays to teach Amara mindfulness mediations to help quiet her mind and increase her positive emotions.
3. Maria will make herself available anytime to Amara to provide support, mediate between her and the parents, and offer her home for time-out periods or to permanently live there if necessary.
4. Hassan and Carmen will commit to ongoing family therapy to work on improving their communications and resolving their conflicts with Amara.
5. Amara will continue to try family therapy, providing she received at least a half hour of individual session time when she requested it.
6. Matthew will continue family therapy to increase positive family interactions between Amara and her parents, attempt to strengthen their relational bonds, and resolve their conflicts over Amara's sexual orientation.

We scheduled our next collaborative team meeting in 2 weeks. Before Amara left, I wanted to meet alone with her to see how she was holding up after our emotionally distressing group ending. Amara said that she was "totally bummed out." She had thought things were improving with her and her parents and in our meeting it had felt like to her "the same old, same old." I provided support and pointed out how her sister had really stood up for her with their parents and to not forget she had a great collaborative team behind her. I reminded Amara about Mr. Slive's words of wisdom regarding maintaining "openness to all possibilities," even during the darkest moments. Amara smiled and looked less down. I encouraged her to use this as her personal mantra and work with him on adopting a daily mindfulness practice. Finally, I stressed that things were tenuous right now in her relationship with her parents and to strive to walk a straight line with them when she returns home from Maria's house. Our next family session was scheduled for the next week.

Crisis Telephone Call from Carmen

Carmen called me 3 days later saying that Amara had run away from home after an "angry screaming match with her father over failing two tests in her English and history classes." She had just received a call from her friend Cindy's mother, Mrs. Stoddard, that Amara spent the night at their home and was hesitant to go back home. Carmen asked me what they should do. Since the situation was so volatile in their home, I felt that they should have a time-out from one another for a few more days until our next family session so things could simmer down. In addition, Amara could still go to school. I encouraged her to take some clothes, other personal necessities, and her school materials over to the Stoddards.

The Second Family Therapy Session

Upon entering this second family session, I felt like I would have to be unusually active and on my toes, cutting off verbal assaults between family members. Amara sat back from us, with her arms folded and head down. Hassan refused to look at or talk to Amara. The tension in the room was unbearable. Carmen's attempts to get family members to talk with one another proved futile. I decided to break up the family session and see the parents alone first. Hassan opened up by saying to me, "I want her out of my house! She's a loser! She has a negative attitude about school! She has no respect for our values and religious beliefs!" Carmen tried to calm Hassan down. I explored with the parents what alternatives Amara had for living arrangements. Hassan abruptly said that he had been told by a "psychiatrist friend" about "a residential treatment center out West that works with problem girls like Amara." This was one of the options he wanted to put on the table. Carmen did not want to send her away but thought that she could live at Maria's until the end of the school year. Hassan chimed in, "And stress out Maria and Trevor! And corrupt their kids!" I asked the parents, "If the Stoddards were willing to take her for the rest of the school year would that be OK?" Carmen said that she did not want to impose on them. I asked if Hassan could entertain this possibility if the Stoddards were OK with it before trying the extreme alternative of shipping Amara off to residential treatment. I went on to say that I would continue to work with her and collaborate with the Stoddards and the rest of our team to try to turn things around with Amara. Finally, Hassan calmed down and said he would be "willing to try the Stoddards first, if they were willing to take her on." I secured a consent form so I could approach the Stoddards about the situation. Carmen said she would call Mrs. Stoddard as well.

I met alone with Amara. She looked extremely depressed and frustrated with her life. She had not seen her partner, Cassie, for 2 weeks. All of the family stress was taking its toll on her. She rolled up one of her long sleeves to show me how she had been carving up and down deeply into her arms, reported smoking weed heavily behind their garage, and having thoughts of taking her life again. I asked whether she had a plan, and Amara said that she had fleeting thoughts of overdosing on her mother's sleeping pills and downing a fifth of vodka. Erring on the side of caution, I told Amara that I wanted her parents to take her to the hospital emergency room immediately so I knew she would be safe. Surprisingly, Amara did not fight me on this and the parents took her to the hospital right away after they heard about her suicide plan and intensified engagement in self-destructive behaviors.

Postsession Reflections

Although I am not a big fan of hospitalizing adolescents, in this case, it was an absolute necessity due to Amara's having a clear suicide plan, the depth of her hopelessness and despair, the multiple stressors she had to contend with, her multiple attempted suicide history, her arm looking like a battlefield of deep gashes and long cuts, her abusing substances, and not being able to count on her parents to be emotionally present and validate her. There were far too many risk factors to mess around. In addition to making sure that Amara was safe, I felt like I needed to reach out to Hassan during the week for fear that he would drop out of treatment. It was clear to me that Carmen was softening and trying to interact differently with Amara. I also wanted to revisit with the parents option of Amara living with the Stoddards after she got out of the hospital. Finally, I needed to collaborate with the psychiatric team working with Amara and her family and make sure we came up with a tight aftercare plan.

Telephone Calls from the Hospital Staff

Two hours after our tumultuous family session, I received a call from the psychiatric resident in the emergency room telling me that he had decided to admit Amara on the adolescent psychiatric unit due to her extensive history of self-harm and past suicide attempts. The emergency room doctor felt she was presently at high risk for another suicide attempt.

Three days later, I finally received a telephone call from Ms. Moran, one of the adolescent unit social workers assigned to Amara. She had a release signed by the parents to talk to me. Ms. Moran had scheduled a family session later in the week, and she said that Amara really wanted me to attend. I also had an opportunity to talk with Dr. Chobani, who happened to be on the unit while I was talking to Ms. Moran. He had diagnosed her with "major depression, recurrent type" and put her on Prozac, since this drug has had some success with patients who self-injure and/or engage in other compulsive behaviors. I learned that Amara was "talkative, cooperative, and seemed to be in better spirits" even though she was still "on suicide precautions." Dr. Chobani was planning to attend the family session as well. What was troubling to both Ms. Moran and Dr. Chobani was the father's decision to drop out of the treatment, not even to visit his daughter. I learned from both Ms. Moran and Dr. Chobani that the parents had been fighting a lot about what to do with Amara when she eventually left the hospital. Apparently, once Hassan had discovered from Ms. Carson that the school would not help pay for residential treatment because Amara did not have an IEP nor did the school district have funds to cover it, he gave Carmen the ultimatum of either choosing between him or Amara. I learned from Ms. Moran that Carmen had told Hassan, "If I have to choose between you and Amara, I have to be there for our daughter." This resulted in Hassan's leaving the family and going to live at his brother's house in a distant suburb. I shared with Ms. Moran and Dr. Chobani that I had spoken to Hassan and tried to set up a meeting with him but he indicated to me that he was "done with" his "family and me."

Next, I discussed with Ms. Moran and Dr. Chobani about the idea of inviting Maria, Ms. Carson, Mr. Slive, and the Stoddards to the family session. I told them that Amara is like family with the Stoddards and they care a lot about her and have consistently been there in the past to support her. In fact, I told them that I had spoken with the Stoddards about Amara living with them and they were totally receptive to the idea. Prior to our Friday scheduled family session at the hospital, Dr. Chobani had written orders in Amara's chart for me, Maria, Ms. Carson, Mr. Slive, and the Stoddards, including their daughter, Cindy, to visit her on the unit.

The Third Family Therapy Session on the Hospital Unit

Maria, Ms. Carson, Mr. Slive, Carmen, Amara, the Stoddard couple, Ms. Moran, and Dr. Chobani attended the third family session. Ms. Moran opened up our meeting by thanking everyone for coming and acknowledged that it was great to see that so many people cared about Amara's well-being. Carmen also thanked everyone for coming. After introductions and rapport building, Ms. Moran and Dr. Chobani updated all of us on how Amara was doing in their adolescent program. Both of them reported that Amara was off suicide precautions and was actively participating in their group and individual therapy sessions. Amara told us that she was "so glad" that she was in the program and that "it was really helping."

The next major subject we covered was the aftercare living arrangement situation. Carmen took the lead here and said that she had a few meetings with Connie and Lester Stoddard and she felt completely OK for Amara to live with them until the end of the school year. The Stoddards said that they were "crazy about Amara and she is like another daughter" to them. Their 16-year-old daughter was also excited about Amara living with them since they were best friends. The other participants supported this idea, including Maria. After there was consensus about the living arrangements following Amara's discharge from the hospital, Carmen asked the adults could meet alone. Amara stepped out for a little while.

Carmen updated the meeting participants about the status of her marriage with Hassan. Apparently, they had "conflicts about and fought for years about Amara." Hassan blamed her for Amara's problems and did not like the fact that she would take her side against him. Recently, he had come by the home to collect his belongings and announced to Carmen that he wanted a divorce. Carmen began to cry about the situation and how her "35 years of marriage was ending." Maria got up and comforted her mother. All of the participants offered empathy and support as well. Maria shared with the group that she had met with her father twice to try talk some sense into him, but she came to the conclusion that he was done with the marriage, her mother, and Amara.

Carmen told us that she had not worked in years but had lined up a couple of interviews for management positions at department stores. She had worked in retail administrative positions in the past. Sadly, Carmen felt that she could not count on Hassan for financial support and she decided to be proactive with securing a job. Carmen turned to the Stoddards and shared how grateful she was that they could help out with Amara and that once she started working, she would drop off money to cover food, school, and other expenses for her. Although the Stoddards told Carmen that they did not think that was necessary, she insisted on doing so.

Prior to the goal setting and action planning portion of our meeting, the Stoddards shared their expectations for Amara while lived with them: accepting their TLC (tender loving care), respecting their household rules, using her coping tools to refrain from substance abuse and self-injuring, attending all of her scheduled counseling appointments, and regularly doing her homework. Amara declared that she would uphold and respect all of the Stoddards' expectations. All members of the group, including Carmen, loved the fact that the Stoddards were going to run both a tight and loving ship with Amara.

Amara rejoined us for the aftercare plans discussion. The collaborative team members shared their goals and action steps they planned to take with Amara:

1. Dr. Chobani will provide medication management and be available to all of the collaborative team members for psychiatric backup and consultation.
2. Matthew will provide a combination of individual sessions with Amara and family therapy with Carmen, Maria, and the Stoddards.
3. Ms. Carson will provide individual sessions at school for Amara and actively collaborate with Amara's teachers to help her turn around her academic situation and gain their support with this process. She also will actively collaborate with Matthew and Connie Stoddard.
4. Connie Stoddard will use her skills and experiences as a learning disability (LD) resource teacher and consultant to help Amara in her weak academic subject areas to improve her executive skills.
5. The Stoddards will attend all scheduled family therapy sessions for Amara and will promptly contact Matthew if they have any concerns.
6. Mr. Slive will resume working with Amara in teaching her mindfulness meditations and related practices.
7. Maria will participate in family therapy and be available for texts, phone calls, and impromptu meetings with Amara. In addition, she hopes that they can get together for dinners and hanging-out time.

Postsession Reflections

I felt our family/collaborative meeting was quite productive. It was nice to know that Amara would be living in a very nurturing yet structured family environment, which would help her to heal, be less compelled to engage in self-destructive behaviors, and be more focused and successful in school. It was also reassuring to me that I had such a solid, committed team backing me up and ready and willing to help out in any way with Amara.

Regarding school, I felt it was critical to collaborate with all of Amara's teachers to gain their support in helping her to get caught up and pick up her grades in their classes. Ms. Carson was going to spearhead our collaborative meetings with the teachers. The biggest stroke of luck was to discover that Connie Stoddard was an LD teacher and consultant. We were blessed with having a built-in tutor in the Stoddard household to spend extra time helping Amara strengthen her executive skills and improve in specific subject areas she was struggling with.

Individual and Family Therapy Session with Amara

One week after Amara's discharge from the hospital, she had requested that Connie Stoddard contact me to set up an individual session for her prior to our next scheduled family therapy session. Amara had much brighter affect and she was feeling much more balanced. She felt that the Prozac was really helping her. She also had had a nice medication management session with Dr. Chobani. Amara was eager to tell me that it had been great living at the Stoddards, particularly doing lots of fun things with her best friend, Cindy. She proudly reported having a strong desire to "quit for good the cutting and substance-abusing" habits. In fact, she had spoken with her mother about wanting to do something about trying to find a product or seeing a doctor who can cover up or remove her "battlefield" cutting scars on her arms and legs. Having worked with self-injuring clients for decades, I have found that wanting to cover up or remove their scars is a rite of passage, of wanting to close the door on what was, and move in a new direction with their lives. Amara confirmed this by sharing with me her goals for herself, such as wanting to quit smoking cigarettes, take yoga classes with Cindy and Connie, eating healthier, and doing better in school. Amara told me how Connie had already been a big help with tough homework assignments and teaching her better study skills. She had also had some nice lunches and "hang-out time" with Maria and her mother. She said that her mother had secured a great management position at a popular department store.

I revisited with Amara her strong desire to see me individually at this time. She shared with me that "the Stoddards were very different than her parents in that they were not super religious and were very liberal." Amara desperately wanted to come out to the Stoddard couple about being lesbian, but wanted my opinion about this. First, I asked her if she had already come out to Cindy. Amara said, "Yes, and she was cool with it." Second, I asked Amara, "Knowing the Stoddard couple, do you think they will embrace you unconditionally about this, or do you think it could backfire for you?" Amara said that maybe she should first try coming out to Connie with me there. She was much more confident that Connie would not have a problem with it because she was "like a second mom." Since Connie was in the waiting room, I asked Amara if she would like me to invite her in and we could try it out. Amara bravely wanted to take the risk. After Connie sat down and got comfortable, Amara courageously came out to Connie, who was completely supportive and open to Amara's sexual orientation. She pointed out to Amara that she cared about her "like a second daughter, unconditionally." Amara sprang out of her chair and hugged and thanked Connie for being so understanding. Connie asked Amara whether she had already come out to Cindy, and Amara said that she already had done so and Cindy was completely fine with it. Next, Amara wanted to let Connie know about Cassie, her partner. She told Connie how she had not seen Cassie in weeks and really missed her. The next courageous step Amara took with Connie was to see whether Cassie could come by their house to visit her or go out with her on a weekend night. Connie was OK with this, but first wanted to discuss this with her husband, Lester, so there were no surprises. I asked Connie, "How do you think Lester will respond to Amara's coming out to him and having Cassie over?" Connie responded, "Lester has always been a bit of a left-winger and radical about things, so I am convinced that he will embrace you unconditionally like me." Amara had a big smile on her face. I asked Connie whether she would be willing to sit down with Lester and Amara when she comes out to him. Connie was happy to do so. Since this session had become like a regular family therapy session, we decided to push the next family therapy appointment back a week. I also thought it would be best to have a meeting the following week with Ms. Carson, all of Amara's teachers, and Connie to strategize about how best to meet her academic needs and optimize her success at school. Connie agreed and committed to joining us. Amara left our session smiling and on cloud nine!

School Collaborative Meeting

Present at the school collaborative meeting were Amara, Carmen, Connie, Ms. Carson, Mr. Slive, Mr. Beech (the history teacher), Ms. Stoughton (the math teacher), and Mr. Krause (the English teacher). Her art and P.E. teachers could not attend. Amara had been failing her history, math, and English classes. On the upside of her academics, Amara's grades were no longer in the failing range. In fact, she had moved up to a D+/C− in all three of these classes. In Mr. Slive's class, she was now getting a B+ and was delighted with how hard she was working on picking up her grade and being disciplined about meditating daily. Amara shared with the rest of the group that Mr. Slive was teaching her mindfulness meditations. She credited Connie's homework and study habit help with completing her past assignments. Carmen, Mr. Beech, Ms. Stoughton, and Mr. Krause all complimented Amara on turning in her past assignments and performing much better on tests in their classes. Carmen told Amara that she was really proud of her. Amara smiled and felt compelled to share with the teachers the problems she had been grappling with. She let them know about being depressed for a long time, her family problems, and why she was living at the Stoddards' house. Everyone around the table was highly supportive and understanding. Prior to ending our meeting, Connie requested that the teachers email her weekly on Amara's progress and any extra help she may need preparing for tests and completing more challenging assignments. We decided to meet again in 3 weeks.

The Fifth Family Therapy Session

Amara, Carmen, Maria, Lester, Connie, and Cindy attended our fifth family therapy session. I decided to divide the meeting in half and begin with the Stoddards and Amara. I wanted to have a progress report from the Stoddards on how things were going with Amara's adjustment living with them and see whether any kinks needed to be ironed out. Both Connie and Lester felt everything was going smoothly and Amara was following their rules. Lester commended Amara on her courage to come out to him in a very mature way. Connie also told Amara how proud she was of her being able to take this big step with Lester and pick up her grades at school. Cindy eagerly shared what a joy it was to have "a friend sister"! Amara reported to me that the Stoddards had invited Cassie over for dinner and she had been over a few times since that night. She thanked again the Stoddard's for being so understanding and supportive of her relationship with Cassie. I complimented the Stoddards on being such a great family fit for Amara and what a super job they had done at being so compassionate and empowering Amara to be all she could possibly become. I thanked Connie for being such a big help in helping Amara come out to her and Lester and paving the way for her dramatic academic turnaround. I complimented Cindy on being such a great "friend sister" to Amara. Amara and Cindy looked at each other and smiled. Finally, Amara wanted to let me know that she had been going to yoga classes with Connie and Cindy and really loving it.

For the second half of the family session, I decided to meet with Maria, Carmen, and Amara alone. Amara opened up the meeting by sharing with her sister and mother how much she had enjoyed her time with them when they had visited. They both acknowledged that they felt the same way. Amara had asked them about how her father was doing. Both Carmen and Maria felt like it was hopeless to try to talk with him. Apparently, he refused to meet with Carmen and occasionally would see Maria but the latter's "conversations would go nowhere with him." Carmen disclosed to Amara that she and her father were pursuing a divorce and that their marital difficulties had long predated her psychological and behavioral problems. Amara started to blame herself for her parents' divorcing. Both Carmen and Maria said to Amara it was not her fault, "there were problems with the marriage for many years." I checked to see if Carmen was still OK with Amara's continuing to live at the Stoddards, and she was fine with it.

Since we were running out of time, I wanted to meet alone with Amara to make sure she was OK after the divorce discussion and offer her some additional relapse prevention and self-control tools and strategies. I complimented Carmen and Maria for being so supportive and loving with Amara.

Although Amara shared that she had felt some guilt about her parents' divorce, I challenged this unhelpful belief by reminding her of Mr. Slive's mantra, "Openness to all possibilities." I reiterated what Maria and Carmen had said about their having had long-standing marital difficulties. I also shared that maybe over time her father would soften up a bit and miss not having contact with her. Amara appeared to cheer up. I introduced her to the important Buddhist principle of *self-compassion*. I offered her as an experiment writing a compassionate letter to herself from the perspective of a good and close friend who embraces her unconditionally, in spite of any personal flaws or big mistakes she thinks she had made in the past (Neff, 2010). I stressed the importance of including in her letter all of her positive qualities, strengths, talents, and everything she was grateful for in her life. After completing her letter, she was to imagine all of her personal goodness and great qualities taking over her mind and body in a calming and relaxing way. Amara liked the experiment and was eager to try it out. Finally, I told her that she should put the letter in a safe place so that if she ever was in a bad place or started to emotionally beat herself up, she could read her letter to quickly elevate her mood and establish inner peace and harmony in her mind.

I wanted to cover the back door with her as far as relapse prevention. We talked about what could trigger her to cave in to cutting and substance abuse again, and she mentioned her mother's referring to her as "a sinner" or "being evil" because of her sexual orientation. Not that she thought it was imminent, but Amara felt that if Cassie broke up with her at this time she could relapse. I taught her *urge surfing* and had her practice accessing triggers for 5 minutes (Bowen et al., 2011; Selekman & Beyebach, 2013). She handled the mindfulness activity really well. I also told her that if she started to feel out of control as she built up time sitting with her triggers, she could stop and seek out Connie or Lester. I encouraged her to practice urge surfing daily and gradually add more time. I loaned her my kitchen timer to use when she was practicing.

Next, we filled out one of my worst-case scenario forms together. In the first column, she listed four worst-case scenarios. In the second column, she listed the steps she would take to not cave in to her old self-destructive habits, such as using Mr. Slive's mindfulness meditations. In the last column of the form, she listed steps the Stoddards or Maria could take to help her not to cave in to her old habits. I encouraged her to go over her filled-out worst-case scenario form with the Stoddards, her mother, and Maria when we reconvened with her families.

Finally, to build off of Amara's positive momentum in turning her life around, I gave her the *plan out your perfect day* experiment (Peterson, 2006; Selekman, 2009) to do over the next few weeks so we could seize other positive steps she was taking to improve her situation. I pointed out that sometimes we shoot for a 7 or 8 day and something unexpected happens that temporarily may derail us. We discussed what steps she could take to get back on track and finish the day with a 6. Amara really liked the experiment and was eager to try it out. I reconvened everyone so we could wrap up the session and have a short discussion about the importance of relapse prevention with the family members. I pointed out to the two families that slips go with the territory of change and that they are an indication that we have already made good headway. I said that triggers for slips can be the reoccurrence of family guilt-inducing or blaming interactions, being invalidated and not listened to, being devalued or disrespected, certain mood states, doing poorly on a test, and so forth. Next, I asked Amara to share with both families what some of her worst-case scenarios were that might trigger her to self-injure or abuse substances again. She courageously mentioned to her mother what she wanted her to avoid saying to her at all costs, which in the past would lead to some "intense cutting." Surprisingly, the mother promised Amara, "I will not say those words to you ever again." All family members listened intently to Amara about what specific steps they could take to help her stay on track if she felt shaky or in an emotionally vulnerable place. They assured Amara that they would be there to help her stay on track and "move upward and onward" with her life. Finally, I alerted the Stoddards about the urge surfing relapse prevention coping strategy I was having her do to help consolidate her gains. I pointed out to them that if at any point Amara felt like she was losing self-control she should stop and come to them for support.

I felt as a vote of confidence to Amara and her two families, and due to all of their progress, I should offer them a vacation from counseling. When asked if they would like to come back in 3 or 4 weeks, they decided that we should meet in a month. I reminded them that there would be a collaborative meeting at Amara's school in 3 weeks.

Postsession Reflections

I was totally blown away by what great shape Amara was in. It was like night and day. Clearly, having her live with the Stoddards was the most therapeutic move we could have made. It was the perfect family fit for what Amara desperately needed in her life. Connie was instrumental in helping Amara dramatically turn around her academic progress. Other important developments was Amara's increased courage to take positive risks and come out to Lester, gently confront her mother about what not to say to her, and being a much better self-advocate both at home and at school. Finally, the quality of her relationships with her mother and sister had greatly improved as well.

With all of Amara's great progress, I felt it was critical to do some relapse prevention work. She did a nice job of identifying and sharing with both families what her major triggers were for cutting and substance abuse. Amara also shared with them concrete steps family members could take to help her to stay on track and prevent slips from happening.

The Final School Collaborative Meeting

Present at our final school collaborative meeting were Carmen, Connie Stoddard, Amara, Ms. Carson, Mr. Slive, Ms. Stoughton, Mr. Krause, and Mr. Beech. The consensus across the board was that Amara had been doing an amazing job in school. All of her former D+ and C− grades were now at a B level and she was getting an A in Mr. Slive's class. When I asked Mr. Slive what his secret was about moving Amara up from a B to an A grade, he told his fellow teacher peers that he was "cheating," in that he had the edge over them because he was spending extra time with her after school teaching her mindfulness meditation. Amara shared with the group that she could see the results of doing mindfulness meditation. She noticed that she could concentrate and focus better, felt that she became a better problem solver, and felt happier and more self-confident. Jokingly, I turned to the other teachers and asked them, "What top personal skills could you teach Amara so that she could make A grades happen in your classes as well?" Everyone laughed. Mr. Krause said, "I do karate and could teach you that!" Amara responded with, "Well, that would be sweet." He added, "If you have time or are interested, please let me know." Ms. Stoughton offered, "Well, I make delicious chocolate chip cheese-cakes." The whole group and Amara responded with, "Wow! That sounds great!" Finally, Mr. Beech added, "Well, I build furniture." We wrapped up our meeting and I commended all of the teachers, Ms. Carson, and her two mothers on a job well done and told them to keep up the great work. Amara had a huge smile on her face and she thanked everyone for all their support. Carmen also told the whole group how proud she was of Amara and thanked them for all of their help. Due to Amara's tremendous progress, the group decided that there was no need to meet again.

The Sixth and Final Family Therapy Session

In attendance for our sixth family session were Carmen, Maria, Amara, the Stoddard couple, Cindy, Ms. Carson, and Mr. Slive. When asked what further progress Amara and the families had made in their relationships, Carmen took the floor first, saying that Amara had transformed into a "dynamic young woman." When asked what she meant by this, she explained that Amara was now "a serious student, is much more confident, not hurting herself, seems happier, and optimistic about her future." I asked Carmen to share some examples of some of these changes she had experienced with her. They had had dinner together with Maria, and apparently Amara dominated the conversation by telling the two of them how "happy and proud of" herself she was about "doing great in school and possibly considering college in the future." She also had told them that her daily meditating, using other coping tools, and yoga had helped her to conquer her cutting and substance-abusing habits. Mr. Slive chimed in to add that Amara had done a fine job of mastering a wide range of mindfulness meditations and practices. Maria also pointed out how she had been "blown away by Amara's amazing changes and growth." Both Lester and Connie had echoed Carmen and Maria's positive feedback about Amara's transformation, particularly with her academic performance. Ms. Carson joined in with compliments for Amara as well.

At this point in the session, I wanted to test the staying power of Amara's changes and played the devil's advocate by asking her and both families, "What would you have to do to make things go backward at this point?" Amara took the floor first and shared, "Well, I could blow off my homework, blame myself for the family problems, stay closeted with my sexual orientation, start cutting and getting stoned and drunk again, stop meditating, not use my coping tools, and run away." Surprisingly, Carmen shared that she would "start laying guilt trips on Amara about being lesbian and how she was sinning." Amara abruptly responded to her mother's words with, "Wow! I can't believe I'm hearing that from you!" She got up and hugged her mother for now accepting her sexual orientation and being more understanding. Maria chimed in to say that she too was "proud of their mother for finally coming around and accepting Amara's sexual orientation.

I shifted gears and met alone with Carmen and the Stoddards. We discussed Amara's tremendous progress and the living arrangement situation. I asked Carmen if she was still OK with Amara's living at the Stoddards, and she said it would be fine. I shared with them the old adage, "If it works, don't fix it." I went on to say that Amara was doing so well that we should not mess with a good thing since she was on a roll with her multitude of positive changes. The Stoddards and Carmen all agreed. The Stoddard's told Carmen that since Amara only had one more school year left that it would be OK with them if she wanted to remain in their home until she graduated. Although Carmen didn't think this was necessary, the Stoddards insisted it would be their great pleasure to have her. Carmen made it clear that she would send them a weekly expense check to cover Amara's food, school lunches, yoga class, and entertainment costs.

I complimented both sets of parents on their great teamwork helping pave the way for Amara's great success in all areas of her life. I particularly wanted to underscore Carmen's coming to grips and change of heart with Amara's sexual orientation. Carmen shared with us that she could not have done this alone if it were not for Maria and Connie's private meetings with her on the side about "the importance of having unconditional positive regard with your children, no matter what they choose to do or believe in." I stressed to Carmen that her acceptance of Amara's sexual orientation was like the icing on the cake for her. I went on to add that her unconditional acceptance would help greatly repair and strengthen their relationship. Next, I took a huge risk with Carmen and asked if she was in a place where she would be willing to meet Amara's partner, Cassie. Connie chimed in to say that "Cassie was a sweet, caring, and responsible young women who got good grades in school and worked at her father's restaurant part time." Carmen was happy to hear this and said, "Maybe I should take the two of them (Cassie and Amara) out for dinner one night." Connie and Lester thought this was a great idea.

Prior to wrapping up the family session, I briefly met alone with Amara to amplify and consolidate her gains and to assess how the *planning out my perfect day* experiment went for her. Amara pulled out her sheets of paper with her daily number ratings and what she found that worked for her. On a daily basis, she was averaging anywhere from 7 to 9 ratings. When asked what specifically she was doing on those days that were rated from 7 to 9, Amara answered, "Staying away from my drug-using partying friends, meditating, using my other coping tools, doing yoga, hanging out with Cindy a lot, not cutting, and having nice conversations and visits with my mother and Maria." I gave her a big high-five for her great work and amazing turnaround. Next, I asked Amara, "If you were to rate today, what number would you give it?" Amara shouted out, "A 10!" When asked why, Amara shared that hearing that her mother finally accepted her sexual orientation was "huge!" I acknowledged how great this was too.

I reconvened the family and complimented everyone on their great teamwork. Again, I underscored Carmen's huge step at coming to grips with Amara's sexual orientation and unconditional acceptance of her. Amara added, "I love you mom and I want you to know that this is huge for me!" She got up and hugged her mother. Carmen then asked Amara to invite Cassie to go out to dinner with them. Amara cried out, "This is awesome!" Just to get a reading on where everyone was in their readiness to terminate due to all of Amara's tremendous changes, I asked the following scaling question, "On a scale from 1 to 10, with 10 being the situation was better enough, and 1 you are on the road to making progress, where would everyone rate the current situation?" Amara shouted, "At a 10!" Cindy said, "A 10." Everyone else rated the situation at a 10 as well. I fell out of my chair out of amazement with the high ratings. Everyone laughed. I pointed out that the positive vibrations and change ratings were so high and strong that they propelled me out of my chair. I told the group that they were like the Marvel comic strip dynamic team *The Avengers!* In a humorous way, the members of the group who were familiar with the Avengers started flexing their muscles and laughing. I asked the group if they wanted to schedule another appointment or should I just leave the door open for a tune-up in the future if necessary, and they felt fine with just calling if they needed further help. Everyone thanked me for my help and I wished Amara and her two wonderful families the best of luck.

Postsession Reflections

Clearly, the biggest critical change that happened was Carmen's finally accepting Amara's sexual orientation, which meant so much to Amara and helped to repair the rupture in their relationship. In fact, it really blew the Stoddards and me away that Carmen wanted to meet Cassie and take her and Amara out for dinner. Another major contributing factor to all of Amara's major changes was the Stoddards' healthy and nurturing family environment and Ms. Carson, Mr. Slive, and the other teachers' tremendous support and great work in the school context. In looking back, there was no way I could have produced such great results with Amara without the help of the caring and committed adults' efforts.

Final Reflections and Case Follow-Up

I spoke with Carmen and the Stoddards at 6 and 12 months. Both times they gave glorious reports of Amara pulling in "A and B grades, she was working at Cassie's father's restaurant part time, no slips with cutting or substance use, and Amara was talking to them about wanting to become a counselor working with lesbian, gay, bisexual, and transgender teens." She had applied to a state university for the next fall to begin pursuing her career goal.

Shortly after my 1-year follow-up call to both sets of Amara's parents, Amara called me out of the blue to meet with her. I was so delighted to have this opportunity to reconnect with her and hear about her life and career plans. Much to my surprise, Amara brought Cassie with her to meet me. They were eager to tell me how strong their relationship was and that Amara was planning to move into Cassie's apartment. Apparently, Cassie was being groomed to take over her father's successful restaurant and she was making enough money to afford a one-bedroom apartment. I really liked Cassie and it was great to see how happy Amara was with her partner. Next, Amara shared with me her career plans of becoming a counselor working with LGBT teens. I told Amara that she would make a great counselor because she could truly empathize with all of the personal challenges, emotional turmoil, and family conflicts that they must endure and the best ways to cope. Amara agreed, and she was eager to get out there and help them.

Two years later, I received a call from Amara wanting to meet with me to discuss her internship options in the community that served LGBT clients. I was so impressed with how responsible and focused she was on becoming the best possible counselor. I loved her thirst for learning and tremendous enthusiasm. Out of her list of internship sites, I pointed out two that I knew about that would be great places for her to learn and develop counseling skills. In addition, she updated me on how Cassie had taken over her father's restaurant and was earning a good income for them. Amara also said that things were going strong with her and her mother but she still had not seen her father. Apparently, she had made numerous attempts to reconcile with him, but he would not respond to her efforts. I empathized with her frustration about this and encouraged her to not let this bring her down and keep focused on her career goals and all of the great things going on in her life. I reminded her about Mr. Slive's words of wisdom about keeping one's mind open to all of the great possibilities awaiting us. Last, Amara mentioned to me that she and Cassie had a nice dinner at the Stoddards and that she continued to hang out with Cindy when she was back in town from the out-of-state college she attended.

CHAPTER 9

Therapeutic Mistakes and Treatment Failures
Wisdom Gained and Valuable Lessons Learned

> Negative results are just what I want. They're just as valuable
> to me as positive results. I can never find the thing that does
> the job best until I find the ones that don't.
> —THOMAS EDISON

The challenging and complex nature of many high-risk adolescent family case situations can make working with them feel like entering a maze in a dark room. We may see a glimpse of light or possibility worth seizing at a distance coming from a slightly open door, but just as we are about to approach it, it slams shut in our faces. In some cases, just as we are starting to make some good headway reducing the adolescent's presenting difficulties, crises occur with two other family members, and he or she suddenly spirals downward out of control with his or her behavior. With the chaotic and unpredictable nature of these complex families, it is highly unlikely that we can avoid making mistakes and experiencing some treatment failures along the way. However, just like when clients have slips or even prolonged relapsing situations, making mistakes and failing every now and then with families provides us with great opportunities for learning and wisdom about what we need to avoid doing when faced with similar stressful and challenging clinical situations in the future. Mistakes also can serve as springboards for brilliant improvisational moves for creating something novel and special or taking us in more meaningful and productive directions with families. In his well-written memoir *Possibilities,* the great jazz pianist Herbie Hancock shares his experience playing with the Miles Davis Quintet in his 20s, in Stockholm, Sweden.

At one point, when his all-star band was really swinging, just as Davis was about to break loose with his solo, Hancock played the wrong chord. He described his chord "like a piece of rotten fruit hanging out there" (Hancock, 2014, p. 1). Inside his mind, he is beating himself up about what he initially thought was a big mistake. Instead of the situation turning out to be disastrous for Hancock, Davis briefly paused and then took their classic tune "So What" that they were playing at the time in an improvised different direction, incorporating his errant chord by blowing notes that made it "sound right." According to Hancock, "The crowd went absolutely crazy" (p. 2).

Within every mistake and failure we make, there are hidden assets and opportunities worth seizing. O'Connor and Dornfield (2014) found in their research on what they call *unignorable moments*, which are costly mistakes, that by making room for storytelling from all parties involved we can track where things went awry, what people were thinking, where they felt stuck, what they desire and think would make a difference, and we can often discover alternative pathways to pursue with similar challenging situations in the future.

Erik Kessels, an advertisement business consultant, once said, "Failure is good. Big failure is better. Big, ignominious failure in front of a lot of people is the best" (in Tyler, 2015, p. 76). Kessels believes that daring to make mistakes is what produces novel ideas and opportunities. In fact, he gives workshops on *forced errors,* which are about the art of making mistakes (Tyler, 2015).

In this chapter, I present how therapeutic mistakes and failures occur, early warning signs, and practical tools and strategies we can employ to help reduce the likelihood of their occurring. Failing fast and well with prototype, co-designed interventions can be useful for co-generating high-quality solutions with families and involved helpers. I also share some of the wisdom I have gained and lessons learned from making mistakes and experiencing treatment failures with complex high-risk adolescent family cases for over three decades in a wide range of practice settings.

Contributing Factors and Key Reasons Why We Make Mistakes and Experience Failures

Under intense physical and emotional duress, our survivalist brains do not function well. They do not like the challenges of uncertainty and of solving abstract and complex problems (DiSalvo, 2011; Schoen, 2013). We tend to rely heavily on our intuition rather than on careful reasoning (Soll, Milkman, & Payne, 2015). Holmes (2015) contends our brain's need for closure makes us more prone to commit to certain ideas, beliefs, and courses of action. When faced with challenging situations in the midst of the therapeutic process in a session or feeling stuck between sessions, warning signals are sent to our amygdalae, our brain's alarm center to either dig in and desperately try to come up with the right set of therapeutic tools and strategies that may eventually work (fight response) or we pursue the flight-or-freeze responses, that is, we are no longer totally present with our clients, we lose our spontaneity, are too much inside our heads listening to our critical voices, we may experience therapeutic paralysis, or distance ourselves from the clients and blame them for being "noncompliant" or "resistant."

The 15 Cognitive Biases and Mental Traps

In addition, our brains encourage us to pursue shortcuts to quick fix solutions for these dilemmas. Unfortunately, our survivalist brains mislead us and we fall prey to one or more of the 15 cognitive biases and mental traps that can ensnare us in their logic. This can result in us making therapeutic mistakes and, worse yet, clients dropping out or treatment failure. Below, I briefly discuss these cognitive biases and mental traps, how to recognize when they are governing our decision making, and recommend steps we can take to liberate ourselves from them.

Affective Heuristic

With this mental trap, we minimize the risks and costs of the decision we make. We tend to be too emotionally attached to the client situation at hand and lose our objectivity because we believe that what has worked for us will be good for the clients; the client's presentation may be a blind spot or vulnerability area for us, in that it mirrors a negative life difficulty that we had experienced and still have not totally resolved; or provocative, hostile, or highly demoralized family members are testing our integrity and abilities as therapists, which is putting us on the defensive. All of the above scenarios have us making decisions under emotional duress, creating a ripe climate for costly therapeutic mistakes (Goleman, 2013; Weisinger & Pawliw-Fry, 2015).

Remedies

We need to operate in a purposeful way with our clients. This means critically reflecting, session by session, on what drives our thinking, the therapeutic actions we choose to take, and whether they help our clients to achieve their goals. We can ask ourselves, "Have I fallen in love with my idea or solution?" Kahneman, Lovello, and Sibony (2015) recommend using a checklist to see if there is anything you may be missing about the case situation. Each session is a unique entity and clients determine their session agendas. It is not about what we think they need to focus on or discuss, or what we think is best for them. We can use *suspension,* as discussed in Chapter 3, when we are having strong emotional reactions to pessimistic helping professionals or parents and critically examine our assumptions, thoughts, and feelings. We can formulate questions to ask ourselves what is going on with us and how can we change or redirect our actions with these challenging family members. We also can use ourselves as emotional barometers and take risks, sharing with family members what we are thinking and feeling to see how that might be related to what is happening in the session, process-wise. If clients' stories, presenting problems, or adverse life situations too closely parallel our own past negative experiences, and we find ourselves not being totally present or experiencing a strong emotional reaction, this needs to be discussed in clinical supervision. It may be helpful to videotape sessions to bring to supervision for input or have an observing team of colleagues sit in and support what we are doing that seems to benefit the clients and what is unproductive. They can identify our emotional hooks and offer the clients and us some fresh ideas.

Salient Analogies and Bias

We make treatment decisions based on our past success stories working with families presenting with similar problems and characteristics. This is one of the dangers of being locked into a particular empirically supported treatment model because of the research imperatives. Just because we have had past emotionally memorable experiences treating similar families with the same types of adolescent problems, the same treatment approach is not guaranteed to work with new families presenting with similar problems and characteristics (Mudd, 2015).

Remedies

We need to ask ourselves, "How is this family case different from similar families I have worked with in the past?" Kahneman et al. (2015) recommend that we think about as many past similar family cases as possible and carefully analyze them for how they were different from the present case. By doing so, we may see that there are clear differences among the families, notice multiple new therapeutic options, and look at the strengths and weaknesses of pursuing any one of these solution strategies. The bottom line is that each adolescent and his or her family is unique and their presenting problems are constantly evolving. We can't be absolutely certain of anything, and more important, we need to tailor what we do therapeutically to the unique needs, characteristics, and goals of our clients.

Confirmation Bias

Sometimes we prematurely lock into one possible explanation, hypothesis, strategy, intervention, or treatment approach (Kahneman, 2011; Mudd, 2015; Nisbett, 2015). We refrain from being curious about what the second, third, or fourth possible explanation could be, what other therapeutic approaches or strategies may work, or what our supervisor or team might recommend trying with the case situation.

Remedies

I am reminded of the French Existential philosopher Emile Chartier's great quote, "Nothing is more dangerous than an idea when it is the only one you have" (Goolishian & Anderson, personal communication, 1988). We can ask ourselves, "How can I be certain that I completely understand the family's problem situation?" "What are two or three other ways of viewing this problem situation?" We need to catch ourselves if we are limiting our focus and the type of information we are gathering from our clients just to support our limited views about their situations. With this bias, we need to use the most versatile tool we have in our therapeutic arsenal, which is *curiosity*. We should ask ourselves, "In what ways could this intervention or my treatment approach fail to work or exacerbate the family's problem situation?" There is always more to know about the client's story and many possible avenues to pursue for client change.

Availability Bias

The mind-set here is "what you see is all there is" (Kahneman, 2011). As we too quickly sift through clients' case complexities to make sense of what we are seeing, hearing, and experiencing with them, our minds have a tendency to construct for us a coherent, albeit limited, narrative based on the evidence we have (Nisbett, 2015). Although there may be holes in families' presenting problem stories, we tend to overlook what is missing. This bias gets us into trouble because we tend to give too much weight to the probability of something occurring if we have seen it recently or if it is vivid in our minds (Mauboussin, 2009). This happens a lot with specialty clinics and programs for particular types of adolescent problems and disorders. For example, if an adolescent is assessed at an ADD specialty clinic because of his or her alleged ADD-like behaviors, more than likely he or she will receive that diagnosis after the assessment is completed. Alternative explanations will be ignored, such as growing up in a chaotic and unpredictable family environment, which certainly could fuel such symptoms and behaviors.

Remedies

We need to be curious with our clients about what is not being talked about, what their theories are about how their problem situations got to this point, and who else is not present in initial family sessions but may be involved in the maintenance of the adolescent's difficulties. How will families know they achieved their ideal outcomes? We need to put families in the expert position regarding what needs to be addressed and what former therapists had missed. Doing so will fill in the information gaps in our case formulations, create a more *thick description* (Geertz, 1973) of the family's story, and help us to better understand where it is most critical for us to intervene.

Representative Bias

Similar to the availability bias, we often rush to conclusions based on representative categories in our minds, neglecting any possible alternatives or explanations for what might be driving high-risk adolescents' intimidating or provocative behaviors (Mauboussin, 2009; Nisbett, 2015). A great example of this is with the popularity of the borderline personality disorder label that adolescents who self-injure frequently get branded with. Since self-injury is a hallmark symptom in the borderline personality disorder symptom constellation, therapists and other helping professionals take this one symptom and leap to the conclusion that they must have this disorder without considering anything else that might be contributing to their self-injuring behavior. According to DSM-5, in order to use this diagnosis with an adolescent, borderline symptomatology must be present continuously since early childhood, which is often not the case for the adolescents wrongly being diagnosed with this disorder (DSM-5; American Psychiatric Association, 2013).

Remedies

Everything that was recommended for countering the availability bias I would employ here as well. Furthermore, never stop being curious and asking questions, because there is always more to know about the adolescents' and their families' stories. We can ask ourselves, "Did I too quickly reject alternative directions or other potential solution strategies because I thought they were bad ideas or because of my confirmation, representative, and availability biases?" (De Brabandere & Iny, 2013). Research indicates that when people think more than once about a problem, they often come at it from a different perspective, which adds valuable information (Soll et al., 2015). Similarly, Spetzler, Winter, and Meyer (2016) recommend that we employ what they call *system 3* thinking, which is to imagine how professionals from different fields and skill sets would view and try to solve your client's problem situation.

Anchoring Bias

With this bias, we have a tendency to buy into our own estimates, hunches, explanations, hypotheses, and associations as gospel. We don't put forth the extra time and effort to search for the hard facts to better ground our positions and explore other possible treatment directions we could pursue with our clients. Kahneman (2011) has observed that we have a tendency to start with a specific piece of information or trait (the anchor) about a client situation and adjust as necessary to come up with a final explanation about it. Our treatment responses are off the mark because our case formulations are too close to the anchor and we still do not know enough about the clients' problem stories. We cling to our initial impressions or hypotheses, which we believe are accurate and based on some higher truth.

Remedies

In countering this bias, recall Emile Chartier's quote and familiarize yourself with the great philosopher Karl Popper's work. He believed that true intellectual honesty meant trying to refute, rather than prove a theory about the world (Holmes, 2015). Popper's (1965) contention was that a scientist could never know for certain whether his or her findings are true, but he or she may sometimes establish with reasonable certainty that a theory is false through rigorous testing. Finally, I would recommend pursuing the suggestions under how to counter the confirmation bias.

Halo Effect

We view clients' stories or presenting difficulties as simpler and more emotionally coherent then they really are. We stop gathering information or are not sensitive enough to the complexities of their stories and presenting difficulties. By keeping things too simple and too narrowly focused in one direction, our approach is destined to produce therapeutic mistakes and possible treatment failures (Kahneman, 2011). Here is where William of Ockham's "keep it simple" logic, "It is vain to do with more what can be done with fewer," can backfire for us (Stokes, 2008, p. 55). With complex family case situations, we have a tendency to simplify, take shortcuts, and be satisfied with quick, *good-enough* therapeutic decisions (Spetzler et al., 2016).

Remedies

We need to ask ourselves, "How can I be absolutely certain that my case formulation is totally accurate and using my choice therapy model is a perfect fit for this family?" It is helpful to keep oneself in check, be curious about what has not been said or what you don't know, gather more information, and leave room for incubating and reflection before jumping into action with your clients. We must steer clear from "one-size-fits-all" thinking with our clients. Kahneman et al. (2015) recommend that we try to identify and eliminate our false inferences by seeking advice from our colleagues. John Frykman, a professional colleague of mine, once shared with me some wise words: "When you know what you already don't know you know, things will happen in even better ways" (Frykman, personal communication, 1996).

Sunk Cost Fallacy/Endowment Effect

Similar to the salient analogies and bias, we are overly attached to past decisions made with similar types of client presentations (Mauboussin, 2009). Unfortunately, history can lead us astray. The past cannot be a starting point for resolving a current client problem situation. Past successful therapeutic and client attempted solutions are not necessarily blueprints for resolving present client difficulties.

Remedies

We can ask ourselves, "Am I being too narrow with my intervention choices here?" What are two or three other possible interventions that might work?" Everything that was recommended for countering the salient analogies and bias I would recommend here.

Optimism Bias

We become too wedded to our choice therapy models or specific sets of tools and strategies for specific types of adolescent and family problems. We view our therapeutic abilities and the particular treatment approaches as panaceas. Since we have such religious fervor about what we believe and do therapeutically, we stop delving into clients' histories to find out about their past attempted solutions. Operating out of this mind-set, we don't seek input from our colleagues about how else to think or what else to try with our clients (Mudd, 2015).

Remedies

We should ask ourselves, "How can I be absolutely certain that my favorite therapy model is a perfect fit for this family?" I also would remind oneself of Emile Chartier's and John Frykman's words of wisdom under the confirmation, anchoring, and halo effect biases and their recommended remedies. Kahneman et al. (2015) recommend that we ask ourselves, "Is the worst case bad enough?" With our colleagues, we can imagine the worst has happened after implementing a particular solution and develop a story about the causes. This helps us to see the dangers of our overconfidence and being too wedded to a particular solution strategy or treatment approach. Checklists also are helpful here to make sure we have covered all of the bases with having a comprehensive understanding about the client's problem situation and, with their guidance, where to intervene first (Gawande, 2010).

Overconfidence

The *overconfidence* mental trap goes hand in hand with the optimism bias (Goleman, 2013; Kahneman, 2011; Nisbett, 2015). We are so certain that our views of our clients' situations and what we try therapeutically is the most perfect fit that we see no need to explore with them barriers to change. Even if the clients make progress, we see no need to do worst-case scenario planning with them because we believe the change process is all set and the likelihood of slips is minimal. This occurs a lot with overzealous and rigid solution-focused therapists who strongly believe in keeping the focus solely on the positive, keeping things simple, and avoiding *problem talk* at all cost. They think there is no need to prepare clients for management of inevitable slips or address any concerns they may have outside of their target goal areas (Nylund & Corsiglia, 1994; Selekman & Beyebach, 2013).

Remedies

Tetlock and Gardner (2015) contend that we need to strike the right balance between over- and underconfidence when it comes to solving complex problems and predicting the outcome of implementing our ideas.

They encourage us to defer judgment; do not prematurely commit to one perspective or one course of therapeutic action. Instead, reflect and incubate before taking decisive action. Everything that was recommended above for the confirmation and optimism biases I would recommend here for countering this mental trap.

Risk and Loss Aversion Bias

This bias fuels our cautiousness and derives from our adopting fixed mind-sets (Dweck, 2006). We find it much more comfortable to play it safe with our clients and stay within our comfort zones. The wish to avoid making mistakes, or upsetting or losing our clients to premature dropout outweighs the desired gains we would like to achieve with them and with our own professional growth as therapists.

Remedies

Unfortunately, by choosing to stay in one's comfort zone with highly complex adolescent high-risk family cases, risk-averse therapists will end up quickly being neutralized and defeated. This will lead to the very negative treatment outcomes they are trying to avoid. We can ask ourselves, "Am I being overly cautious with this family?" With support from their supervisors or consultation teams they need to be encouraged to lighten up, take the plunge, step outside of their comfort zones, and try something daring or surprising with their clients. These experiences will help liberate them from therapeutic complacency and fixed mind-sets, particularly when they start to feel more self-confident, playful, and enjoy their work more with families. Therapeutic change often occurs when we operate outside of our comfort zones and embrace novelty.

Superiority Bias

When we start afresh with a new high-risk adolescent family case that has had multiple treatment experiences or when other therapists may still be involved with other family members, we can have a tendency to privilege our key assessment findings and performance over what other therapists and helping professionals have tried. With the superiority bias, we tend to focus only on the strengths of our case formulations and what we plan to do therapeutically. We overlook the weaknesses in our case analysis and therapeutic decision making. Conversely, we have a tendency to focus on the weaknesses of other therapists' clinical opinions and approaches, ignoring the strengths in their perspectives and what they have to contribute to us treatment-wise for our mutual clients. We will only agree with other therapists and involved helping professionals if they see eye to eye with us in our case formulations and treatment approaches.

Remedies

Everything that has been recommended under the overconfidence, optimism, confirmation, anchoring, and halo effect biases and mental traps I would recommend here. This kind of professional arrogance will end up costing us big time with our clients and colleagues. Inspired by the work of Karl Popper, the philosopher Bryan Magee (1985) speaks to the benefits of welcoming the input from others:

> No one can possibly give us more service than by showing us what is wrong with what we think or do; and the bigger the fault, the bigger the improvement made possible by its revelation. The man who welcomes and acts on criticism will prize it almost above friendship: The man who fights it out of concern to maintain his position is clinging to non-growth. (p. 37)

We need to view other involved therapists and professionals from larger systems as potential allies who can help us better understand our clients' presenting problems and who we can tap to bring fresh and creative ideas to our work with our clients.

Predictive Bias

Although we may have many years of clinical experience and do quite well with particular types of client difficulties, this does not mean we are experts and God-like. No matter how skilled we are with our beloved treatment approaches, successful outcomes are not guaranteed. As Mudd (2015) points out, "Deep expertise leads us to assume that we can predict the future. It's this confusion between expertise and the ability to see tomorrow that we need to avoid" (p. 195).

Several studies have indicated that we have a tendency to overestimate our performances and the outcomes of others (Kahneman, 2011).

Remedies

Gilbert (2007) and Gilbert and Ebert (2002) have found in their research that we have a strong tendency to imagine future success based on past emotionally memorable successes at solving particular types of problems. However, these are illusions about our abilities to predict the future. They cause us to misconstrue and underestimate the complexity of the clients' presenting problems. We then are off the mark for selecting and tailoring the most appropriate treatment approaches. Tetlock and Gardner (2015) recommend that we look for clashing causal forces at work and adopt a "dragonfly-eye view," that is, be open to how one causal explanation can lead to another and another. We should attempt to synthesize them into one multifaceted explanation. Everything I recommended under the overconfidence, optimism, confirmation, anchoring, and halo effect biases and mental traps I would recommend here as well.

Post Hoc, Ergo Propter Hoc

With this mental trap, which means *after this, therefore because of this,* we have a strong tendency to seek simple explanations for clients' presenting difficulties and family dynamics that are much more complex than we think (Mudd, 2015). Often, we are missing huge amounts of important data about the family's story and the adolescent's difficulties. This mental trap is also due to the fact that our brains do not like struggling with complex and abstract problems, and so the simple and the coherent explanation often wins out to give us relief.

Remedies

Everything I recommended under the halo effect and many of the aforementioned biases and mental traps applies here.

Reasonable Man or Woman Bias

Our ways of viewing the world are based on our personal life experiences, professional training and experiences, our values, and so forth. Because we consider ourselves *reasonable* in terms of our beliefs and abilities to solve problems, we have a strong tendency to assume that others (our clients and involved helping professionals) think like us (Mudd, 2015).

Remedies

We have to be careful not to impose our own values on our clients and involved helping professionals or assume that they will agree with us regarding what may be most useful to them. The bottom line is that the clients' preferences, theories of change, and goals should drive the treatment process and we need to respectfully follow their lead. They are the true experts on their life situations and unique needs!

Self-Imposed Constraints
That Can Contribute to Mistakes and Failures

In addition to the 15 cognitive biases and mental traps discussed above, there are nine self-imposed constraints that can contribute to our making mistakes and possibly lead to client premature dropout or treatment failures. I describe each one below.

Therapy Is Serious Business!

When therapists adopt a humorless demeanor and mind-set that "therapy is serious business," it is a big turnoff for high-risk adolescents. What I have learned over the past 30-plus years of working with challenging, high-risk therapy-veteran adolescents is that they tend to warm up to and like therapists who are playful, funny, have a little bit of wild and coolness to them, and who talk straight with them. We also have to be highly active in sessions working both sides of the generational fence, disrupting parental blaming and invalidating in sessions. We can't just sit there in the thinking position as passive observers studying the therapeutic process like scientists. We also need to be able to connect with powerful adolescents and find out what is in it for them in terms of the changes they want to see happen with their parents' most "annoying" behaviors and what privileges they desire and wish for us to advocate for them with their parents. When we fail to deliver on these fronts, they may decide to drop out or their parents will discontinue family therapy because their kids either don't like us or think it is a waste of their time.

Weak Therapeutic Alliances

As mentioned in Chapter 2, if we fail to establish strong alliances with the parents or legal guardians and the adolescents, therapy is destined to fail. This is why it is so critical to secure feedback every session from each member of the family on the quality of our therapeutic relationships with them (Lambert, 2010; Norcross & Lambert, 2013). When family members report having weak alliances or were upset by certain therapeutic moves we made in sessions, it behooves us to find out from them what specifically we need to do differently. We then need to change our behavior to better accommodate family members' unique needs so that they are more satisfied with the treatment experience (Norcross & Wampold, 2013). Having strong therapeutic relationships with our clients is highly predictive of positive treatment outcomes (Norcross & Lambert, 2013). Along these same lines, having strong alliances with challenging adolescents in

family therapy is also highly predictive of positive family treatment outcomes (Diamond et al., 2014; Diamond et al., 2006; Robbins et al., 2006;
Santisteban et al., 1996). Parents will commit to the family therapy when
they feel that their kids liked and connected well with their therapists.
Finally, research indicates that if clients do not feel satisfied with the
treatment they are receiving by the third session, they are more likely to
drop out (Lambert, 2010).

The Fear Factor

When we are under emotional duress due to fear, we are highly likely to
make mistakes in our sessions. Fear kills curiosity. Once we stop asking
questions and cling to narrow, unhelpful ideas about the clients' presenting problems, it can lead to a loss of focus in sessions and the treatment
process can run astray (Kashdan, 2010). For many of us, fear can be triggered when we are faced with highly intimidating and provocative clients
presenting with serious and chronic DSM-5 disorders (American Psychiatric Association, 2013). For example, in our first family therapy sessions,
during our one-on-one time with self-injuring adolescents, some of these
youth may spontaneously choose to show us their scars and recent cut
marks up and down their arms. Fueled by anxiety, we may jump to the
conclusion that these are suicidal gestures and they want to die. We may
encourage them to sign a no-suicide contract before we have gathered sufficient information about this behavior, how it is connected to their family
environments, and before we have built a safe and trusting relationship
with them. Therapists who react this way toward therapy-veteran self-
injuring adolescents indicate to them that they may be too much for the
therapist to handle, and that it is not safe to reveal anything private about
themselves. They lose their faith in the therapist's ability to help them.
Along these same lines, we had a self-injuring client who was bulimic in
our qualitative study who told the researcher, "Freaking out when I show
my cut marks and scars. One of my doctors was so uptight about my cutting that I wanted to give him some of my meds he was prescribing to me
to chill him out." This client stopped going to this psychiatrist. Another
psychiatric evaluation determined that she should not have been placed
on antidepressant medication in the first place (Selekman & Schulem,
2007).

The bottom line is that if you feel uncomfortable working with certain types of challenging adolescent presenting problems or feel you lack
the knowledge and skills to do a competent job, you should get written
consent from the clients to videotape sessions, have supervisors sit in
on sessions with you, or arrange for a consultation team of trustworthy

colleagues to observe and intervene with you and the family. This kind of support and access to multiple perspectives and fresh ideas will help you feel more confident and comfortable working with tougher treatment populations.

Another reason for our fear may be that we have already experienced some treatment failures with clients. According to Kahneman (2010), when we experience failures they become imprinted into our subconscious minds and our memories of these failures can reinforce our fear of it happening again in the future. However, being too cautious and second-guessing our abilities will not fly with therapy-veteran high-risk adolescents and their families who may be feeling a strong sense of hopelessness and despair. We have to give ourselves permission to venture out of our comfort zones. One strategy I like to recommend to my supervisees and trainees is first to think about a tough case they are struggling or feeling stuck with. They are then to ask themselves, "If I were to do something really daring and surprising in my next session with the _____ family, what would it be?" They are next to commit to trying out one or two surprising therapeutic moves and evaluate how it worked for the clients and them. This can be discussed in the next supervision or training meeting. Once supervisees, trainees, and therapists discover the freedom and joy of working outside their comfort zones with families, there is no turning back.

Too Much of a Focus on Problems

Challenging therapy-veteran high-risk adolescents and their families are often quite tired of having to tell and retell their problem-saturated stories. Therefore, we must strive to make enough room for family members' sharing their presenting difficulties, history and past treatment experiences, those times when problems were not occurring, and what specifically works during those times. We need to read family members' nonverbal and verbal indications that it is time to move off the problem talk and pursue a new journey to possibility land; we need to immediately shift gears and ask questions like the miracle and presuppositional future-oriented questions that help tell us their desired ideal treatment outcome. If we fail to do this, and the problem stories go on too long, the session begins to digress into possible blame–guilt cycles of negative interactions. Some family members may start to feel that we are no different than the other therapists they have seen in the past and decide to drop out. We want our clients to leave our first family sessions feeling hopeful, not thinking that they were big downers and deciding not to come back.

The Treatment Goals
Are Too Vague, Unrealistic, or Therapist-Driven

Often when we are feeling stuck with high-risk adolescents and their families the treatment goals are too vague, unrealistic, or the therapists' goals
are driving the treatment. Back in 1995, the great cognitive therapist Art
Freeman shared with our training group the following: "Vague goals
leads to vague therapy" (Freeman, personal communication, 1995). Yes,
it leads to a vague therapy that drifts along aimlessly until the clients say,
"Enough is enough; we're exiting from this therapy." Our job is to invite
the clients to decide what they see as the right problem to begin with and
take the lead in clearly and specifically defining their initial treatment
goals. As collaborators, we need to help them get to their destinations in
the most efficient way possible. Two other ways treatment can end up at
a standstill are when the treatment goals are too big or unrealistic and
when we decide what they should work on changing.

We try to be like Hercules and try to change all symptom-bearing
family members at once, despite the fact that they may be highly emotionally disconnected from one another and most may be in the *precontemplative* stages of change, which means they don't think they have problems
(Prochaska, Norcross, & DiClemente, 2006). This is a highly unrealistic
treatment objective and goal. When faced with these kind of clinical
dilemmas, simplifying the situation can make it much more workable. See
individual family members or subsystems separately, with separate goals
and work projects. Also, parents or legal guardians in these families who
are burned out with their kids may try get us to buy into their highly unrealistic goals, like changing their "temperaments," "make them smarter
in school," or changing several of their kids' problems all at once. With
parents or legal guardians who want to see multiple problem behaviors
changed all at once, we can establish *multiple scales* with the goal setting
process as described in Chapter 4 (George et al., 1999). As we make progress in each of these problem goal areas, the parents will start to see how
they are interconnected.

We Are Prisoners in the Boxes of Our Choice Models

Due to our practice setting mandates, we may be locked into practicing a
particular empirically supported family therapy approach. We also may
be too wedded to our choice family therapy models. The danger with
taking either position is that we limit ourselves theoretically and therapeutically to what we will be able to see and do with families. As Milton
H. Erickson once said, "Yes, therapy should always be designed to fit the

patient and not the patient to fit the therapy" (Erickson & Rossi, 1979, p. 415). The following will help us to reduce the likelihood of making mistakes and prevent treatment failures from happening: recognizing the limitations and weaknesses of the treatment models we are mandated to use or are well versed in; allowing our models to evolve; integrating ideas from other approaches when necessary; and carefully tailoring what we do to the unique needs, characteristics, and preferences of our clients to help them achieve their goals.

We Are Too Preoccupied with Performance

When we are too preoccupied with our therapeutic performance, either trying to emulate one of our favorite family therapy pioneers or trying to do a particular model the so-called *right way,* we will inevitably make mistakes because we are so much in our heads and not totally present with the family. In addition, when we are under duress or put too much pressure on ourselves, it limits our cognitive functioning and downgrades our behavioral skills (Sukel, 2016; Weisinger & Pawliw-Fry, 2015). Not only will we miss great opportunities in the midst of the therapeutic process in sessions, but also we may focus too sharply on certain dynamics or places we need to target in a given session. This can lead to costly blunders that family members were ill prepared for, were not in the right stage of change for, or find so upsetting enough that they drop out.

The Treatment Focus Is Too Narrow

Another way we get into trouble is when there is a mismatch between the unique needs, characteristics, and preferences of the family, and the treatment protocol's focus in sessions. We may focus too much on the positive (what is working) or too much on problem behaviors and interactions in the here and now, when certain family members would like to share their past painful traumatic experiences and stories (Nylund & Corsiglia, 1994). When we block clients from sharing their long stories, they may feel invalidated, and we have become narrative editors. We also may spend too much time in family therapy sessions working with particular subsystems, such as devoting an inordinate amount of session time to the parents and needlessly antagonizing and shortchanging the adolescents. We have to use ourselves like wide-angle and telephoto lenses, zooming in family members' needs to seize specific opportunities in sessions, and zooming out to gain a broad perspective to observe and reflect on the outcomes of our actions across the family system and other systems they interface with.

Strong Aversion to Uncertainty and Silence

As I mentioned earlier in the chapter, our brains do not like uncertainty and not knowing. We like to have control and understand or think we understand what is going on with our clients. We often do not cope very well with silent family members. These situations often make us feel anxious because we may not know exactly why that person is shut down and not talking, even after our efforts to engage him or her in the conversation. When we become excessively anxious, we may end up talking too much, which has been found to be one of the reasons why clients prematurely drop out of therapy (Beyebach & Carranza, 1997). Family members may sometimes sit in silence because they are sizing us up and trying to determine whether they like or can trust us; they're trying to see whether we are different from the other therapists they have seen before us; it is not safe to open up in their family or no one will listen to them anyway; or silence is a powerful weapon for frustrating another family member or a therapist, for that matter. We can ask, "What's not being talked about that may need to be talked about?" Sometimes this question will open the door for family members to talk about the *not yet said* (Anderson, 1997). We also can view uncertainty as a positive opportunity to create something new together with families and to explore different avenues for therapeutic change.

Guidelines for Preventing Therapeutic Mistakes and Failures

In this section, I present practical guidelines for how we can reduce the likelihood of making mistakes, prevent premature dropout, and avoid treatment failures. I describe below seven different strategies that can be employed throughout the therapeutic process to help optimize treatment success.

Key Drivers to Explore and Focus Our Attention On

With complex, high-risk adolescent family cases, it is very easy to get lost in a sea of information about their problems and their extensive treatment histories. To help them achieve their goals and address their session-by-session agendas, we need to limit our focus to some key *drivers* (critical areas of concern for the clients) and determine with them what specific relationships we should focus on first. John Mudd, a former deputy director for the FBI and counterterrorism analyst for the CIA and author of *The Head Game: High-Efficiency Analytic Decision-Making and the Art of Solving Complex Problems Quickly,* recommends that we sort key drivers into categories. These become "go-to" bins to help us make better sense of the complexities of our clients' presenting problems (Mudd, 2015). To get started with the driver identification process, we need to first strive to ask good questions from a position of curiosity, such as:

"What is this problem a solution for?"
"How is the adolescent's presenting problem connected to the family drama and politics?"
"What is still unclear about the family's presenting problem?"
"What is the question that must be answered about this problem situation?"
"What am I still missing about the client's and former therapist's attempted solutions?"
"When the problems are absent, how do the family members account for that?"
"What else do I need to know about the spaces in between problems [non-problem times] that may be worthwhile harnessing and increasing?"
"What key resource people do we need to engage from the family's social network who could make a big difference in optimizing treatment success?"
"Is there more I need to know about key barriers to change, so we can intervene and begin to remove those obstacles?"

Once we have answers to the above questions, they can become our primary drivers to focus on and help us steer away from an unproductive previous treatment course.

Reflection-in-Action and Reflection-on-Action

Schon (1983) has observed that expert practitioners from a wide range of professional disciplines practice both *reflection-in-action* while engaging in a problem-solving task and *reflection-on-action* upon its completion. With reflection-in-action, we are stepping outside of ourselves in the midst of the therapeutic process and carefully observing and listening to family members' nonverbal and verbal responses to determine the effects our therapeutic moves have on them. If we see head nods, smiles, moving forward toward us, listening intently to us, it could be that they found a good fit in what we were saying and doing. Reflection-on-action, on the other hand, involves our reflecting on the following question: "If I had another shot of conducting this family therapy session all over again, what would I have done differently?" In response to this question, we can prepare the following checklist:

- Specific questions for further inquiry about the presenting problem and/or the family drama that we are still puzzled by or need more information about.
- Key family members we need to strengthen our alliances with.
- Have the family identify key resource people from their social network who may make a big difference with the solution construction process and between-session support.
- Other than the referral source, find out if there are any key helping professionals you need to collaborate with.
- Write down a few therapeutic tools or strategies you think may have a great shot at working and helping the family to achieve their goals.

Through reflection-in-action and reflection-on-action, we can keep an open and curious mind; catch ourselves when we prematurely lock into one or two ways of viewing the presenting problems and family; and be curious about the third, fourth, or fifth possible explanations. The same therapeutic flexibility occurs with intervention design and selection. Critical reflection is used to determine what may have the best shot at working.

Wu Wei and Incubating

When we are feeling stuck with our clients, they are having slips, or things are starting to unravel in goal areas, we can become anxious and scramble for the *right* interventions to try with them. Unfortunately, this will only make matters worse. Instead, we need to step back and adopt the Taoist position of *wu wei,* or not doing. The key to enlightened wu wei is to abandon doing or having others tell you what to do. This creates a receptive space and openness to learning. This worldview is that our unconscious mind is going to lead us in the right direction because it possesses sacred quality. By not doing and engaging in quiet reflection, we shut down our mind's cognitive controls in the brain's prefrontal cortex and let our adaptive unconscious mind take over. Once this happens, it is *qi* (chee), which provides us with a direct connection to our true heavenly natures, the sacred power within the self (Slingerland, 2014).

Some of the greatest historic figures, artists, architects, authors, musicians, and so forth used *incubating* to give themselves time to step back from the projects they were working on, engage in some other relaxing activities, collaborate with others to get their input, and reflect further on their projects after having downtime. For example, not only would the great artist Vincent van Gogh incubate but also he would routinely write letters with detailed sketches of a new art piece he was working on to his brother, Theo, Victor Hugo, Voltaire, and others to get feedback on his work (Bakker, Jansen, & Luijten, 2010). Kahneman (2011) believes that incubation is a critical activity in what he calls *system 2* thinking. With highly complex problem situations, he recommends that we pursue system 2 thinking, which involves incubating and carefully reflecting on all of our options and, based on the information we have, pursue the solutions that logically have the best shot at working. However, he cautions us to not decide too quickly or be swayed by one or more of the cognitive biases, and make sure we have sufficient information or support for the solutions we have selected, as discussed earlier in this chapter.

Premortems

For decades, Klein (1998, 2002) has studied professionals who work in settings where they have to make quick decisions or manage crisis situations, like emergency room doctors and nurses, police officers, firefighters, military personnel, air traffic controllers, and so forth. Across the board, Klein and his colleagues found that these professionals conducted *premortems.* Prior to resolving a complex problem or crisis, they would project themselves through visual simulations into the future, seeing them solving or stabilizing the problem or crisis at hand. While walking back from the future to the present, they would carefully look for loopholes or flaws in their plans of action. When they identified loopholes or flaws in a plan that were deemed problematic, they would come up with a plan B or C until they came up with a nearly foolproof strategy to pursue. Using premortems in our therapeutic work with tough, high-risk adolescent family cases can be most advantageous in helping us to be much more mindful about the interventions we co-design or select to offer our clients. This is why it is so important that we have clients identify not only small, realistic behavioral goals but also obstacles that might get in the way of achieving them. This provides us with valuable information about what may interfere with the implementation of selected therapeutic experiments.

Checklists and Going Back to Basics

In his best-selling book *The Checklist Manifesto: How to Get Things Right,* Atwul Gawande (2010) shows how using checklists can help us conduct much more thorough and comprehensive assessments of complex problem situations, reduce costly errors, and improve the quality of care and service for clients. In addition to regularly reflecting on our actions after each family session and putting together checklists, we still may be missing something critical that is keeping the treatment at a standstill or the clients are getting worse. This is when I conduct my *going back to basics* troubleshooting analysis. I ask myself the following questions:

"Do we have a well-formulated behavioral goal?"

"Is the goal still too big and needs to be broken down further into smaller pieces?"

"Do we know who the true customer(s) for change are in the family or in their social network?"

"Have we carefully matched our questions and interventions with each family member's unique stage of change?"

"Do we know family members' theories of change?"

"Have we honored family members' unique preferences, theories of change, and expectations?"

"Do we know which key resource people in the family's social network we need to engage who could make a big difference in the solution construction process and with relapse prevention?"

"Are there any other key helping professionals involved who I need to begin to collaborate with?"

"Are there any powerful reluctant nonattending family members or key members from their social network that I need to reach out to and engage?"

Once we are able to answer the above questions and take appropriate actions, we will be able to get unstuck and move the treatment process in a more productive direction.

Session-by-Session Client Feedback

Another great way we can avoid making mistakes and getting stuck and prevent premature client dropout and treatment failures is by soliciting feedback from our *clients about the quality of our relationships with them at the end of every session* (Duncan, 2010; Lambert, 2010; Norcross & Lambert, 2013; Norcross & Wampold, 2013). We can learn the high points for them in a given session in terms of what ideas they found most useful; whether there were specific aspects about the presenting problem that they were surprised I had not asked them more about and they may wish to explore in future sessions; find out from any of the family members whether I said or tried something that they wish me to stop doing; and find out if they are feel like they are getting their needs met and making progress. Across the course of family therapy, even when things are going well, make room in sessions to find out any concerns family members have or recent crisis events that occurred outside of their target goal areas and address them. Unless we take care of them, they could come back to haunt us. As the great family therapy pioneer Harry Goolishian once said, "If we expect our clients to change, we too have to be willing to change our thinking and behavior" (Goolishian & Anderson, personal communication, 1988). By taking care of our therapeutic relationships with each family member in this way, we will increase their satisfaction with us.

Deliberate Practice

Throughout our professional careers, we may have periods when we become complacent with how we practice our therapeutic crafts. We may neither critically evaluate our work with our clients nor seek to improve our weaker skill areas through further training or close supervision. Furthermore, we have a tendency to overinflate our therapeutic talent and skills, particularly when we develop expertise with certain types of presenting problems and feel no need to refine our beloved therapeutic tools and strategies and formulaic way of doing things (Miller, Hubble, & Duncan, 2007). We can greatly improve our therapeutic technical skills and improve our treatment outcomes with our most challenging clients through *deliberate practice* (Ericsson, 2008; Ericsson & Pool, 2016). Deliberate practice consists of picking specific therapeutic skills we wish to strengthen or learn outside of our comfort zones, setting clear and realistic goals for skill mastery, and working closely with a supervisor or trainer who will offer us immediate feedback while we hone or attempt to master a new therapeutic skill. The immediate feedback from a supervisor or a trainer helps us produce *mental representations*; as our performance improves, these representations become more detailed and effective in helping us further enhance our skills (Ericsson & Pool, 2016). This is why it is so helpful to videotape family therapy sessions or receive live supervision so we can see the specific skill areas where we are good and where we need further improvement. Periodically, having a team of trustworthy colleagues observe us work or sitting in with a stuck family case can provide us with multiple sources of constructive feedback. Robert Bjork, a renowned memory researcher, found that we learn better when the learning is hard, which he referred to as "desirable difficulties." For him, skill development comes from struggle and eventual mastery (Benjamin, 2010).

Failing Fast and Well?: The Upside of Failure

Up to this point in the chapter, I have spent a lot of time discussing how mistakes and failures occur and constructive steps we can take to both remedy and learn from them. In addition to gaining valuable practice wisdom from our mistakes and failures, I now discuss how we can use failure as a resource to add to our therapeutic armamentarium. According to Danner and Coopersmith (2015), "Failure is today's lesson for tomorrow. It contains the secrets that can show you what you will need to know and how you need to change your strategy. Managed correctly, it can be a vital resource for resiliency" (p. xviii). These organizational consultants have developed a highly practical framework for anticipating, constructively managing, and learning from failures called the *failure value cycle framework*. It consists of the following steps: *respect, rehearse, recognize, react, reflect, rebound,* and *remember.* I briefly describe each of these steps below.

1. *Respect*: We need to come to grips with the fact that we are fallible and failures will inevitably occur. Failures should not be considered taboo subjects to avoid thinking or talking about but are opportunities for learning, resilience, and professional growth.
2. *Rehearse*: Practice using whatever appropriate adaptive action steps, checklists, and protocols best fit the type of failure scenario.
3. *Recognize*: Identify any warning signals (changes or unusual patterns out of the ordinary) of a potential failure looming on the horizon as early as possible to buy time to strategize and minimize its long-term effects.
4. *React*: When failure does occur, respond effectively, whether unexpected or self-initiated, when and as it happens.
5. *Reflect*: Reflect thoughtfully, thoroughly, and with an open mind to clearly understand the factors that led to the failure, and develop your action plan for bouncing back.
6. *Rebound*: Bounce back from the effects of the failure, and apply its lessons to improve your post-recovery performance.
7. *Remember*: With all failures, share mutual stories about them and establish rituals with your colleagues about the hard work and the challenging journeys involved in the process. Failures are like sages offering you and your collaborative team valuable wisdom (Danner & Coopersmith, 2015, p. 101).

With the help of the above framework, we can now view failures in a much more positive light, as great opportunities for improving our therapeutic crafts and treatment outcomes.

Failing Fast and Better

When working with complex and challenging high-risk adolescent family cases, it is best to jump right in co-generating many ideas and potential solutions and test them as early in the treatment process as possible. By doing so, we will learn what potential solutions are to be discarded and those that, with further refinement, might be more on target. Sastry and

Penn (2014) contend that "thinking combined with action" provides an antidote to working with challenging, nonlinear complex systems. Joe Kraus of Google Ventures had the following to say about failing fast:

> The best way to integrate failure positively is to fail fast. Run many experiments quickly. If you develop a strong foundation and tradition of rapid experimentation, then you can deal with small failures much more effectively, in part because you know you will be running another experiment very soon. If you do not run many experiments, then you can become more invested in the success or failure of any one, and it may take on an unreasonable importance. (cited in Danner & Coopersmith, 2015, p. 128)

Lessons Learned and Wisdom Gained from Treatment Failures

Over my three decades of clinical work with high-risk adolescents and their families, I have made my share of therapeutic blunders, lost family members to premature dropout, and experienced treatment failures. In wrapping up this chapter, I share below some of the valuable lessons and wisdom gained from these experiences. Some case examples are provided, with posttherapy analyses and hindsight reflections about what I could have done therapeutically that might have helped and produced better outcomes.

Sometimes We Need to Slow Down

Often we get off to a great start in our first sessions with families and our enthusiasm and optimism can lead us to moving too quickly and trying to do too much too soon. What may be operating here are the cognitive biases and mental traps that can fuel poor clinical decision making. We need to slow down, give ourselves time to incubate and reflect, and based on our clients' guidance and feedback, determine with them what they are ready to try. What specifically are we doing with them that has been helpful and where do we need to make adjustments so that they are more satisfied with our work together? It is important that we strive to empower our clients to be collaborators.

Alicia, a white 16-year-old, was brought in by her parents for anorexia nervosa and self-injury. Over the past 5 years they had seen six therapists for the same presenting problems, with four of those therapists seeing Alicia individually. I noticed in the first and second family sessions that the parents' conflicts would surface around how best to get Alicia to stop starving and cutting herself. They had completely different ideas about what could work. In session two, I decided to take a gamble and cross the bridge to the marital subsystem to address the parenting conflict and had Alicia step out. Suddenly, the couple became a united front, offended by my implying that they were not working well together as a parenting team. Together, they pointed out that they were not in my office to work on their marriage but for me to help them help their daughter. They further added that they do work well together as a parenting team. When I met alone with Alicia, I could tell that she was upset with me. Alicia let me know that she felt shortchanged with not getting enough session time. Needless to say, after the family left I was not confident they would return. The mother called me 2 days later to say that they found a new therapist.

Case Analysis: "If I could rewind the clock and see this family afresh for the first time, what would I do differently?"

In reflecting back on this case, I would have remembered an important family therapy rubric, which is our job is to empower parents as consultants to help them resolve their adolescents' difficulties first. Once we help the parents to accomplish this goal, then if, and only if, they want to contract to work on marital issues we can pursue that therapeutic direction with them. If we prematurely address the parental relationship conflicts, we run the risk of offending the parents and losing them to future family therapy. The other therapeutic blunder I made was not finding the balance in how session time was used with parents and adolescent. Alicia was quite angry with me about not leaving her with enough session time. Since she had tremendous power in her family with two dramatic and provocative self-destructive habits and was a therapy veteran, I should have met with her first to set in motion an alliance before seeing the parents. My family therapy rubric is when adolescents wield the most power in their families we should meet with them first. If we meet with the parents first, the powerful adolescents will think we are plotting with the parents behind their backs and may question whether they can trust us.

The Shortcomings of Keeping Things Simple: Failure to Engage the Most Powerful People in the Family's Social Ecology

Therapists operating from pure solution-focused (de Shazer et al., 2007) and MRI brief problem-focused therapy (Fisch & Schlanger, 1999) models believe it is important to keep things simple, that is limiting their work to the nucleus of family members that originally present for treatment, such as the most motivated parent (the true customer for change) and, if possible, the adolescent. They would view absent fathers, powerful reluctant adolescents, their siblings, and sabotaging extended family members not even window-shoppers for counseling (precontemplators), and typically they do not reach out to or chase after them.

In many cases, the fathers are in the *precontemplative* stage of change. If they are traditional, they may believe it is up to mother to solve their children's problems and go to therapy (Prochaska et al., 2006). Sometimes the mothers, in an effort to not rock the boat with their male partners, will not let them know about going for therapy or not ask the father to attend with them. It can be problematic not having the fathers present in family sessions because the biggest source of conflicts and problem-maintaining interactions may be left untouched. In addition, I believe that we should reach out to these fathers and attempt to engage them, as discussed in Chapter 2. I have made the mistake in the past of not being sensitive enough to the role of fathers in different cultures and angered the fathers, which in turn led to their yelling and arguing with the mothers and some crisis occurring with their adolescents. In some cases, I have been able to engage the fathers to attend, but their presence in sessions contributed to the adolescents being silent and withholding. Over time, by making it safe for the adolescents, I have been able to do meaningful father–son or father–daughter connection building work.

Other powerful people we may need to engage and intervene directly with are adult siblings of parents and grandparents who have strong grips on the mothers or fathers, blaming them for their kids' difficulties or sabotaging their parental authority. Noncustodial divorced or separated parents who refuse to communicate or collaborate with us to help their adolescents can be a powerful disruptive force that can have a negative effect on our family work. Tyrannical and powerful adolescents who refuse to attend sessions with their parents will need to be intervened with directly if seeing the parents alone and their attempts to implement change strategies proved to be futile. Finally, we need to consider the adolescents' peer group as an important place to intervene, particularly when they have more leverage and power than the adolescents' parents do.

No Ripple Effect: Extreme Emotional Disconnection and Untreated Multiple Symptom Bearers in the Family

With some of the high-risk adolescents and their families we work with, there may be a Grand Canyon of emotional distance between them and their parents. This may be due to their having serious physical, mental health, and substance-impaired difficulties. So the family system concept of *holism* does not apply here. A ripple effect does not occur—when one member makes a change, the other members do not respond by changing their problem-maintaining behaviors. I have mistakenly assumed otherwise and worked with the whole group together, rather than breaking them up and working with them separately, to establish separate goals and work projects. We need to walk side by side with each family member at his or her unique pace through the stages of change. This creates a much more workable reality for them and us. Once each member is making great progress and we have consolidated their gains, it may be possible to bring them back together to establish mutual goals and work with them to co-create the kind of compelling future reality they would like to have together.

Failed to Advance the Adolescent to the Next Stage of Readiness for Change

The majority of high-risk adolescents referred to us would be considered *precontemplators* (Prochaska et al., 2006). Just because we establish good rapport with them in our initial family therapy sessions does not mean they are customers for change armed with goals and ready do work. Sometimes we make the mistake of offering them tools to experiment with well before they are either in the *preparation* or *action* stages of change. They will not use them because they think they don't have a problem (Prochaska et al., 2006). We need to slow down and meet these adolescents where they are at and gradually raise their consciousness through the use of the *two-step tango* (see Chapter 2). This helps them arrive at the conclusion that maybe they do have a problem to take a look at. Once this occurs, they have moved into the *contemplation* stage of change (Prochaska et al., 2006). If we fail to make it to this second stage with the adolescents, the treatment may be destined to fail unless collateral changes with their parents and/or their powerful peer groups occurs and propels them onto the road to change.

I once worked with a single-parent Mexican American family where the mother had absolutely no leverage with her twin 16-year-old gang-involved sons. Not only were they failing in school but also they spent all of their free time running with their gang and sneaking out at night to attend rave parties. The father had abandoned the family when the boys were toddlers. Although I had thought I had connected well with them in the first family session and they both voiced a strong desire not to end up back in the "juvie" (juvenile detention center) again, outside of our sessions they refused to cooperate with their mother's rules and expectations. Neither one of the boys had an adult inspirational other or a strong male extended family member who could have join us in sessions to offer the mother and me added leverage with them. Even when their probation officer would join us and try enforcing his probationary contract with them, it seemed to go in one ear and out the other. Eventually, they refused to come with their mother to our sessions. Finally, the mother got so frustrated and demoralized coming alone for our sessions that she dropped out of therapy.

Case Analysis: "If I could rewind the clock and see this family afresh for the first time, what would I do differently?"

In reflecting back on this case, there were a number of adjustments that might have made a difference with the treatment outcome. First, I would have seen the boys separately with the mother in an effort to strengthen her relational bonds with each one with the hope that this would help generate more respect for her authority and respect from them. Second, I would have seen each boy separately in an attempt to build stronger alliances and gain more leverage with them. Third, I might have tried to introduce them to two of my former gang-involved clients who were 18 and 19 years old, who had turned their lives around with school, work, kicking drug habits, and steering clear from police involvement. They could have been a positive influence in the boys' lives. The other thing I failed to do was construct with the mother a solution-determined collaborative team involving the school social worker, the high school dean, an involved youth officer, and the probation officer. Although the probation officer was actively involved, having more creative brainpower and people join us to co-generate ideas or potential solutions and provide more support outside family therapy sessions could have been helpful.

Lack of Leverage and Strong Working Alliances with Involved Therapists and Other Helping Professionals from Larger Systems

Often high-risk adolescent cases attract an army of helping professionals from multiple larger systems. If we fail at the beginning of the treatment process to secure signed client consent forms and collaborate with the involved helpers, the latter may have concerns about whether the clients are coming to treatment, want to know our case impressions, and may be eager to share their concerns with us. When we fail to regularly communicate and collaborate with these powerful representatives from larger systems, they may become increasingly alarmed and persist in unproductive interactions with the clients that can contribute to the maintenance of the adolescent's difficulties. They may be totally oblivious to the fact that their attempted solutions are having a deleterious effect on the clients because they are just trying to do their jobs of monitoring them to make sure they are taking responsibility and complying with the treatment mandate.

Ideally, we want to establish strong partnerships with all of the involved helping professionals, tap their expertise, and gain their allegiance in the client change effort. Ultimately, they can serve as key members of the solution-determined collaborative treatment team, as discussed in Chapter 4.

Jacintha, a 17-year-old non-Muslim Tunisian American female, was brought for therapy due to depression, family conflicts, and academic decline. From the first session, I witnessed intense conflict between the parents and between Jacintha and her mother. Each parent blamed the other for Jacintha's problems. Jacintha also was sitting on her father's shoulders in a cross-generational coalition against the mother. When meeting alone with the parents, I could never get them to agree on anything. The mother had her own therapist whom she had been seeing for a while, and she would bring her therapist's recommendations into our sessions about what I should be addressing in our family therapy sessions. In particular, I should be changing the father's behavior of being allegedly "too permissive and undermining her." Although I had built solid alliances with Jacintha and the father, I never could get any semblance of an alliance going with the mother. I also failed to secure written consent from her to collaborate with her therapist. The next session only the father and Jacintha showed up, and they told me the mother was not coming back. In spite of persistent outreach efforts to re-engage the mother, she refused to come back in for family therapy. For our remaining time together, I only saw Jacintha and her father. Although Jacintha had made some progress by the end of our work together, the conflict between the parents and in the mother–daughter relationship was left untouched.

Case Analysis: "If I could rewind the clock and see this family afresh for the first time, what would I do differently?"

In reflecting back on this case, I should have worked much harder to build a stronger alliance with the mother. The mother needed a lot more support from me because she had little power and control in the family. I also could have tried *unbalancing*, a structural therapy strategy for trying to better balance the power and control dynamic in the marital subsystem (Fishman & Minuchin, 1981). Another failure on my part was my poor salesmanship with the mother to gain her trust and support with collaborating with her therapist, possibly including her in our family sessions. This therapist had a very strong alliance with the mother, and I could have greatly benefitted from her support and expertise. I also had fallen prey to the *superiority* cognitive bias by privileging my treatment plan and not considering at the time the importance of collaborating with the mother's therapist and welcoming her therapeutic input. After the mother dropped out, it was like there were two warring factions, the mother and her therapist versus the father and Jacintha. At times, I too got sucked into taking sides by allying myself more with the father and daughter, which obviously posed a threat to the mother.

From Potential Allies to Outlaws: The Power and the Strong Grip of the "Second Family"

With high-risk adolescent family cases, we must intervene with the adolescents' peer group, particularly when it is a street gang or an unsavory group of friends who are heavily into substance abuse, disordered eating, and self-injuring behaviors. We can work wonders in our family sessions and make some good headway in improving family relationships, but everything can quickly unravel when the adolescents' peer groups sway them to engage in risky behaviors outside their homes. When adolescents have to contend with the threat of being yelled at or worse, being harmed in some way, and when they can't count on their parents to soothe, listen to, or respect them, then it is more likely they will gravitate toward negative peers who become their *second families* (Taffel & Blau, 2001). In their second families, they feel a strong sense of belonging, personal power, and being valued and respected.

The way that we can positively infiltrate our adolescents' second families is to begin by asking them in the first session, "When you are really stressed out or need some good advice, which one of your friends will you turn to first for support?" After finding out from the adolescents what is special about these two or three friends and how they have been able to count on them in the past, we can ask them if they may be willing to bring them in for you to meet. If they agree to do so and they and their parents sign off on my significant other consent form (see Chapter 4), we also need to secure signatures on the consent form from the friends' parents and the friends. Once the friends come in, we need to treat them like royalty so that they feel comfortable with us, think we are nice, and "cool to chill" with. Not only will they be more likely to want to attend future sessions but also they may start to look out for their friends (our adolescent clients) in terms of trying to prevent them from ending up having to do juvenile detention time, being locked up in a psychiatric hospital, or sent to a residential treatment center. The clients and their friends may also choose to bring in some additional members of their peer groups for the parents and us to meet. One client brought in eight friends to meet the parents and me—a house record!

When we are unable to get adolescent clients to agree to bring in friends for us to meet or they continue to experience serious consequences as a result of their continued involvement with them, I will explore with them whether they would be willing to meet adolescent alumni I used to work with who are now upstanding citizens and gave up gang life or conquered their serious self-destructive habits. The alumni can serve as a positive influence for them by sharing their wisdom and expertise about how they conquered their problems and stayed on track. In some cases, our adolescent clients may build meaningful friendships with the alumni outside of our sessions.

Failure to Securely Cover the Back Door: Lack of a Highly Structured Relapse Prevention Plan Sets the Stage for Disaster

When we fail to develop a highly structured relapse prevention plan in the early stages of the treatment process, adolescent behavioral slips and prolonged relapsing crisis situations will occur on a regular basis, which can have a demoralizing effect on the clients and lead to their dropping out of treatment. Whether we are pursuing harm reduction goals or not with the clients, we need to have them identify potential obstacles to achieving their goals. Having representatives from all of the adolescents' social contexts can give kids easy access to support people. Finally, we need to make sure that we have conducted worst-case scenario planning with the solution-determined collaborative team and armed the adolescents with an arsenal of coping tools and strategies that they can use when they experience negative emotions, high stress, or negative life events.

In summary, it is important that we carefully examine our errors behind the mistakes we make and the treatment failures we experience with our clients by asking ourselves, "Where exactly did I go wrong?" In addition to critically examining our thinking and actions that led to our therapeutic blunders and failures, we should carefully analyze our successes as well. Tetlock and Gardner (2015) contend that we may have been successful with a particular intervention or sets of interventions with an adolescent and his or her family because of luck, not our reasoning. Furthermore, they believe if you adopt the same rationale for why you did what you did with similar clients in the future, sooner or later we will be met with "a nasty surprise."

CHAPTER 10

Therapeutic Artistry

Finding Your Creative Edge

I really like to play out on the edges. It is a really exciting place to be.
It is where something special is about to happen!
—CYRUS CHESTNUT

Working with high-risk adolescents and their families successfully is all
about a high level of versatility and flexibility. We have to be on our toes
constantly and ready to change position like a ballet dancer or jazz musi-
cian and willing to move in any direction family members wish to take us.
Along the way, we need to seize opportunities as they emerge to co-create
something special and novel with them. We also have to be courageous
and daring with our risk taking and allow our curiosity to run wild, particularly when the pathways to change are unclear or our integrity and
competency as family therapists is being tested with our toughest therapy-
veteran families. Donald Schon (1983), author of the thought-provoking
book *The Reflective Practitioner: How Professionals Think in Action,* had the
following to say about the management of complex and challenging problem situations:

> In each instance, the practitioner allows himself to experience surprise, be
> puzzled, or confused in a situation he finds uncertain and unique. He is
> not dependent on categories of established technique, but constructs a new
> theory of the unique case. He does not keep means and ends separate, but
> defines them interactively as he frames a problematic situation. (pp. 16–17)

Schon makes some important points that are quite applicable for our
family therapy practices. First, we should not allow uncertainty to ruffle

our feathers, but instead welcome it both as a surprising and unique experience. Second, we should not rigidly adhere to the rules, formulas, and procedures of any one family therapy approach, but tailor what we do to the unique needs and characteristics of each family we work with.

In this chapter, I present the family therapist artist's palette, which is a strategic use of self-framework that offers us 12 different ways to use ourselves in the therapeutic process in response to the climate in the therapy room. Finally, I provide 32 practice guidelines for how we, as family therapists, can increase our inventiveness and hone our therapeutic artistry skills.

The Family Therapist Artist's Palette: A Strategic Use of Self-Framework

Curiosity

Curiosity is one of the most versatile tools we have for gaining a deeper understanding of a particular event or chapter of a family's story. It invites family members to identify their key strengths, share their expertise, and guide us when puzzled. It is a way to help open up space for more workable future realities with families. Sternberg (1981) has found in his research that individuals who entertain multiple ways of viewing a problem situation prior to beginning the problem-solving process perform much better at solving difficult problems than those who do not.

There are four types of curiosity we can use: *emotional, empathic, diversive,* and *epistemic* (Grazer & Fishman, 2015; Leslie, 2014). For 35 years, Brian Grazer, the producer of many highly successful movies and TV shows has conducted what he calls *curiosity conversations* with highly successful thought leaders representing a wide range of professional disciplines outside of the entertainment business. These conversations provided a source of inspiration and new ideas to pursue in his work. He was particularly interested in learning from his renowned interviewees what made them tick, that is, connecting a person's attitude and personality with their meaningful and important work. Grazer refers to this as *emotional curiosity* (Grazer & Fishman, 2015). Empathic curiosity has to do with our genuine and deep interest in the thoughts and feelings of the people we are working with, which occurs when we are truly present and our clients feel felt by us.

The case example below illustrates the use of *empathic curiosity* with Brenda, a Nigerian mother, and her white husband, Henry, who had been struggling for years with George, their 16-year-old son.

George had been exhibiting poor academic performance, school disruptive behaviors, chronic lying, and more recently, substance abuse. Brenda felt that she had been constantly stuck having to discipline him alone most of the time. Brenda and Henry also had an 11-year-old son, Keenan, who was an A student with no behavior problems. George used to bully him. A few weeks back, the mother had requested marital therapy for her and her husband but she had not followed up with me nor defined the primary issue she wanted resolved in their relationship.

I was picking up on some tension and disagreement between Brenda and Henry and decided to have both of their sons step out so I could meet alone with their parents. George had just failed math for the fourth time after performing extremely poorly on his final exam. For years, Brenda had been the lead parent monitoring his homework and calling his teachers. She absorbed the brunt of George's verbal abuse, lying, and manipulations. Brenda looked totally exhausted and beside herself. From a position of curiosity I asked her, "Is this the biggest issue for you with Henry, that because you have had to work overtime putting out fires with George that you feel like you have been shortchanging Keenan's special time with you?" Brenda cried for the first time ever in family therapy and nodded vigorously that I was on target and understood her frustration. She said, "That's it, you got it! I feel like I have let Keenan down." Next, I asked Brenda, "What do you need from Henry that can free you from this predicament?" Brenda responded, "For Henry to step up more and take over with George for a while." It turned out that Henry spent very little time with George due to a heavy workload and his chronic difficulties with depression. Brenda thought it would be great if Henry would set aside some time each week to do high-quality activities with George and take over the schoolwork monitoring duties. Henry agreed to step up more to free Brenda up so she could spend more time with Keenan. Next, I had Brenda step out so I could have some father–son session time to come up with ideas for activities they could do together and for George to come to know his father better as a person. Since there was a history of Henry stepping up for a short time and then vanishing from his co-parental role, I gently and empathically predicted that as much as I wanted to see Henry to set a house record in this role for extended period of time, things might snap back to square one quickly for him. This could happen if the stress level gets too high trying to manage George and to protect himself from another depressive episode. The good news was that Henry accepted this challenge and ended up spending a lot of time over the next week with George on schoolwork and spending quality time by going out to a movie and to a couple of hobby shops. They were looking for and eventually purchased balsa wood World War II airplanes they could build together. George was very interested in World War II history, particularly air warfare. We used worst-case scenario planning in future sessions as a way to keep Henry on his toes and for protecting his newfound co-parental leadership role, no matter what challenges George threw his way.

With curiosity, we have to be totally absorbed and listen generously to our clients' responses to our questions. We have to allow the answers to inspire us and provide us with the courage to take what we have learned, and risk creating something new and special out of what we learned from them. Curiosity also allows us to see that the ways we had been operating in a session or two with a particular family are not the only way, or even the best way. Therefore, curiosity can help us to maintain an open mind and be therapeutically flexible.

According to Leslie (2014), "curious learners go deep, and they go wide, they make creative connections between different fields and/or subjects to lead to new ideas" (p. xvi). This is what he refers to as *diversive curiosity*, which is our attraction to novelty and adopting an explorer's mind. When we take diversive curiosity to an even deeper level, *epistemic curiosity* kicks in, which is a relentless thirst for new knowledge, sensations, experiences, and challenges. All we are curious about within family sessions and outside the therapeutic arena is grist for the mill and can tapped for sparking new ideas, pursuing new therapeutic directions, and co-designing therapeutic experiments with our clients.

Perceptual Acuity: Scanning and Seizing Opportunities and Being Prepared to Be Surprised in Every Session!

In every family session we conduct, there are unlimited opportunities worth seizing. We need to constantly zoom in and zoom out while observing around the room full circle how family members' style of interacting with one another either opens up or closes down conversation. Observe their nonverbal responses to one another and with us, how unified the parents appear to be as a team, who speaks for whom, who dominates the floor the most, who is sitting on whose shoulders, who takes whose side. Look for and lock into choice places to challenge and intervene. At the same time, we need to listen generously to how family members describe their presenting dilemmas and concerns, their theories about why they exist, how they think they will change, their preferences and expectations of us. We need to listen for deeper meanings of family members' words by asking open-ended questions from a position of curiosity like cultural anthropologists visiting a tribal group's village for the first time. In addition, we need to both look and listen for the following opportunities worth seizing: poetic and inspirational themes in the clients' stories that can be utilized with the co-construction of solutions; wisdom they gained from their reported epiphanies; key serendipitous practices that tend to bring them good luck and produce positive outcomes; times when they are getting along better and the problem behaviors are absent both in and out of sessions. Determine with them like detectives joining forces on the same case what specifically contributes to these sparkling moments when things are going well. This includes family members' positive ways of thinking, feeling, and doing.

Stephanie, a 16-year-old white girl, came to our family therapy consultation with her mother, Barbara, and two sisters, Alison and Belinda, ages 14 and 12, respectively. What brought them in was that Stephanie and Belinda were talking more about their sexual victimization by their father. That had occurred a few years back and the child protection and legal systems had let the family down by dropping charges against him. The parents are now divorced. Stephanie has full-blown posttraumatic stress symptoms, including self-injury, cleansing rituals, and severe anxiety and depressive symptoms. Belinda was reported to child protection and placed on probation for 1 year after sexually offending with her cousin. Alison was having major problems with her school, including academic decline and disruptive behavior. Barbara was an adult sex abuse survivor and had had quite a lot of therapy to come to grips with her past victimization. Apparently, Barbara had no idea that behind the scenes when she was not around her ex-husband had been sexually abusing their children. I found Barbara not only to be an incredibly resilient person but also very inspirational. She had plans to go to law school and specialize in family law so she could champion the cause of other families like hers that were let down by both the child protective and legal systems. Her present work was joining forces with agencies and programs for youth in her community to start a family drug court program, so that youth could be legally ordered for treatment rather than being incarcerated. While listening attentively to and being emotionally moved by how inspiring Barbara was, a question started to materialize in my mind that I wanted to ask the daughters: "In what ways has your mother inspired each of you as young women to be all that you can possibly become?" Each daughter shared how their mother was "like a mother and father" to them, that she encouraged them "to set big goals" for themselves, telling them that unlimited possibilities awaited each of them, and two of the daughters had strong desires to work with their mother some day in her future law practice firm. While listening to her daughters, Barbara was smiling and laughing. I shared with the family how I could picture in my mind seeing these "three strong women who had overcome adversity making a difference in our society." Following this discussion about how inspiring their mother was to them, Barbara told each daughter how much she appreciated and loved them and was blessed having them as her daughters. It was both an emotionally moving and uplifting consultation session for all of us.

Sharing Gut Hunches

In the midst of therapeutic action or when stuck, something in our guts will tell us that we should take a risk and ask a specific question, share a great quote or story that mirrors the family's dilemma, or try out a particular therapeutic strategy we think will have a great shot at working. The decision to make a particular therapeutic move is sparked by pattern recognition. Certain types of questions or therapeutic tools that we have used in the past with similar families fit nicely like a lock and a matching key to produce a positive outcome either in the session or between sessions. Klein (1998, 2002) did research with highly skilled professionals in occupations regularly requiring quick decisions. He found that across the different professions, they relied on *action scripts* in their minds about what works best with specific types of crises based on successful management of these situations in the past. These skilled professionals also had tended to have back-up plans if the remedy looked problematic or required further refinement. As family therapists, it is always good clinical practice to be armed with a plan B, C, or D if what we choose to try out is completely off the mark or not potent enough to disrupt a particular problem-maintaining pattern.

Gigerenzer (2007, 2014) found in his research on the management of complex tasks across a wide range of professional disciplines that having too much information about them led to poor decision making and negative outcomes. He contends that better results occur when we listen to our guts.

The case example below with 13-year-old Luis, a Mexican American only child, illustrates how going with my gut and sharing a quote from a well-known comedian was right on target with how he was feeling about his destructive interactions with his divorced parents and successfully broke his silence in the session.

Luis was brought for our live family consultation in the context of a workshop I was giving with his mother and two staff members from his therapeutic day school. The father failed to show up. Luis had a long history of fighting with his peers, had assaulted his mother in the past, had severe anger management difficulties, and had been arrested for vandalizing buildings. The parents had been divorced for 5 years and they had joint custody. Throughout most of the consultation, Luis was reluctant to talk while his mother spent a lot of session time complaining about his problematic behavior. No matter what I tried to do to cut the mother off and get Luis to talk, it proved to be futile. Finally, I asked the mother to step out so I could meet alone with Luis. I asked Luis what his father was like as a person. He responded, "He is an upsetting and annoying troll!" When asked about what he meant by that, Luis said, "He thinks because he's an adult he can talk to me any way he wants. He complains to me about his economic problems and how his car needs a new engine et cetera, et cetera, and I have to get in his face and tell him, 'You're not going to talk that way to me!'" I took a risk by sharing with him comedian Rodney Dangerfield's famous line, "I don't get no respect!" I asked Luis if that was how he felt, and he vigorously nodded and said, "Uh huh!" I then got him pumped up about how his parents needed to "get their acts together!" He agreed and got highly animated and shouted, "Yeah!" I gave him the brother handshake and he smiled. At the end of our session, Luis shared that he felt like I "understood" him and his difficult family situation. Once the treatment team pulled Luis out of the middle of the parents' long-standing postdivorce battles, he started doing much better.

Transparency

One way we can level the playing field with our clients and humanize our experiences with them is through sharing our thoughts, feelings, gut hunches, and our reactions to a tense, gloomy, or uncomfortable therapeutic climate. A rise in our emotional discomfort may be a signal that what we are doing is not working. We need to redirect the session with the clients and take the lead in deciding what they think is most pressing.

Another important way we can be transparent with our clients is to share ideas or therapeutic experiments that pop into our heads during a session. They may be worthwhile for clients to try out over the next week. We can let them know the rationales for experiments and how they are in line with clients' key strengths and treatment goals. They will have the opportunity to choose which ones they wish to experiment with, further refine, or discard. The case below illustrates how I took a big risk with Anna, an Italian 15-year-old, and her family by sharing how I was feeling a heavy gloominess in the room and exploring with them what it might be about. Anna was brought for family therapy due to her problems with bulimia.

In our third session, the family came into my office as if thick gray storm clouds were hovering over their heads. I noted that I felt like they had just come from a funeral. There was dead silence in the room. I asked them, "OK, what's not being talked about that you think we need to address?" The mother shared that her father was just diagnosed with advanced pancreatic cancer. Apparently, he had been sick for the past 3 years with unidentified digestive problems and she had been quite worried about him. I offered empathy and support. Anna started to cry and shared how painful it would be to lose her grandfather. She also was worried that her binge–purge cycles may increase as a result of finding out about this sad news. I validated her thoughts and feelings and acknowledged that this situation is very difficult to process, but now that it is out in the open she could talk with her mother and siblings about it. They could support one another, rather than Anna trying to rid herself of bad thoughts and feelings by bingeing and purging. I asked Anna, "What could your mother do that could help you not to cave in to 'bulimia's' attempts to brainwash you into increasing your binge–purge cycles?" Anna looked at her mother and replied, "For you to make yourself available to listen to and support me when I want to talk about Grandpa and other things stressing me out." One of Anna's biggest complaints about her mother was her not being very present and invalidating her a lot, which had fueled her bulimia. I had learned this important information after I had asked Anna, "Has something happened to you in the past or more recently that has been difficult for you to stomach or digest?" I have found this question to be very useful to ask clients with eating disorders because such disorders often stem from some relationship conflict with a particular family member or significant other. The mother tearfully shared with Anna and her siblings that she had felt so guilty about having withdrawn from them and not being available to them emotionally because of her excessive worries about her father's health problems. She had lost her mother 2 years earlier to cancer. Anna and her siblings told their mother that they would be there to support her and it was helpful for them to find out from her why she had become so emotionally distant from them.

Storytelling

The purposeful use of engaging personal stories, such as how former clients overcame adversity, can offer our clients hope, new ways of looking at their situations, and possible solutions to consider. We also can share our own personal stories about how we overcame adversity and performance challenges throughout our lives that parallel the clients' situations. Milton H. Erickson used stories to offer clients new ways of looking at their problem situations, to capture their undivided attention, harness and utilize their strengths and resources, evoke abilities, and intersperse suggestions (O'Hanlon, 1987; Rosen, 1991).

Listening deeply and generously to our clients' stories, problem crises, and attempted solutions inevitably will remind us of other stories that we found insightful, meaningful, and potentially transformative. It may be worth sharing these in the midst of our conversations with our clients. As suggested earlier, it is quite helpful to put parents in charge of sharing with their adolescents their stories as teenagers of failing, making mistakes, and how they bounced back and gained wisdom from these experiences.

When working with adolescents who are not keen about doing relapse prevention work and overconfident about their willpower, I often share the story (or remind them) of Odysseus and the island of the Sirens, whose beautiful voices lured sailors to their deaths on the island's rocks. Odysseus had his sailors tie him tightly to the ship's mast and put beeswax in their own ears so they could not hear the alluring voices, which would prevent them from crashing their ship into the rocky coast. Once they were safely past the Sirens' island, he had his sailors untie him from the mast (Homer, 2006). He had the insight to know that his willpower alone would not have produced a successful outcome in the high-risk situation.

The case example below illustrates how we can use a personal story that closely mirrors the client's dilemma to help them to bounce back from adversity.

Terrence, 17 years old, was brought to see me by his parents for marijuana and alcohol abuse, academic decline, and for breaking their rules. His top strength was tennis. He was the number-one singles player on his high school varsity team and was on the road to qualify for the state championship. Terrence also was a great team leader. In his district tournament, he had lost in the finals to his nemesis, whom he had beaten a year earlier as a sophomore. This had emotionally devastated Terrence to such a degree that he drank so much hard liquor with friends the evening of his loss that he ended up in the emergency room. We had a family therapy session the next day.

Present in the family session were Terrence and his parents, Bill and Margaret. Needless to say, the parents were considering placing Terrence in an adolescent chemical dependency program out of state because they felt he had lost control of his drinking. Bill had shared that his paternal grandfather, father, and one of his brothers had died from alcohol-related health conditions and he was very worried about his son. He had decided that he would refrain from drinking due to the history of alcoholism problems on his side of the family. The parents really clamped down on Terrence, taking way all of his privileges and grounding him for 2 full weeks. Terrence was quite sullen and agreed to work with me to abstain from alcohol and marijuana. The parents shared with us that they would be willing to give Terrence another chance to refrain from using substances, but "one more major slip-up would result in residential treatment." As a family, we did relapse prevention work, which included identifying worst-case scenarios and helpful action steps for everyone to take. I also gave Terrence the *positive trigger log* to fill out and use to help stay on track. The good news was although it was clear that Terrence was genetically set up for failure with alcohol, in the past he had had no blackouts, shakes, intense craving to drink, and had gone for long stretches of time without drinking. I had Bill share with Terrence some past stories about how alcohol problems had wrought havoc in his family growing up and generations back. This was the first time Bill had shared these horrendous stories with Terrence and his wife, which consisted of seeing his "brother and father passing out in their vomit, coughing up blood," both he and his mother being beaten by his father when he was intoxicated, and so forth. Terrence was shocked by these stories and thanked his father for making him more aware of what could potentially happen to him if he kept drinking. I met alone with Terrence to deepen my alliance with him. Knowing that he had still qualified for the state tennis championship as a top seed and might have to play his nemesis again, I decided to share my personal story of overcoming adversity in tennis. When I was a high school senior, although our tennis team was undefeated, as a second team doubles player my partner and I were not afforded the opportunity to play in the state tournament. However, I had fought my way into the singles finals of our racquet club and ended up having to play the reigning champion who had won the club championship for the past 3 years. My opponent, Ben, could run

10 miles and bike another 20 miles daily. He was in incredible shape! I was 19 at the time and he was in his early 40s. The first set he beat me 6–0. Rather than giving in to adversity and feeling humiliated, I had channeled all of this negative energy into getting fired up to bounce back and beat Ben. Over the next 2 hours, I eventually beat him 0–6, 6–2, 6–1, and won the club championship. Terrence was in awe that I was able to pull off what appeared to be an impossible task. I told Terrence that whenever I am feeling down or need to get fired up, I play a movie in my head of seeing myself win this championship match against Ben at the racquet club. I encouraged him to think the same way and find the strength within himself to bounce back and be fired up when he plays in the state championship and more than likely will face his rival again. In building off of this theme, I had Terrence practice using my *visualizing a movie of success* where he had won a big tournament championship match in the past. With his eyes closed, Terrence was smiling because he had transported himself back to winning a big out-of-state tennis tournament a year ago where he had beaten the state champion, who also was a nationally ranked player. I had him share with me his thoughts and feelings watching himself beat this guy during the match. I encouraged Terrence to practice accessing this movie of success daily to not only put him in great spirits but also to boost his confidence and to fire him up for the upcoming state championship tournament. Terrence thought this was a "cool idea" to try out. Two weeks later, not only had Terrence maintained abstinence from alcohol and marijuana but also he had beaten his crosstown rival, landing him a second-place finish in the state tournament.

Humor, Absurdity, and Playfulness

There is no better way to take the sting out of clients' problem-saturated situations and lighten up the atmosphere in the therapy room than injecting humor, absurdity, and playfulness into our sessions with them. It is helpful to listen carefully in the initial session for humorous and absurd twists to the family members' problem descriptions, explanations, and attempted solutions that we can tickle them with or exaggerate in a playful way. Humor helps us all to gain distance from our worries and provides us with strong doses of positive emotion and endorphins. I always know that I have got off to great start when adolescents at the end of first sessions tell me, "That was fun!" Through the use of humor and absurdity, we can help family members attain a meta-view of their problems and their problem-maintaining patterns of interaction. They can then see more clearly how they keep themselves stuck and eventually arrive at the conclusion that it is time for a dramatic change. Ultimately, we want family members to view each session with us as a playground for fun, joy, and possibilities.

Solomon, a 16-year-old African American boy, was referred to me by his school social worker for ADD, poor grades, and going for the school record of earning the most detentions with his disruptive classroom behaviors, such as clowning around in class. Apparently, in one semester he had received 20 detentions. I had done some research with the school social worker and we discovered that in the history of the high school the house record for the most detentions was 50, achieved in 1982. The parents were deadlocked in a battle of wills over Solomon's grades and frequent detentions. This would result in his losing his privileges and being grounded for weeks. I sensed that the more the parents dished out punishments, the more Solomon would get even with them through underachieving and acting out. Efforts to get the parents to be less rigid and fairer with their consequences went absolutely nowhere. Although I had a good relationship with Solomon and there had been some progress in his raising his grades in some of his classes, he continued his protest and crusade against the parents by getting detentions and getting poor grades in the rest of his classes.

I decided to adopt a paradoxical approach to Solomon's skill at getting detentions. I told him and his parents that the house record for the most detentions at his high school was 50 by a student in 1982. I asked Solomon if he thought he could break this record. He looked at me perplexed and both the parents chuckled. I went on to say that he was currently on pace to break this record but that he needed to step up his detention snagging speed in the upcoming semester. We discussed the art and skill involved in earning detentions. I asked Solomon what his secret was and whether he had a special training regimen to increase the likelihood of earning detentions. Again, Solomon was quite confused by my questions and interest in detentions. The parents were at their wits' end with Solomon and ready to try anything. Together, the parents and I created a game with Solomon where they would predict privately each day in what class their son would be most likely to earn a detention. If their predictions were on target, Solomon would be submitted to harsh consequences like having to clean the garage, the cellar locker floors, or pick weeds in his backyard for a few hours. Solomon did not like the sound of the hard labor he could potentially receive if his parents were talented and accurate forecasters. The parents also made it clear to their son that going a whole week with no detentions could earn him some rewards, like being treated to a movie with a friend, ordering pizza from his favorite restaurant, and so forth. If he went a whole semester without a detention and picked up his grades, he could earn the privilege of getting his driver's license. All of his teachers were notified of what we were doing, as well as the school social worker. I met alone with Solomon and told him that my mind was split over the detention situation. I said that one part of my mind thought he would keep striving to break the 50 detentions record. The other part of my mind was thinking that he had such a great opportunity to earn such wonderful rewards and ultimately, the privilege of driving. I wondered aloud with Solomon if it was worth the risk of sabotaging all of this by getting more detentions. He agreed with me and made it clear that his parents were very intelligent people and might prove to be quite accurate with their predictions. I told him that it would be a real drag to have to clean the garage and cellar lockers or to pick weeds for hours every time he got detentions. Solomon also brought up how cool it would be to get his driver's license. I recalled with him how cool it was when I got my driver's license at age 16 and could take my girlfriend out on dates without my parents' driving us. Solomon responded, "That sounds sweet!" We discussed steps he thought he could take to avoid getting detentions, such as moving up in the front row of his classes and not sitting next to his troublemaking friends. Finally, we discussed the subjects at school he had the most difficulty with and if there were any specific teachers he needed me to collaborate with so he could raise his grades. Once I got this important information from Solomon, I could be his advocate at school and help him to get the resources that he needed in order to do better academically. Solomon decided to err on the side of caution and avoid the ordeals he would have to submit himself to. The best news was that Solomon decided to set a new record, going a whole semester without a detention and earning the biggest prize, which was getting his driver's license.

Improvisation and Surprise

There is no other art form that captures improvisation and surprise better than jazz music. As jazz pianist Cyrus Chestnut aptly points out in the chapter opening quote, the "something special" of excitement and therapeutic breakthroughs happens out on the edges, not in a model's formulaic scheme. Since each therapy session is a unique entity and the clients take the lead in setting the agenda, it is a quest into the unknown. We may start off playing the family's problem "melody" or central theme in a straightforward manner, carefully and respectfully making sure that we are clear on what they consider the *right problem* to work on changing first is. As we continue to strengthen our alliances and they have identified their goals, the sky is the limit in terms of our improvisational moves, such as *quoting*, which consists of introducing novel ideas, reframing, asking a bold and intriguing question, and sharing an engaging story or joke that parallels the family's problem story but with a positive and surprising twist to the outcome.

Another way we can improvise with our clients is through the use of *time bombs*. Time bombs are used by jazz drummers for not only keeping the time, but also for marking a transition into something new, and to provide irregular bass drum accents. We can use time bombs to punctuate, underscore, and celebrate positive growth steps and sparkling moments by giving family members high-fives, providing a timely "Wow!" and inviting them to share their motivational inner self-talk, and how they achieved their positive steps. We can fall out of our chairs with shock and amazement in response to how family members courageously pulled off their changes. When family members report the huge steps they took and how they pulled them off, we are inviting them to take the lead as proud *soloists* sharing their musical magic with us and to compliment themselves on their resourcefulness.

The case example below illustrates the use of an improvisational move with a severely depressed self-injuring and substance-abusing boy.

For most of the session, Jacob had his head down and remained quiet. I was having difficulty getting him to talk in the session. Since he had become a teenager he had started experimenting with marijuana and had police involvement. His father would verbally put him down and go through his bedroom without permission looking for drugs. In our session, his father openly admitted that he was like a "puffy chested rooster," an ogre-like dad at times, but wanted to change. The father's past actions had not only been emotionally upsetting to Jacob but also to his mother and 14-year-old sister, Kirsten, who typically would defend him. Jacob was a talented guitarist and had a band that regularly performed in his town. Surprisingly, the father also played guitar, but the two men never jammed together. Something in my gut told me that it might be worthwhile trying to bring the two men together around their mutual love for music.

In the midst of the miracle question conversation, in my efforts to surprise Jacob and get him to laugh, I asked, "Would you recruit your dad to join your band?" He laughed and shared, "That would be hard!" I then asked, "If there were a song that you would wish to teach him, a song that means a lot to you, what would it be?" Jacob responded, "Probably Papa Roach's 'Broken Home.'" All of a sudden the father chimed in, "I knew that was coming. The music is really hard. But after you listen to the words and don't just hear the music, he had a point." To take advantage of this opportunity to propel Jacob and his father's relationship into a positive future reality, I proposed that Jacob experiment with my *adolescent mentoring his parent* ritual. Over the next week, he and his father would set aside 45–60 minutes daily for guitar lessons in which Jacob would teach him on his acoustic guitar how to play Papa Roach's "Broken Home." Jacob thought this would be "sweet"! When I met alone with his father to help facilitate the connection building process, I offered him the *secret surprise* experiment, which involved him pulling two secret positive surprises over the next week that Jacob would notice and really appreciate. I asked the father what surprises he had in mind and he said he would check in daily with him to get feedback on how well he was doing avoiding the temptation to be the puffy-chested rooster ogre dad with him and seeing if he could get two tickets for a Papa Roach concert so that he could take Jacob to the show. One week later, not only was the father highly complimentary of Jacob's excellent teaching abilities and patience with him when hitting the wrong notes, but he contracted with him for another week of lessons. In addition, the father was able to secure two tickets for a Papa Roach concert that was a 4-hour drive from where they lived. Jacob was thrilled, and this combination of all of these positive experiences that helped these two to grow closer.

Weaving Tapestries of Metaphors and Analogies

The family therapy pioneer and arguably the master tapestry weaver of metaphors is Salvador Minuchin. In 1986, I was blessed with the opportunity to participate in a weeklong live supervision training with him and bring in for a live consultation with him one of the toughest families I had ever worked with (Minuchin, 1986). The family consisted of a 17-year-old boy named Tim and his father who were highly enmeshed. Tim had an extensive treatment history for psychotic symptoms, hallucinogen abuse, running away from home, and school failure. His mother had abandoned the two of them when Tim was 7. Throughout the session, the father would think and talk for Tim and the latter would passively accept this without confronting him. Minuchin did not waste any time challenging the following with this family: (1) the enmeshed family structure, (2) the rigid and destructive family interactions that maintained Tim's symptoms and bizarre behaviors and squelched his healthy attempts to become more independent, and (3) the role of Tim as the symptom bearer in the family.

Minuchin did a brilliant job of weaving together a tapestry of metaphors and provocative analogies to challenge all of the above in order to create a crisis and make the family more malleable and receptive to changing its destructive ways and to propel Tim out of the long-standing patient role. The metaphorical images he used included a newspaper headline for them that read "The Yuppie and the Hippie" (the father used to have long hair before he became a businessman and Tim had long hair); he referred to them as being like Corsican twins; he said that Tim reminded him of the lead character in the Woody Allen movie *Zelig*, a human chameleon who could be a woman, a historic figure, an African American person, and so forth, to underscore how Tim had no identity and was an "empty vessel"; he pointed out how when Tim used LSD his father experienced his hallucinations to underscore how enmeshed they were; and finally, Minuchin found a palmistry hand on the table in the therapy room and used it with Tim to show him on his hand that he lacked "the separate line of life" and therefore would never be able to separate from his father. By the end of the session, Tim became quite angry with Dr. Minuchin's provocative accusations about his inability to set personal goals and ever become an independent person. Thanks to this consultation and seven more sessions, Tim successfully graduated high school and secured a job (Selekman, 2013).

We too can string together metaphors and analogies triggered in our minds in response to hearing the families' presenting problem stories, resiliencies, and observing their problematic and positive interactions. There are many rich sources for metaphors and analogies we can draw from and apply to our clients' situations: nature, philosophy, religion, science, anthropology, history, art, architecture, literature, theater, film, popular TV shows and characters, music, dance, sports, and so forth. According to Pollack (2014, p. 67), the most persuasive analogies do the following:

- Use the familiar to explain something less familiar.
- Highlight similarities and obscure differences.
- Identify useful abstractions.
- Tell a coherent story.
- Resonate emotionally.

The case example below of Jeff, a Chinese American 16-year-old, illustrates the use of metaphors from the popular science fiction movie *Inception,* which he loved.

Jeff was the only one of three siblings who was underachieving in school. This drove his high achievement-oriented parents crazy throughout his middle school and high school years! His older brothers were attending top-notch academic institutions and one of them was entering medical school. Although Jeff was deemed a gifted student, he got excellent grades only in math, science, and English. He tended to get D's in all other subjects that "bored" him. During his free time, he read science fiction books, played hours of action-packed video games and watched movies alone and with his friends, and communicating with friends on social media sites.

Jeff was referred to me by his school social worker. It had been very difficult to set realistic treatment goals with the parents because for them it was all or nothing, either Jeff gets all A's or he loses all of his privileges, which included all of his technology, video games, and time with friends. They were locked in a major power struggle—the more the parents demanded A's, the more Jeff would resist doing homework and preparing for tests in subjects like history, art, music, and health. He would either blow off going to gym or put little effort in it. Knowing that Jeff loved the movie *Inception,* I took a risk and asked him, "If you were 'Dom' Cobb [the lead character in the movie, played by Leonardo DiCaprio] and could perform an *extraction* from your parents' minds while they are asleep, what unhelpful views or ideas about you would you remove?" Jeff responded, "That I don't care about school and that I don't want to go to college and make something out of my life." Next, I asked, "If you could perform an *inception* with your parents and plant in their minds while they are asleep the kind of vision and dream you would like them to have for you and your future, what would that be?" Jeff replied, "For my parents to know that I am different than my brothers but that I do want to be successful one day in a career, maybe seeing me work as an engineer for a major tech company out in Silicon Valley." Surprised, his father chimed in, "You have that goal for yourself? I was beginning to think that you didn't care about going to college and trying to get a good job." The mother added, "I would love to see you take your math and science smarts and put them to good use pursuing an engineering career." I turned to Jeff and asked him, "What do you need from your parents at this time that could make a big difference for you with them and put you on that pathway to pursuing an engineering degree at a college?" Jeff replied, staring at his parents, "For you to stop putting all of the pressure on me to get straight A's! To be happy with who I am and believe in me." I asked, "How will you know that they really believe in you more; how can they show that?" Jeff replied, "Well stop contacting all of my teachers and checking up on me like I'm 6 years old! It's really embarrassing! Take an interest in what I'm passionate about and ask me questions about my future goals." The parents were very pleased to discover in this session that Jeff did have goals for himself and did want to make something out of his life. They agreed to begin a fresh start with Jeff, which included backing off with the academic achievement pressure, stop communicating with his teachers all of the time, giving him back his technology and privileges, and giving him an opportunity to take responsibility for his schoolwork.

_____

Embracing Uncertainty, Unpredictability, and Chaos: Stepping into the Unknown with Excitement

Our survivalist brains do not handle uncertainty and unpredictability very well (DiSalvo, 2011; Schoen, 2013). We want to have control at all costs. For some of us, not having control when working with challenging families can trigger anxiety and fear, which can contribute to poor therapeutic decision making and costly blunders. Highly complex therapy-veteran high-risk adolescent family cases may not be able to identify where we should begin or offer us a clear picture of what treatment outcomes will look like. Since these families are random, nonlinear dynamic systems, we need to match what we do therapeutically with their unpredictable nature without being too attached to outcome. This means we have to drum up the courage to dive into the unknown with excitement and anticipation that something special will eventually happen in our work together. Live in the immediacy of the moment; court and welcome surprises, pursue ends and means interdependently; and take risks to allow action to generate outcomes in and out of our sessions. We need to adopt a *flexibly purposive* stance, that is, we need to be prepared that where we are headed with and how we will get there will continually shift in our work with them (Austen, 2010).

Two beautiful examples of diving into the unknown and co-generating exciting possibilities are the jazz recording *Streams of Consciousness* and the *Dis-Diseasing of Mental Health* conference put on by the Galveston Family Institute (Goolishian & Anderson, 1991). The first example illustrates how two virtuoso musicians—the great jazz bebop drummer Max Roach and the highly talented South African pianist Abdullah Ibrahim, who had never played together—could sit down in a studio with no written music and produce inventive solos and a completely improvised musical conversation that covered the whole history of jazz in 40.39 minutes (Roach & Ibrahim, 2003)!

The Dis-Diseasing of Mental Health Conference, co-facilitated by the family therapy pioneers Harry Goolishian and Harlene Anderson, was one of the best conferences I had ever attended. In attendance were nationally and internationally renowned family therapy pioneers and therapists. It was like the Hall of Fame of Family Therapists. The radical theme of the conference was to co-generate innovative ways of successfully empowering clients and their families to resolve their difficulties without resorting to applying DSM labels or institutionalizing their members. There was very little structure to the conference. Unlike most conferences, participants did not sign up for workshops or panel discussions. Instead, as a larger group, they identified several topic areas regarding family work, and participants could choose a topic that interested them and participate in smaller working groups of 12 to 15 people. The small-group discussions were rich and meaningful, sparking many interesting and novel ideas. On the last day of the conference, a spokesperson representing each small interest group reported their key ideas to the larger group. In some cases, implementation steps were recommended. Many highly creative and innovative ideas grew out of this conference. Going into this event, none of us knew what was going to happen after the opening-day plenary by Harry Goolishian. Both of these examples illustrate the importance and the benefits of embracing uncertainty, unpredictability, and chaos as exciting challenges that offer us unlimited possibilities for creating workable realities with our colleagues and our toughest families.

Marilyn, a 17-year-old white girl, and her family were referred to me by a social worker at an inpatient psychiatric program for aftercare family therapy for her self-injuring, bulimia, substance abuse, and sexually acting-out behaviors. Although I thought I had established good working alliances with all family members and we had realistic treatment goals, both Marilyn's and the parents' goals were constantly shifting from one week to the next. In addition, every week I saw this family there was some new crisis we were trying to stabilize. For example, after stabilizing her self-injuring and bulimic behaviors, one early Saturday morning Marilyn ended up in the emergency room after drinking too much and taking four Ecstasy tablets at a rave. Another week, I found out from the mother that Marilyn's father had an extramarital affair and a gambling problem. These were hot conflict areas in their marriage. When we began family therapy, the parents wanted to see Marilyn change all four of her problematic behaviors immediately. We had established four corresponding scales as problem target goal areas and appeared to get off to a good start, in that we were able to reduce the frequency of these problem behaviors. However, the parents' marital conflicts would surface in our sessions and suddenly overshadow our main focus on stabilizing Marilyn's self-destructive behaviors. This demanded separate session time for the parents, to put out their relationship fires, leading to a loss of focus on Marilyn's goals. It was unclear where we were heading in the treatment process.

After three sessions of one crisis after another, I decided to embrace the family in this random nonlinear family system. I opted to tinker with the family's entrenched crisis-prone pattern that appeared to have a life of its own. I had them forecast what their next crisis would be, who would be involved with it, and where and when it would occur. Next, we talked about the steps each family member would take to defuse it. Marilyn brought up that her parents would probably have a big argument about something at home one evening, which would stress her out to such a degree that she would return to cutting and bulimia. When asked what she would need her parents to do to prevent her from resorting to cutting and bulimia again, Marilyn replied, "Stop arguing and see what it is doing to me. Instead, be there to comfort and listen to me when I am worried about slipping back into cutting and bulimia again." I asked her what her catastrophic fear was about her parents' situation and she disclosed, "That they will divorce." Next, I asked her, "What would that mean for you if that would happen?" She responded, "I would probably not see my father again." I asked, "Why do you think that?" Marilyn answered, "Well, he has had an affair before and will probably find another woman. Also, he always puts his gambling before us anyway." The father protested, "That is not true; I do love you, Marilyn, and will never check out of your life." Marilyn looked very surprised to hear that. Her mother added, "Honey, it's true, your dad does love you very much." I then asked Marilyn, "What's missing in your relationship with your father that would make a difference for you if it were present?" Marilyn responded, "Well, when I was much younger my dad used to bike with me, play Ping-Pong with me, and we used to go to the movies together." I asked her, "If your father were more present in your life and offered to do those activities with you again, what affect would that have on your self-injuring, bulimia, substance abuse, and engaging in sexually risky activities?" Marilyn replied, "Yes, all of that would help, but for me what would make the biggest difference would be for them to work on improving their marriage." I turned to the parents and solicited their feedback on what Marilyn just said. The parents looked at each other and agreed to work with me on trying to save their marriage. The father told Marilyn that he would work on being more available to reinstate the fun activities he used to do with her. They picked a weekend day to go for a long bike ride and play Ping-Pong together. I asked them who usually wins and Marilyn chimed in, "I do!" The father agreed, saying Marilyn used to beat him a lot when she was 12.

With this family, there was a clear-cut relationship between Marilyn's self-destructive behaviors increasing, sometimes to a crisis level, as the parents' conflicts surfaced and arguing intensified. In some ways, Marilyn was like a modern-day Joan of Arc, sacrificing herself like a noble heroine defending her family castle. Once I was able to help the couple resolve their long-standing conflicts, which included the father's rebuilding trust with the mother, committing to being faithful to her and their marriage, and addressing his gambling problem, Marilyn no longer had to rely on high-risk behaviors to distract her parents from their marital problems. She could count on them to be more present in her life and soothe her when necessary.

Confusion and Incompetence

When we are faced with ambiguous and confusing client situations, we can feel at a loss for what to do. We feel incompetent as family therapists. We want our clients to have faith in our knowledge, competence, and expertise to empower them to resolve their most pressing difficulties. Some therapy-veteran high-risk adolescent families can be quite vague or unrealistic with their goals and expectations of us. We may feel like every therapeutic move we make both in and out of sessions is a dead-end street. Rather than throwing up our hands, we can allow our incompetency to shine through and get clients to feel sorry for our bungling ways. The case below of Peter, a white 17-year-old, illustrates how making strategic use of incompetence can invite clients to feel sorry for us and want to help us out by giving us the gift of change.

I had seen Peter for 10 family therapy sessions. His maternal aunt and uncle became his legal guardians after his mother had died from a heroin overdose. The family had seen eight therapists before me, dating back to when Peter was 13. Since that age, he had heavily abused alcohol, marijuana, stimulants, heroin, and a variety of hallucinogens. With the support of his aunt and uncle and Peter's hard work, we were able to get him to achieve abstinence from every drug except marijuana. He was now smoking marijuana three to four times per week with friends, and his aunt and uncle were threatening to place Peter in a residential chemical dependency program if he did not quit his marijuana use. At the time, I was the assistant director of a youth service program, which was a five-person job at times and quite stressful. The Monday I had seen Peter I came into the office and had lots of messages in my mailbox about crises with both my families and my staff's crisis cases that needed my attention. Also, my boss wanted to meet with me in the afternoon and after reading her note, I was thinking, "This is not going to be good!" I was feeling so confused by this family because we had strong working alliances and there had been considerable changes. Why, then, was Peter continuing to smoke marijuana? I told the family what a stressful morning it had been and how this day was the worst day of my professional career. I added that I was even considering hanging up my counseling career to go to cooking school! Peter exclaimed, "Don't do it, Matthew! You're not a bad counselor!" I replied, "I know, but I feel like I am really blowing it with you and your family. In fact, later on when I have to meet with my boss and have supervision with her, she is not going to like hearing that your parents now want to ship you off to a drug rehab program. I will feel really horrible if this happens!" His aunt said, "Would you like us to talk to your boss for you to help you out? We like you!" Later in our session we had a breakthrough when Peter announced that he did not want to go to rehab and he did want to get his driver's license. Apparently, he now had a girlfriend and he thought it would be cool to be able to take her out. His legal guardians and Peter contracted to honor his wishes once he achieved abstinence from marijuana and had a month of clean random hair follicle analyses. Peter, his legal guardians, and I did more intense relapse prevention work together in subsequent sessions to optimize his success. The aunt also let me know that if I had any future bad days at work, she would be happy to be my advocate with my boss.

Humility, "Brilliant Ignorance," and Inviting Clients to Speculate about the Therapist's Unsaid

Inevitably, we will all have those challenging and complex high-risk cases where we feel completely stuck and at a loss for what to do. To top it off, we may not have the luxury of a team of colleagues to observe us and offer fresh ideas or have the equipment to videotape our sessions and present them in supervision. What are we to do when faced with these treatment dilemmas? Since our clients are our partners in the treatment process and are quite resourceful and perceptive, expressing one's humility and tapping our clients' expertise to get unstuck can be a productive pathway to pursue. Renowned Israeli conductor Itay Talgam (2015) coined the term *brilliant ignorance,* which results in the understanding that creating new, unpredictable knowledge is achieved by combining existing knowledge, will, and making the conscious decision to be ignorant, to not know the answers, not even try and come up with them. We need to let go of our pride and egos and be willing to bravely put ourselves on the line with our clients. Next, we can *invite clients to speculate about the therapist's unsaid,* that is, what courageous questions, critically necessary conversations, and therapeutic moves have we held back from might be contributing to the treatment impasse. We can ask families the following questions:

"What questions do you think I have avoided asking you about your situation that are really meaningful to you and important for me to ask?"

"Do any of you have any hunches about why you think I have held back from asking those questions?"

"What courageous steps do you think I have held back from taking with you in our sessions together that would make you feel that we were more on the same page with meeting your expectations and give you more faith in my ability to help you in the best way possible?"

"What unhelpful thoughts and uneasy feelings do you think I am reacting to that have prevented me from taking those steps?"

"What do you think I am missing or did not hear you say that is really important that we need to revisit and do something about that could make a big difference with your situation?"

"I would like all of you to pretend here. Let's say you were my family therapy supervisor observing us work together. What unproductive thoughts or ways of interacting with you would you have me abandon?"

"What new ways of viewing your situation and new directions would you encourage me to pursue that would be much more productive in helping a family like you?"

"What else would you encourage me to ask them or try with them that you think could really make a difference?"

Once we have alliances with our clients, they will be more likely to want to help us become aware of our blind spots, how treatment stalled, and what constructive steps we can take to move the therapeutic process forward.

Kelsey, a depressed 13-year-old white girl, often threw severe temper outbursts, had crying spells, disordered eating, would not do her chores, argued and fought intensely with her "angelic" 11-year-old brother, and had poor grades in school. Apparently, Kelsey used to be a straight-A student and was the best female long-distance runner in her school. The parents had a tendency to kick off every session with a litany of complaints about Kelsey's behavior. My attempts to disrupt their rigid complaint pattern proved to be futile, even after I tried to cooperate with their pessimism using both the *coping* and *pessimistic sequence questions* (de Shazer et al., 2007; Selekman & Beyebach, 2013). The parents also could not identify any triggering events for Kelsey's dramatic behavioral decline. I also had trouble trying to build an alliance with Kelsey and kept getting met with dead-end street responses from her, like "I don't know" or "I don't want to talk about it." My gut was telling me that there was a missing piece or pieces of the family puzzle that I needed to find out about, but I was at a loss for where to probe and what questions to ask.

In my third session with the family, I changed the format by first meeting alone with Kelsey and tapping her expertise as a family therapy consultant. I asked her, "If you were my family therapy consultant observing me working with a family like yours, what would you encourage me to ask the daughter that I failed to ask her in earlier sessions?" Kelsey shared the following questions: "Why do you suppose your parents don't see how depressed you are?"; "Which one of your parents' 'most annoying' behaviors would you like to see changed first?"; "Do your parents favor your younger brother over you?"; "How do your parents get along with each other?" After thanking Kelsey for being such a great family therapy consultant to me in opening up new pathways to pursue with her and her family, we discussed each of her questions. I found out that she had felt depressed since age 11, but her parents would never take her seriously or do anything about it. When I asked, "What depresses you the most?" Kelsey shared that she is so used to her parents putting pressure on her "to get good grades and perform well in running races," particularly her father, who used to be a track star in college, that she had become a perfectionist. This would fuel what she described as rumination and beating herself up emotionally when she would not get an A on a test or paper or coming in second in a race. Kelsey also was depressed and stressed out by her brother being favored and getting away with pushing her buttons behind the scenes. Finally, another major stressor was her parents' incessant arguing and her father's explosive temper, which frightened her at times. The latter was a red flag for me, so I asked Kelsey if he had ever laid a hand on her or her mother. She replied, "He just roars like a lion but never tries to hurt anybody physically." Again, I thanked Kelsey for being such an excellent family therapy consultant to me. Like Colombo, the TV detective, I asked Kelsey, "One more question: Where do you think I should begin first with your parents?" Without hesitation, Kelsey responded, "Work on their arguing problem." Before I met alone with her parents, I asked Kelsey if she would prefer this new session format where we would meet alone and I would see her parents separately for a while to work on their "arguing problem." Kelsey thought this would be a great idea. I finally felt like an alliance was set in motion with Kelsey.

When I met alone with the parents I told them how well my mini-meeting went with Kelsey and that it seemed to be a good idea for us to meet separately.

I took a risk with the parents and asked them a provocative question: "Do the two of you argue enough?" The mother reported that they argued all of the time because they had different parenting styles and were not a unified team. The father chimed in, blaming his wife by saying, "Yes, she is the problem! She's a softy and always gives in to Kelsey, never enforces my consequences." The mother countered with, "Well, you're too extreme! You take away her privileges and try to ground her far too long!" I disrupted this blame–counterblame exchange and asked them, "How would the two of you like to learn how to become a dynamic duo as parents?" They both agreed that this needed to happen. We contracted to work separately on improving their parental teamwork and resolving other conflicts they were having. Once the parents improved their parental teamwork and stopped arguing, Kelsey started doing much better at home and in school.

Using the Future for Co-Creating Compelling Family Realities

Science fiction writer William Gibson once said, "The future has arrived—it is just not evenly distributed" (Gibson, 1999). This is so true. Bits and pieces of our families' desired future outcome pictures are already appearing in their minds and during times when problems are absent. They arrive well before we see them for the first time because clients collectively possess the necessary strengths and resources to make their desired futures realities. However, clients may have difficulty identifying any past successes or noticing pretreatment changes because they do not fit with their oppressive dominant stories. In these clinical situations, we need to propel the treatment to where the future becomes the present. We can do this one of three ways: using future-oriented questions, using the imaginary time machine to co-create future selves and relationships minus problems (see Chapter 5), or using the *can–if* strategy with families discussed in Chapter 4 (Morgan & Barden, 2015; Selekman, 2009; Selekman & Beyebach, 2013).

The following case illustrates how to use the imaginary time machine to co-create future selves and relationships with a family that had experienced several unsuccessful treatment experiences in both inpatient and outpatient mental health and substance abuse treatment settings.

Zachary, a 16-year-old white boy, had been abusing marijuana, heroin, alcohol, and a variety of over-the-counter cold remedies. He also had been dealing drugs on and off for 2 years. Zachary was pulling in D's and F's in school, which really upset his mother, Cindy, who wanted to see him go to college and make something out of his life. Zachary had several strengths: deep knowledge of classic and alternative rock music, playing electric guitar with his band, and writing his own music. Cindy had been divorced from Zachary's alcoholic father since Zachary was 2 years old, and he has not seen his father since they split up.

After three sessions, family therapy had reached a standstill. Even though I had gotten Zachary to stop dealing and achieve abstinence from heroin and over-the-counter cold remedies, he was still breaking his mother's rules and not doing well in school. Cindy was experiencing a great deal of hopelessness and despair about Zachary, because he was still smoking marijuana, drinking, and appeared to her to not think about his future. I decided to propel our stuck treatment system into a compelling future reality.

Zachary liked reading science fiction books and was into fantasy video games and movies. I decided to introduce my trusty imaginary time machine and have Zachary take it into the future. Upon stepping out of the time machine, he is now 24 years old, completed a community college associate's degree program, was working, had his own studio apartment, and came over for Sunday night dinner with his mother. I asked Cindy what her first response would be to her transformed son. Cindy first shared that she would "probably faint" and after awakening, "give him a big hug and let him know how proud" she was of him. Zachary smiled. Next, I asked him what he would be most excited to share with his mother that was going on his life. Zachary said that he was pursuing a career in broadcasting and had applied to a local college program to get a bachelor's degree in this area and land a better-paying and fun disc jockey job. He also would tell his mother about his new girlfriend whom he was eager for her to meet. In addition, Zachary also would tell his mother that he was earning extra money performing gigs at local music clubs with his band. Cindy was blown away by all of Zachary's accomplishments. I asked Zachary to slowly walk his way back from the future and tell us what his thinking and action steps were to pick up his grades high enough to get into both the community college and eventually into the university. He said first he would stop ditching his classes, complete his past-due and current homework assignments, and study and better prepare for tests. Acting as if this had already happened, I asked Zachary to tell me about the useful self-talk that got him fired up to turn his school situation around. Zachary said that he told himself he will never make it as a disc jockey unless he improved his grades, completed a college education, and stopped doing drugs. I responded with a big "Wow! What great wisdom and insight you have about the roadmap for your future success!" I asked Cindy if this was the first time she had heard this from Zachary. Apparently, Cindy had no idea that he wanted to go to college and become a disc jockey. She told Zachary how happy this positive vision of the future had made her feel and gave her hope. Next, we used the back from the future strategy with both his landing a job and with quitting drugs. With landing his job, he had cut his long hair, dressed nicer, and came armed with questions to ask employers. When it came to quitting drugs, he cut his contacts with drug-using friends, places where he used to party, and told himself, "There is no place for drugs when I start working." I asked him what he meant by this. Zachary pointed out that "a lot of places drug test these days" and he wanted "to do well at the job and protect it at all costs." I responded with another big "Wow!" Looking over at Cindy, who was all smiles, I asked if she was ready to faint again after hearing that from her son. Both Zachary and Cindy laughed. One day after our session, I arranged a school meeting with all of Zachary's teachers to talk about this family session and to develop a catch-up plan with his schoolwork to optimize his school success. With the help of the imaginary time machine, his compelling future reality became his new present, which he could clearly picture and embody, and served as the driving force for turning things around both at school and at home with his mother.

Guidelines for Cultivating an Inventive Family Therapy Mind

In this section, I provide 32 guidelines, which include intriguing questions and hypothetical scenarios, to aid in cultivating an inventive family therapy mind. They are designed to spark creative ideas, help us to keep an open mind, be more playful, be therapeutically flexible, and be more daring risk-takers and better dance partners with even the toughest high-risk adolescents and their families.

1. Fertilize your brain by re-reading the classics by some of the greatest authors and poets; read more science fiction, philosophy, detective mystery books; nonfiction books on recent and historical accounts of important national and world events and movements and biographies on famous artists, scientists, and historic figures; and business books on leadership, organizational change, collaboration, sales and persuasion, and effective teamwork.

2. Browse through your old *Dr. Seuss* books.

3. Go to jazz concerts of top players to experience improvisation at its best.

4. Go to art museums and pay close attention to the artists whose unique styles, themes, and techniques intrigues and inspires you the most.

5. Build mindfulness meditation and related practices into your daily routine.

6. Infuse more rhythm into your sessions and into your daily regimen by listening to different types of music, playing an instrument, dancing, engaging in artwork, and being more adventurous in the kitchen by combining different cuisines and coming up with your own tasty new creations.

7. Practice stretching the boundaries of your comfort zone daily; outside of work, try new activities that require mastering specific skills, and be more courageous and daring in your family sessions.

8. Every day, be on the lookout for anomalies, meaningful coincidences, good-luck events, and epiphanies worth seizing both in and outside of our family sessions.

9. View every problem with a beginner's mind.

10. Don't allow yourself to drown in a sea of client problem talk because the solutions lie outside of problem explanations in the spaces in between and out on the edges.

11. Ask yourself, "What do I find most aesthetically pleasing and intriguing about this family's problem story?"

12. Ask yourself, "If I were to create a delicious gourmet three-course meal out of this family's presenting problem, what type of appetizer would I prepare? What type of entrée would capture the core elements of this problem? What type of dessert would go best with my appetizer and main course and why?"

13. Think and play with new ideas with childlike curiosity. Keep asking questions.

14. Think and experiment with opposites.

15. View your mistakes and blunders as an indication that you are on to something.

16. The mysterious holds many possibilities.

17. Look to nature for ideas and metaphors.

18. When a family session feels too humdrum, ask yourself, "How can I really shake things up in here? What would really surprise them?"

19. Let's say that during your intersession break, a miracle happened and all of your client family's difficulties are now solved when you reconvene the family. What will they say that you had been doing differently with them that helped pave the way for their miraculous changes? What else will they be eager to share with you that helped transformed their situation?

20. When feeling stuck or highly challenged by a really tough family, spontaneously step out of the session, reflect, and incubate on any emerging ideas. Once the bulb lights up over your head, go back into the therapy room and give it a test run.

21. Ask yourself, "What would be a song title or newspaper headline that best captures this challenging new family I am working with?"

22. When faced with a challenging family, hop into your imaginary helicopter to gain an aerial view. From this perspective, look for what you may be missing.

23. Let's say Pablo Picasso, Miles Davis, and Thomas Edison visited you during your intersession break with this difficult family. What recommendations would each of them have for you to think about and try out?

24. Complete the following statement with as many ideas you can think of that have a shot at working in your next session: "It would be really crazy if I . . . ."

25. What if your success was completely guaranteed with your toughest family? What would you try to pull off in today's session?

26. With your most challenging family, ask yourself, "How can I bungle more and fail better with them?" Now, get to work!

27. What if you woke up today with amnesia and had completely forgotten how to conduct your choice family therapy approach with your clients. What would you do? How would you manage? What would you do next?

28. When you run into a therapy dead end, ask yourself, "What bold and intriguing question could I ask?"

29. Ask yourself the *five whys* (five "why" questions back to back) when you're stuck, until you generate new meaning about or new directions to pursue with a family's challenging presenting problem.

30. A *New York Times* reporter interviews you right after you succeed in helping the toughest therapy-veteran family on your caseload resolve their difficulties. The reporter asks, "What was the first courageous step you took that put you on the road to treatment success with them? What early obstacles did you have to overcome, and how did you get past them? What advice would you give another therapist who had to work with a similar family?" Now ask yourself, "What new directions and potential solution strategies have been sparked for the clients and for myself?"

31. Keep a personal *hall of fame quotations log* for sources of good wisdom, inspiration for new ideas, and to make timely use of them in family therapy sessions.

32. Keep a *successful ideas box* to store therapeutic ideas and strategies that have consistently worked with particular types of adolescent and family difficulties. This can come in quite handy when we are feeling stuck.

Although this is not a definitive list of how best to cultivate our family therapy artistry skills, I hope that these ideas will inspire you to be more daring, inventive, and improvisational in your family therapy practices with high-risk adolescents and their families.

References

Alexander, J. F., Waldron, H. B., Robbins, M. S., & Neeb, A. A. (2013). *Functional family therapy for adolescent behavior problems.* Washington, DC: American Psychological Association.

American Psychiatric Association. (2013). *Diagnostic and statistical manual of mental disorders* (5th ed.). Arlington, VA: Author.

Andersen, T. (1991). *The reflecting team: Dialogues about the dialogues about the dialogues.* New York: Norton.

Andersen, T. (1995). Reflecting processes: Acts of informing and forming: You can borrow my eyes but you must not take them away from me. In S. Friedman (Ed.), *The reflecting team in action: Collaborative practice in family therapy* (pp. 11–38). New York: Guilford Press.

Anderson, H. (1997). *Conversation, language, and possibilities: A post-modern approach to therapy.* New York: Basic Books.

Anderson, H., & Gerhart, D. (Eds.). (2007). *Collaborative therapy: Relationships and conversations that make a difference.* New York: Routledge.

Anderson, H., Goolishian, H., & Winderman, L. (1986). Problem-determined systems: Towards transformation in family therapy. *Journal of Strategic and Systemic Therapies, 5*(4), 1–14.

Andolfi, M., Angelo, C., Menghi, P., & Nicolo-Corigliano, M. (1983). *Behind the family mask: Therapeutic change in rigid family systems.* New York: Brunner/Mazel.

Andreas, S. (2012). *Transforming negative self-talk: Practical, effective exercises.* New York: Norton.

Andreas, S. (2014). *More transforming negative self-talk: Practical effective exercises.* New York: Norton.

Anthony, E. J. (1987). Risk, vulnerability, and resilience: An overview. In E. J.

Anthony & B. J. Cohler (Eds.), *The invulnerable child* (pp. 3–48). New York: Guilford Press.

Austen, H. (2010). *Artistry unleashed: A guide to pursuing great performance in work and life.* Toronto: University of Toronto.

Bakker, N., Jansen, L., & Luijten, H. (2010). *The real van Gogh: The artist and his letters.* London: Royal Academy of Art.

Baumeister, R. F., & Tierney, J. (2011). *Willpower: Rediscovering the greatest human strength.* New York: Penguin.

Benjamin, A. S. (Ed.). (2010). *Successful remembering and successful forgetting: A festschrift in honor of Robert A. Bjork.* Hove, UK: Psychology Press.

Berg, I. K., & Miller, S. D. (1992). *Working with the problem drinker: A solution-focused approach.* New York: Norton.

Beutler, L., Harwood, T. M., Michelson, A., Song, X., & Holman, J. (2011). Reactance/resistance level. In J. C. Norcross (Ed.), *Psychotherapy relationships that work: Evidence-based responsiveness* (pp. 261–279). New York: Oxford University Press.

Beyebach, M. (2009). Integrative brief solution-focused family therapy: A provisional roadmap. *Journal of Systemic Therapies, 28,* 18–35.

Beyebach, M., & Carranza, V. E. (1997). Therapeutic interaction and drop-out: Measuring relational communication in solution-focused therapy. *Journal of Family Therapy, 19*(3), 173–213.

Bohart, A. C., & Tallman, K. (1999). *How clients make therapy work: The process of active self-healing.* Washington, DC: American Psychological Association.

Bohart, A. C., & Tallman, K. (2010). Clients: The neglected common factor in psychotherapy. In B. L. Duncan, S. D. Miller, B. E. Wampold, & M. A. Hubble (Eds.), *The heart and soul of change: Delivering what works in therapy* (2nd ed., pp. 83–113). Washington, DC: American Psychological Association.

Bohm, D. (1996). *On dialogue.* London: Routledge.

Boscolo, L., & Bertrando, P. (1993). *The times of time: A new perspective in systemic therapy and consultation.* New York: Norton.

Boscolo, L., Cecchin, G., Hoffman, L., & Penn, P. (1987). *Milan systemic family therapy: Conversations in theory and practice.* New York: Basic Books.

Bowen, S., Chawla, N., & Marlatt, G. A. (2011). *Mindfulness-based relapse prevention for addictive behaviors.* New York: Guilford Press.

Brandeau, G. (2014). Creative abrasion. In L. A. Hill, G. Brandeau, E. Truelove, & K. Lineback (Eds.), *Collective genius: The art and practice of leading innovation* (pp. 121–147). Boston: Harvard Business Review Press.

Branzei, O. (2014). Cultivate hope: Found, not lost. In J. E. Dutton & G. M. Spreitzer (Eds.), *How to be a positive leader: Small actions, big impact* (pp. 115–126). Oakland, CA: Berrett-Koehler.

Brier, N. B. (2010). *Self-regulated learning: Practical interventions for struggling teens.* Champaign, IL: Research Press.

Brier, N. B. (2014). *Enhancing self-control in adolescents: Treatment strategies derived from psychological science.* New York: Routledge.

Brisken, A., Erickson, S., Ott, J., & Callanan, T. (2009). *The power of collective wisdom and the trap of collective folly.* San Francisco: Berrett-Koehler.

Cade, B., & O'Hanlon, W. H. (1993). *A brief guide to brief therapy.* New York: Norton.

Camillus, J. (2015, Winter). Feed-forward systems: Framing a future filled with wicked problems. *Rotman Management*, pp. 52–60.

Caspersen, D. (2014). *Changing the conversation: The 17 principles of conflict resolution*. New York: Penguin.

Chodron, P. (2010). *Taking the leap: Freeing ourselves from old habits and fears*. Boston: Shambhala.

Coleman, P. T., & Ferguson, R. (2014). *Making conflict work: Harnessing the power of disagreement*. Boston: Houghton Mifflin.

Connell, G., Mitten, T., & Bumberry, W. (1999). *Reshaping family relationships: The symbolic therapy of Carl Whitaker*. New York: Brunner/Mazel.

Coughran, B. (2014). Creative resolution. In L. A. Hill, G. Brandeau, E. Truelove, & K. Lineback (Eds.), *Collective genius: The art and practice of leading innovation* (pp. 169–197). Boston: Harvard Business Review Press.

Cramer, K. D. (2014). *Lead positive: What highly effective leaders see, say, and do*. San Francisco: Jossey-Bass.

Creed, T. A., & Kendall, P. C. (2005). Therapeutic alliance-building behavior within a cognitive-behavioral treatment for anxiety in youth. *Journal of Consulting and Clinical Psychology, 73*, 498–505.

Csikszentmihalyi, M. (1990). *Flow: The psychology of optimal experience*. New York: Harper & Row.

Csikszentmihalyi, M. (1997). *Finding flow*. New York: Basic Books.

Cytowic, R. E. (2002). *Synesthesia: A union of the senses* (2nd ed.). Cambridge, MA: MIT Press.

D'Angelli, A. R., Grossman, A. H., & Salter, N. P. (2005). Predicting the suicide attempts of lesbian, gay, and bisexual youth. *Suicide and Life-Threatening Behavior, 35*(6), 646–660.

Danner, J., & Coopersmith, M. (2015). *The other "f" word: How smart leaders, teams, and entrepreneurs put failure to work*. Hoboken, NJ: Wiley.

De Brabandere, L., & Iny, A. (2013). *Thinking in new boxes: Five essential steps to spark the next big idea*. New York: Random House.

De Dreu, C. K., Baas, M., & Nijstad, B. A. (2008). Hedonic tone and activation level in mood-creative link: Toward a dual pathway to creativity model. *Journal of Personality and Social Psychology, 94*(5), 739–756.

De Frain, J. (2007). *Family treasures: Creating strong families*. Lincoln: University of Nebraska.

de Shazer, S. (1985). *Keys to solutions in brief therapy*. New York: Norton.

de Shazer, S. (1988). *Clues: Investigating solutions in brief therapy*. New York: Norton.

de Shazer, S. (1991). *Putting difference to work*. New York: Norton.

de Shazer, S., Dolan, Y., Korman, H., Trepper, T., McCollum, E., & Berg, I. K. (2007). *More than miracles: The state of the art of solution-focused brief therapy*. Binghamton, NY: Haworth Press.

Diamond, G. S. (2014). Returning home: Reflections on research in family therapy. *Family Therapy Magazine, 13*(5), 14–20.

Diamond, G. S., Diamond, G. M., & Levy, S. A. (2014). *Attachment-based family therapy for depressed adolescents*. Washington, DC: American Psychological Association.

Diamond, G. S., Liddle, H. A., Wintersteen, M. B., Dennis, M. L., Godley, S. H., & Tims, F. (2006). Early therapeutic alliance as predictor of treatment outcome for adolescent cannabis users in outpatient treatment. *American Journal on Addictions, 15,* 26–33.

Diamond, G. S., & Stern, R. (2003). Attachment-based family therapy for depressed adolescents: Repairing attachment ruptures. In S. Johnson & V. E. Whiffen (Eds.), *Attachment process in couple and family therapy* (pp. 191–212). New York: Guilford Press.

DiSalvo, D. (2011). *What makes your brain happy and why should you do the opposite.* Amherst, NY: Prometheus.

Dodge, K. (2006). Translational science in action: Hostile attributional style and the development of aggressive behavior problems. *Developmental Psychopathology, 18*(3), 791–814.

Dodson-Lavelle, B., Ozawa-de Silva, B., Negi, G. L. T., & Raison, C. L. (2015). Cognitively-based compassion training for adolescents. In V. M. Follette, J. Briere, D. Rozelle, J. W. Hooper, & D. I. Rome (Eds.), *Mindfulness-oriented interventions for trauma: Integrating contemplative practices* (pp. 343–359). New York: Guilford Press.

Donohue, B., & Azrin, N. H. (2012). *Treating adolescent substance abuse: Using family behavior therapy.* Hoboken, NJ: Wiley.

Duncan, B. L. (2010). *On becoming a better therapist.* Washington, DC: American Psychological Association.

Duncan, B. L., Hubble, M. A., & Miller, S. D. (1997). *Psychotherapy with "impossible" cases: The efficient treatment of therapy veteran.* New York: Norton.

Duncan, B. L., & Miller, S. D. (2000). *The heroic client: Doing client-directed, outcome-informed therapy.* San Francisco: Jossey-Bass.

Duncan, B. L., Miller, S. D., Wampold, B. E., & Hubble, M. A. (Eds.). (2010). *The heart and soul of change: Delivering what works in therapy* (2nd ed.). Washington, DC: American Psychological Association.

Durrant, M., & Coles, D. (1991). The Michael White approach. In T. C. Todd & M. D. Selekman (Eds.), *Family therapy approaches with adolescent substance abusers* (pp. 135–175). Needham Heights, MA: Allyn & Bacon.

Duval, J., & Beres, L. (2011). *Innovations in narrative therapy: Connecting practice, training, and research.* New York: Norton.

Dweck, C. (2006). *Mindset: The new psychology of success.* New York: Ballantine.

Dyer, J., Gregersen, H., & Christensen, C. M. (2011). *The innovator's DNA: Mastering the five skills of disruptive innovators.* Boston: Harvard Business Review.

Elliott, R., Bohart, A. C., Watson, J. C., & Greenberg, L. S. (2011). Empathy. In J. C. Norcross (Ed.), *Psychotherapy relationships that work: Evidence-based responsiveness* (2nd ed., pp. 132–153). New York: Oxford University Press.

Emmons, R. A. (2007). *Thanks!: How the new science of gratitude can make you happier.* Boston: Houghton Mifflin.

Erickson, B. A., & Keeney, B. (2006). *Milton H. Erickson, M.D.: An American healer.* Sedona, AZ: Ringing Rocks Press.

Erickson, M. H., & Rossi, E. L. (1979). *Hypnotherapy: An exploratory casebook.* New York: Irvington.

Ericsson, A., & Pool, R. (2016). *Peak: Secrets from the new science of expertise.* Boston: Houghton Mifflin.

Ericsson, K. A. (2008). Deliberate practice and acquisition of expert performance: A general overview. *Academic Emergency Medicine, 11,* 988–994.

Escudero, V., Heatherington, L., & Friedlander, M. L. (2010). Therapeutic alliances and alliance building in family therapy. In J. C. Muran & J. P. Barber (Eds.), *The therapeutic alliance: An evidence-based guide to practice* (pp. 240–263). New York: Guilford Press.

Eubanks-Carter, C., Muran, J. C., & Safran, J. D. (2010). Alliance ruptures and resolution. In J. C. Muran & J. P. Barber (Eds.), *The therapeutic alliance: An evidence-based guide* (pp. 74–97). New York: Guilford Press.

Farber, B. A., & Doolin, E. M. (2011). Positive regard and affirmation. In J. C. Norcross (Ed.), *Psychotherapy relationships that work: Evidence-based responsiveness* (2nd ed., pp. 168–187). New York: Oxford University Press.

Firstenberg, I. R., & Rubinstein, M. F. (2014). *Extraordinary results: Shaping an otherwise unpredictable future*. Hoboken, NJ: Wiley.

Fisch, R., & Schlanger, K. (1999). *Brief therapy with intimidating cases: Changing the unchangeable*. San Francisco: Jossey-Bass.

Fisch, R., Weakland, J. H., & Segal, L. (1982). *The tactics of change: Doing therapy briefly*. San Francisco: Jossey-Bass.

Fisher, H., & Rainbird, S. (Eds.). (2006). *Kandisnsky: The path to abstraction*. London: Tate.

Fishman, H. C., & Minuchin, S. (1981). *Family therapy techniques*. Cambridge, MA: Harvard University Press.

Franklin, C., Trepper, T. S., Gingerich, W. J., & McCollum, E. (Eds.). (2012). *Solution-focused brief therapy: A handbook of evidence-based practice*. New York: Oxford University Press.

Fredrickson, B. L. (1999). *Positivity: Groundbreaking research reveals how to embrace the hidden strength of positive emotions, overcome negativity, and thrive*. New York: Crown.

Freeman, A. (1995). *Working with difficult clients: A cognitive-behavioral therapy approach*. One-day workshop sponsored by MCC Behavioral Care, Inc., Rosement, IL.

Freeman, J., Epston, D., & Lobovits, D. (1997). *Playful approaches to serious problems: Narrative therapy with children and their families*. New York: Norton.

Friedlander, M. L., Escudero, V., & Heatherington, L. (2006). *Therapeutic alliances in couple and family therapy: An empirically informed guide to practice*. Washington, DC: American Psychological Association.

Friedlander, M. L., Escudero, V., Heatherington, L., & Diamond, G. (2011). Alliance in couple and family therapy. In J. C. Norcross (Ed.), *Psychotherapy relationships that work: Evidence-based responsiveness* (2nd ed., pp. 92–110). New York: Oxford University Press.

Friedman, S. (Ed.). (1995). *The reflecting team in action: Collaborative practice in family therapy*. New York: Guilford Press.

Froh, J. J., & Bono, G. (2014). *Making grateful kids: The science of building character*. West Conshohocken, PA: Templeton.

Galinsky, A., & Schweitzer, M. (2015). *Friend and foe: When to cooperate, when to compete, and how to succeed at both*. New York: Crown Business.

Gawande, A. (2010). *The checklist manifesto: How to get things done right*. New York: Picador.

Geertz, C. (1973). *The interpretation of cultures: Selected essays*. New York: Basic Books.

George, E., Iveson, C., & Ratner, H. (1999). *Problem to solution: Brief therapy with individuals and families* (2nd ed.). London: Brief Therapy Press.

Germer, C. K., Siegel, R. D., & Fulton, P. R. (2013). *Mindfulness and psychotherapy* (2nd ed.). New York: Guilford Press.

Gerzon, M. (2006). *Leading through conflict: How successful leaders transform differences into opportunities.* Boston: Harvard Business School.

Gibson, W. (1999, November 30). The science of science fiction. *Talk of the Nation,* National Public Radio. Retrieved from *www.npr.org/templates/story/story. php?storyId=1067220.*

Gigerenzer, G. (2007). *Gut feelings: Short cuts to better decision-making.* New York: Penguin.

Gigerenzer, G. (2014). *Risk savvy: How to make good decisions.* New York: Viking.

Gilbert, P. (2007). *Stumbling on happiness.* New York: Viking.

Gilbert, P., & Ebert, J. E. (2002). Decisions and revisions: The affective forecasting of changeable outcomes. *Journal of Personality and Social Psychology, 82,* 503–514.

Gilligan, S. (2002). *The legacy of Milton H. Erickson: Selected papers of Stephen Gilligan.* Phoenix, AZ: Zeig, Tucker, & Theisen.

Goldstein, T., Fersch-Podrat, R., Rivera, M., Axelson, D., Brent, D. A., & Birmaher, B. (2012, November). *Is DBT effective with multi-problem adolescents?: Show me the data!* Paper presented at the annual meeting of the Association of Behavioral and Cognitive Therapies, National Harbor, MD.

Goleman, D. (2013). *Focus: The hidden driver of excellence.* New York: Harper.

Goolishian, H., & Anderson, H. (1988). *The therapeutic conversation.* Three-day intensive training sponsored by the Institute of Systemic Therapy, Chicago, IL.

Goolishian, H., & Anderson, H. (1991, October). *The dis-diseasing of mental health.* Galveston Family Institute Conference II, San Antonio, TX.

Gordon, D., & Meyers-Anderson, M. (1981). *Phoenix: Therapeutic patterns of Milton H. Erickson.* Cupertino, CA: Meta.

Grazer, B., & Fishman, C. (2015). *A curious mind: The secret to a bigger life.* New York: Simon & Schuster.

Gregerman, A. (2013). *The necessity of strangers: The intriguing truth about insight, innovation, and success.* San Francisco: Jossey-Bass.

Haley, J. (1973). *Uncommon therapy: The psychiatric techniques of Milton H. Erickson, M.D.* New York: Norton.

Haley, J. (1983). *Ordeal therapy.* San Francisco: Jossey-Bass.

Hancock, H. (2014). *Possibilities.* New York: Penguin.

Hanh, T. N. (1998). *The heart of Buddha's teaching: Transforming suffering into peace, joy, and liberation.* New York: Broadway Books.

Hanh, T. N. (2001). *Anger: Wisdom for cooling the flames.* New York: Riverhead.

Hanson, R. (2013). *Hardwiring happiness: The new brain science of commitment, calm, and confidence.* New York: Harmony.

Hanson, R., & Mendius, R. (2009). *Buddha's brain: The practical neuroscience of happiness.* Oakland, CA: New Harbinger.

Hardy, K., & Laszloffy, T. A. (2006). *Teens who hurt: Clinical intervention to break the cycle of adolescent violence.* New York: Guilford Press.

Havens, R. A. (2003). *The wisdom of Milton H. Erickson: The complete volume*. Williston, VT: Crown House.

Hawton, K., & Rodham, K. (2006). *By their own young hand: Deliberate self-harm and suicidal ideas in adolescents*. London: Jessica Kingsley.

Hayes, J. A., Gelso, C. J., & Hummel, A. M. (2011). Managing counter-transference. In J. C. Norcross (Ed.), *Psychotherapy relationships that work: Evidence-based responsiveness* (2nd ed., pp. 239–261). New York: Oxford University Press.

Henggeler, S. W., & Schaeffer, C. (2010). Treating serious antisocial behavior using multisystemic therapy. In J. R. Weisz & A. E. Kazdin (Eds.), *Evidence-based psychotherapies for children and adolescents* (pp. 259–277). New York: Guilford Press.

Henggeler, S. W., Schoenwald, S. K., Borduin, C. M., Rowland, M. D., & Cunningham, P. B. (2009). *Multisystemic therapy for antisocial behavior in children and adolescents* (2nd ed.). New York: Guilford Press.

Henggeler, S. W., & Sheidow, A. J. (2011). Empirically supported family-based treatments for conduct disorder and delinquency in adolescents. *Journal of Marital and Family Therapy, 38*(1), 30–58.

Hill, L. A., Brandeau, G., Truelove, E., & Lineback, K. (2014). Why collective genius needs leadership: The paradoxes of innovation. In L. A. Hill, G. Brandeau, E. Truelove, & K. Lineback (Eds.), *Collective genius: The art and practice of leading innovation* (pp. 25–45). Boston: Harvard Business Review Press.

Hodges, S. D., Clark, B., & Myers, M. W. (2011). Better living through perspective-taking. In R. Biswas-Diener (Ed.), *Positive psychology as a mechanism for social change* (pp. 193–218). Dordrecht, The Netherlands: Springer.

Hoffman, L. (1988). A constructivist position for family therapy. *Irish Journal of Psychology, 9*, 110–129.

Hoffman, L. (2002). *Family therapy: An intimate journey*. New York: Norton.

Hollis, J. F., Gullion, C. M., Stevens, V. J., Brantley, P. J., Appel, L. J., Ard, J. D., et al. (2008). Weight loss during the intensive intervention phase of the weight-loss maintenance trial. *Journal of Preventative Medicine, 35*(2), 118–126.

Holmes, J. (2015). *Nonsense: The power of not knowing*. New York: Crown.

Homer. (2006). *The Odyssey* (B. Knox, Ed.). New York: Penguin Classics.

Hubble, M. A., Duncan, B. L., & Miller, S. D. (1999). *The heart and soul of change: What works in therapy*. Washington, DC: American Psychological Association.

Hysing, M., Pallesen, S., Stormark, K. M., Jakobsen, R., Lundervold, A. J., & Sivertsen, B. (2015). Sleep and use of electronic devices in adolescence: Results from a large population-based study. *BMJ Open, 5*(1), e006748.

Isaacs, W. (1999). *Dialogue and the art of thinking together*. New York: Currency.

Isen, A. M., Daubman, K. A., & Nowicki, G. P. (1987). Positive affect facilitates creative problem solving. *Journal of Personality and Social Psychology, 52*(6), 1122–1131.

Iveson, C. (2003). Solution-focused couples therapy. In B. O'Connell & S. Palmer (Eds.), *Handbook of solution-focused therapy* (pp. 61–74). London: Sage.

James, C., & Jenkins, H. (2015). *Disconnected: Youth, new media, and the ethics gap*. Cambridge, MA: The MIT Press.

Joiner, T. (2005). *Why people die by suicide*. Cambridge, MA: Harvard University Press.

Joiner, T., Petit, J. W., Walker, R. L., Voelz, Z. R., Cruz, J., & Rudd, M. D. (2002). Perceived burdensomeness and suicidality: Two studies on the suicide notes of those attempting and completing suicide. *Journal of Social and Clinical Psychology, 21*, 531–545.

Justus, P. (2014). Creative agility. In L. A. Hill, G. Brandeau, E. Truelove, & K. Lineback (Eds.), *Collective genius: The art and practice of leading innovation* (pp. 147–169). Boston: Harvard Business Review Press.

Kahneman, D. (2010, February). The riddle of experience vs. memory. TED Talk. Retrieved from *www.ted.com/talks/danilel_kahnemanthe_riddle_of_experience_vs_memory*.

Kahneman, D. (2011). *Thinking fast and slow*. New York: Farrar, Straus & Giroux.

Kahneman, D., Lovallo, D., & Sibony, O. (2015, Winter). Before you make that big decision. In *Leadership: The art of decision-making. Harvard Business Review OnPoint*, pp. 31–41.

Kashdan, T. B. (2010). *Curious?: Discover the missing ingredient to a fulfilling life*. New York: Harper Perennial.

Kauffman, C., Grunebaum, H., Cohler, B. J., & Gamer, E. (1979). Superkids: Competent children of psychotic mothers. *American Journal of Psychiatry, 136*, 1398–1402.

Kegan, R., & Lahey, L. L. (2001). *Seven languages for transformation: How the way we talk can change the way we work*. San Francisco: Jossey-Bass.

Klein, G. (1998). *Sources of power: How people make decisions*. Cambridge, MA: MIT Press.

Klein, G. (2002). *Intuition at work*. New York: Currency/Doubleday.

Klein, G. (2013). *Seeing what others don't: The remarkable ways we gain insights*. New York: Public Affairs.

Koch, R., & Lockwood, G. (2010). *Superconnect: The power of networks and the strength of weak links*. London: Little, Brown.

Kross, E., Bruehlman-Senecal, E., Park, J., Burson, A., Dougherty, A., Shablack, H., et al. (2014). Self-talk as a regulatory mechanism: How you do it matters. *Journal of Personality and Social Psychology, 106*(2), 304–324.

Krystal, H. (1982). Alexithymia and the effectiveness of psychoanalytic treatment. *International Journal of Psychoanalytic Psychotherapy, 9*, 353–388.

Lambert, M. J. (2010). *Prevention of treatment failure: The use of measuring, monitoring, and feedback in clinical practice*. Washington, DC: American Psychological Association.

Lambert, M. J., & Shimokawa, K. (2011). Collecting client feedback. In J. C. Norcross (Ed.), *Psychotherapy relationships that work: Evidence-based responsiveness* (2nd ed., pp. 203–224). New York: Oxford University Press.

Lax, W. D. (1995). Offering reflections: Some theoretical and practical considerations. In S. Friedman (Ed.), *The reflecting team in action: Collaborative practice in family therapy* (pp. 145–167). New York: Guilford Press.

Lebow, J. (2014). *Couple and family therapy: An integrative map of the territory*. Washington, DC: American Psychological Association.

Le Grange, D. (2011). Family-based treatment for bulimia nervosa: Theoretical model, key tenets, and evidence base. In D. Le Grange & J. Lock (Eds.),

Eating disorders in children and adolescents: A clinical handbook (pp. 291–305). New York: Guilford Press.

Le Grange, D., & Loeb, K. L. (2014). Family-based treatment of adolescent eating disorders. In J. Ehrenreich-May & B. C. Chu (Eds.), *Transdiagnostic treatments for children and adolescents: Principles and practice* (pp. 363–385). New York: Guilford Press.

Leslie, I. (2014). *Curious: The desire to know and why your future depends on it.* New York: Basic Books.

Liddle, H. A. (2010). Treating adolescent substance abuse using multidimensional family therapy. In J. R. Weisz & A. E. Kazdin (Eds.), *Evidence-based psychotherapies for children and adolescents* (pp. 416–435). New York: Guilford Press.

Liddle, H. A., & Diamond, G. (1991). Adolescent substance abusers in family therapy: The critical initial phase of treatment. *Family Dynamics of Addiction Quarterly, 1*(1), 55–69.

Linehan, M. M. (1993). *Cognitive-behavioral treatment in borderline personality disorder.* New York: Guilford Press.

Lipchik, E. (1988). Purposeful sequences for beginning the solution-focused interview. In J. C. Hansen (Ed.), *Interviewing* (pp. 105–119). Rockville, MD: Aspen.

Lock, J., & Le Grange, D. (2005). *Help your teenager beat an eating disorder.* New York: Guilford Press.

Lopez, S. J. (2013). *Making hope happen: Create the future you want for yourself and others.* New York: Atria.

Lopez, S. J., & Snyder, C. R. (Eds.). (2009). *Oxford handbook of positive psychology* (2nd ed.). New York: Oxford University Press.

Lyotard, J.-F. (1996). *Just gaming.* Minneapolis: University of Minnesota.

Lyubomirsky, S. (2007). *The how of happiness: A scientific approach to getting the life you want.* New York: Penguin.

Magee, B. (1985). *Philosophy and the real world: An introduction to Karl Popper.* Chicago: Open Court.

Maisel, R., Epston, D., & Borden, A. (2004). *Biting the hand that starves you: Inspiring resistance to anorexia/bulimia.* New York: Norton.

Malchiodi, C. A. (Ed.). (2003). *Handbook of art therapy.* New York: Guilford Press.

Malchiodi, C. A. (2006). *Expressive therapies.* New York: Guilford Press.

Malchiodi, C. A. (Ed.). (2008). *Creative interventions with traumatized children.* New York: Guilford Press.

Marguc, J., Forster, J., & Van Kleef, G. A. (2011). Stepping back to see the big picture: When obstacles elicit global processing. *Journal of Personality and Social Psychology, 101*(5). 883–901.

Marlatt, G. A. (Ed.). (1998). *Harm reduction: Pragmatic strategies for managing high-risk behaviors.* New York: Guilford Press.

Marlatt, G. A., & Donovan, D. M. (2005). *Relapse prevention: Maintenance strategies in treatment of addictive behaviors* (2nd ed.). New York: Guilford Press.

Mauboussin, M. J. (2009). *Think twice: Harnessing the power of counter-intuition.* Boston: Harvard Business.

Mayer, B. (2015). *The conflict paradox: Seven dilemmas at the core of disputes.* San Francisco: Jossey-Bass.

McDermott, D., & Snyder, C. R. (1999). *Making hope happen: A workbook for turning possibilities into reality.* Oakland, CA: New Harbinger.

McKeel, J. (2012). What works in solution-focused brief therapy: A review of change process research. In C. Franklin, T. S. Trepper, W. J. Gingerich, & E. E. McCollum (Eds.), *Solution-focused brief therapy: A handbook of evidence-based practice* (pp. 130–144). New York: Oxford University Press.

Michalko, M. (2006). *Tinker toys: A handbook of creative-thinking techniques* (2nd ed.). Berkeley, CA: Ten Speed Press.

Miles, B. (2015). *Call me Burroughs.* New York: Twelve.

Miller, A. L., Rathus, J. H., & Linehan, M. M. (2007). *Dialectical behavioral therapy with suicidal adolescents.* New York: Guilford Press.

Miller, G. (1997). *Become miracle workers: Language in meaning in brief therapy.* New York: Aldine de Gruyter.

Miller, L. (2015). *The spiritual child: The new science on parenting for health and life-long thriving.* New York: St. Martin's.

Miller, S., Hubble, M., & Duncan, B. (2007, November/December). Super shrinks: What's the secret of their success? Retrieved from *http://psycho-therapynetworker.org/component/content/article/85-2007-novemberdecember/175-supershrinks.*

Miller, W. R., & C'de Baca, J. (2001). *Quantum change: When epiphanies and sudden insights transform ordinary lives.* New York: Guilford Press.

Miller, W. R., & Rollnick, S. (2013). *Motivational interviewing: Helping people change* (2nd ed.). New York: Guilford Press.

Minuchin, S. (1974). *Families and family therapy.* Cambridge, MA: Harvard University Press.

Minuchin, S. (1986). *Four-day live supervision training in structural family therapy.* Clinical intensive training at the Gestalt Integrated Family Therapy Institute, Chicago, IL.

Minuchin, S., & Fishman, H. C. (1981). *Family therapy techniques.* Cambridge, MA: Harvard University Press.

Minuchin, S., Reiter, M. D., & Borda, C. (2014). *The craft of family therapy: Challenging certainties.* New York: Routledge.

Minuchin, S., Rosman, B. L., & Baker, L. (1978). *Psychosomatic families: Anorexia nervosa in context.* Cambridge, MA: Harvard University Press.

Moffitt, P. (2012). *Emotional chaos to clarity: Move from the chaos of the reactive mind to the clarity of the responsive mind.* New York: Plume.

Morgan, A., & Barden, M. (2015). *A beautiful constraint: How to transform your limitations into advantages, and why it is everyone's business.* Hoboken, NJ: Wiley.

MST Services. (2014). 2014 MST data overview report. Retrieved from *www.msinstitute.org.*

Mudd, P. (2015). *The head game: High-efficiency analytic decision-making and the art of solving complex problems quickly.* New York: Liveright.

Mueller, M., & Pekarik, G. (2000). Treatment duration prediction: Client accuracy and its relationship to dropout, outcome, and satisfaction. *Psychotherapy: Theory, Research, Practice, Training, 37,* 117–123.

Muff, K. (2015). Defining the collaborator. In K. Muff (Ed.), *The collaboratory: A co-creative stakeholder engagement process for solving complex problems* (pp. 11–15). Sheffield, UK: Greenleaf.

Muir, J. A., Schwartz, S. J., & Szapocznik, J. (2004). A program of research with Hispanic and African American families: Three decades of intervention development and testing influenced by the changing cultural context of Miami. *Journal of Marital and Family Therapy, 30*(3), 285–303.

Muran, J. C., & Barber, J. P. (Eds.). (2010). *The therapeutic alliance: An evidence-based guide to practice.* New York: Guilford Press.

Myers, M. W., & Hodges, S. D. (2013). Perspective taking and prosocial behavior: Caring for others like we care for self. In J. J. Froh & A. C. Parks (Eds.), *Activities for teaching positive psychology* (pp. 77–85). Washington, DC: American Psychological Association.

Neff, K. (2010). *Self-compassion: The proven power of being kind to yourself.* New York: HarperCollins.

Nisbett, R. E. (2015). *Mindware: Tools for smart thinking.* New York: Farrar, Straus & Giroux.

Nolan, C. (2010). *Inception* [Film]. Warner Brothers.

Norcross, J. C. (Ed.). (2011). *Psychotherapy relationships that work: Evidence-based responsiveness.* New York: Oxford University Press.

Norcross, J. C., Krebs, P. M., & Prochaska, J. O. (2011). Stages of change. In J. C. Norcross (Ed.), *Psychotherapy relationships that work: Evidence-based responsiveness* (2nd ed., pp. 279–301). New York: Oxford University Press.

Norcross, J. C., & Lambert, M. J. (2011). Evidence-based therapy relationships. In J. C. Norcross (Ed.), *Psychotherapy relationships that work: Evidence-based responsiveness* (pp. 3–25). New York: Oxford University Press.

Norcross, J. C., & Lambert, M. J. (2013). Compendium of evidence-based relationships. *Psychotherapy in Australia, 19*(3), 22–26.

Norcross, J. C., & Wampold, B. E. (2013). Compendium of treatment adaptations. *Psychotherapy in Australia, 19*(3), 34–37.

Nylund, D., & Corsiglia, V. (1994). Becoming solution-focused forced in brief therapy: Remembering something important we already know. *Journal of Strategic and Systemic Therapies, 13*(1), 5–13.

O'Connor, M., & Dornfield, B. (2014). *The moment you can't ignore: When big trouble leads to a great future.* New York: Public Affairs.

Oettingen, G. (2014). *Rethinking positive thinking: Inside the new science of motivation.* New York: Current.

O'Hanlon, W. H. (1987). *Taproots: Underlying principles of Milton Erickson's therapy and hypnosis.* New York: Norton.

O'Hanlon, W. H., & Weiner-Davis, M. (1989). *In search of solutions: A new direction in psychotherapy.* New York: Norton.

Omer, H. (2004). *Nonviolent resistance: A new approach to violent and self-destructive children.* Cambridge, UK: Cambridge University Press.

Pahl, K. M., & Barrett, P. M. (2010). Interventions for anxiety disorders in children using group cognitive-behavioral therapy with family involvement. In J. R. Weisz & A. E. Kazdin (Eds.), *Evidence-based psychotherapies for children and adolescents* (pp. 61–80). New York: Guilford Press.

Papp, P. (1983). *The process of change.* New York: Guilford Press.

Pascale, R., Sternin, J., & Sternin, M. (2010). *The power of positive deviance: How unlikely innovators solve the world's toughest problems.* Boston: Harvard Business Review.

Peele, S. (2014). *Recover!: An empowering program to help you stop thinking like an addict and reclaim your life.* New York: Da Capo Lifelong.

Peltz, L. (2013). *The mindful path to addiction recovery: A practical guide to regaining control over your life.* Boston: Shambhala.

Pennebaker, J. W. (2004). *Writing to heal: A guided journal for recovering from trauma and emotional upheaval.* Oakland, CA: New Harbinger.

Pentland, A. (2014). *Social physics: How good ideas spread–the lessons from a new science.* New York: Penguin.

Perkins, S. J., Murphy, R., Schmidt, U., & Williams, C. (2006, July 19). Self-help and guided self-help for eating disorders. *Cochrane Database of Systematic Reviews, 3,* CD004191.

Peterson, C. (2006). *A primer in positive psychology.* New York: Oxford University Press.

Peterson, C., & Seligman, M. E. P. (2004). *Character strengths and virtues: A handbook and classification.* New York: Oxford University Press.

Pinsof, W. M. (1995). *Integrated problem-centered therapy: A synthesis of biology, individual, and family.* New York: Basic Books.

Pittampalli, A. (2016). *Persuadable: How great leaders change their minds to change the world.* New York: Harper Business.

Pollack, J. (2014). *Shortcut: How analogies reveal connections, spark innovation, and sell our greatest ideas.* New York: Gotham.

Pollak, S. M., Pedulla, T., & Siegel, R. D. (Eds.). (2014). *Sitting together: Essential skills for mindfulness-based psychotherapy.* New York: Guilford Press.

Popper, K. A. (1965). *Conjectures and refutations: The growth of scientific method.* New York: Harper & Row.

Post, S., & Niemark, J. (2007). *Why good things happen to good people: The exciting new research that proves the link between doing good and living a longer, healthier, and happier life.* New York: Broadway.

Prochaska, J. O., Norcross, J. C., & DiClemente, C. C. (2006). *Changing for good: A revolutionary six-stage program for overcoming bad habits and moving your life positively forward.* New York: HarperCollins.

Rathus, J. H., & Miller, A. L. (2015). *DBT skills manual for adolescents.* New York: Guilford Press.

Ratner, H., George, E., & Iveson, C. (2012). *Solution-focused brief therapy: 100 key points and techniques.* East Sussex, UK: Routledge.

Ray, W. A., & de Shazer, S. (Eds.). (1999). *Evolving brief therapies: In honor of John H. Weakland.* Galena, IL: Geist & Russell.

Ricard, M. (2015). *Altruism: The power of compassion to change yourself and the world.* New York: Little, Brown.

Roach, M., & Ibrahim, A. (2003). *Streams of consciousness.* Piadrum Records 0301.

Robbins, M. S., Horigian, V., Szapocznik, J., & Ucha, J. (2010). Treating Hispanic youths using brief strategic family therapy. In J. R. Weisz & A. E. Kazdin (Eds.), *Evidence-based psychotherapies for children and adolescents* (pp. 375–391). New York: Guilford Press.

Robbins, M. S., Turner, C. W., Dakof, G. A., & Alexander, J. F. (2006). Adolescent and parent therapeutic alliances as predictors of dropout in multidimensional family therapy. *Journal of Family Psychology, 20,* 108–116.

Robin, A. L., & Le Grange, D. (2010). Family therapy for adolescents with anorexia nervosa. In J. R. Weisz & A. E. Kazdin (Eds.), *Evidence-based psychotherapies for children and adolescents* (pp. 345–359). New York: Guilford Press.

Rohrbaugh, M., Tennen, H., Press, S., & White, L. (1981). Compliance, defiance and therapeutic paradox. *American Journal of Orthopsychiatry, 51,* 454–467.

Roland, J. (1985). Question storming: Outline of the method. Retrieved from *www.pynthan.com/vri/questionstorm.htm.*

Rollnick, S., Mason, P., & Butler, C. (1999). *Health behavior change: A guide for practitioners.* Edinburgh, UK: Churchill Livingstone.

Rosen, S. (1991). *My voice will go with you: The teaching tales of Milton H. Erickson.* New York: Norton.

Rothstein, D. (2011). *Make just one change.* Cambridge, MA: Harvard Education Press.

Rowe, C. L. (2012). Family therapy for drug abuse: Review and updates 2003–2010. *Journal of marital and Family Therapy, 38*(1), 59–81.

Safran, J. D., Muran, J. C., & Eubanks-Carter, C. (2011). Repairing alliance ruptures. In J. C. Norcross (Ed.), *Psychotherapy relationships that work: Evidence-based responsiveness,* (2nd ed., pp. 224–239). New York: Oxford University Press.

Sales, N. J. (2016). *American girls: Social media and the secret lives of teenagers.* New York: Knopf.

Santisteban, D. A., Szapocznik, J., Perez-Vidal, A., Kurtines, W. H., Murray, E. J., & LaPerriere, A. (1996). Efficacy of intervention for engaging youth and families into treatment and some variables that may contribute to differential effectiveness. *Journal of Family Psychology, 10,* 35–44.

Sastry, A., & Penn, K. (2014). *Fail better: Design smart mistakes and succeed sooner.* Boston: Harvard Business Review.

Satir, V. (1983). *Conjoint family therapy.* Palo Alto, CA: Science & Behavior Books.

Satir, V. (1988). *The new people-making.* Palo Alto, CA: Science & Behavior Books.

Savage, J. (2013). Oh! You pretty things. In V. Broackes & G. Marsh (Eds.), *David Bowie is inside* (pp. 100–103). London: V&A Publishing.

Scharmer, C. O. (2007). *Theory U: Leading from the future as it emerges.* Cambridge, MA: Society for Organizational Learning.

Scharmer, C. O. (2013). *Leading from the emerging future: From eco-system, to eco-system economies.* San Francisco: Berrett-Hoehler.

Schoen, M. (2013). *Your survival instinct is killing you: Retrain your brain to conquer fear, make better decisions, and thrive in the 21st century.* New York: Hudson Street Press.

Schon, D. (1983). *The reflective practitioner: How professionals think in action.* New York: Basic Books.

Schwartz, J. M., & Gladdding, R. (2011). *You are not your brain: The 4-step solution for changing bad habits, ending unhealthy thinking, and taking control of your life.* New York: Avery.

Selekman, M. D. (1991). "With a little help from my friends": The use of peers in the family therapy of adolescent substance abusers. *Family Dynamics of Addiction Quarterly, 1*(1), 69–77.

Selekman, M. D. (1995). Rap music with wisdom: Peer reflecting teams. In S.

Friedman (Ed.), *The reflecting team in action: Collaborative practice in family therapy* (pp. 205–223). New York: Guilford Press.

Selekman, M. D. (2005). *Pathways to change: Brief therapy with difficult adolescents* (2nd ed.). New York: Guilford Press.

Selekman, M. D. (2006). *Working with self-harming adolescents: A collaborative strengths-based therapy approach.* New York: Norton.

Selekman, M. D. (2009). *The adolescent and young adult self-harming treatment manual: A collaborative strengths-based therapy approach.* New York: Norton.

Selekman, M. D. (2010). *Collaborative brief therapy with children.* New York: Guilford Press.

Selekman, M. D. (2013). Therapeutic artistry: Finding your creative edge with difficult couple and family practice situations. *Family Therapy Magazine, 12*(6), 22–26.

Selekman, M. D., & Beyebach, M. (2013). *Changing self-destructive habits: Pathways to solutions with couples and families.* New York: Routledge.

Selekman, M. D., & Schulem, H. (2007). *The self-harming adolescents and their families as expert consultants project: A qualitative study.* Unpublished manuscript.

Seligman, M. E. P. (2002). *Authentic happiness: Using the new positive psychology to realize your potential for lasting fulfillment.* New York: Free Press.

Seligman, M. E. P. (2011). *Flourish: A visionary new understanding of happiness and well-being.* New York: Free Press.

Shapiro, D. (2016). *Negotiating the nonnegotiable: How to resolve your most emotionally charged conflicts.* New York: Viking.

Sheinberg, M. (1985). The debate: A strategic technique. *Family Process, 24*(2), 259–271.

Sheinberg, M., & Fraenkel, P. (2001). *The relational trauma of incest: A family-based approach to treatment.* New York: Guilford Press.

Short, D., Erickson, B. A., & Erickson-Klein, R. (2005). *Hope and resilience: Understanding the psychotherapeutic strategies of Milton H. Erickson, MD.* Norwalk, CT: Crown House.

Siegel, D. J. (2014). *Brainstorm: The power and purpose of the teenage brain.* New York: Tarcher.

Siegel, R. D. (2009). *The mindfulness solution: Everyday practices for everyday problems.* New York: Guilford Press.

Simpkins, C. A., & Simpkins, A. M. (2009). *Meditations for therapists and their clients.* New York: Norton.

Slingerland, E. (2014). *Trying not to do: The ancient art of effortlessness and the surprising power of spontaneity.* Edinburgh, Scotland: Canongate.

Smith, D. K., & Chamberlain, P. (2010). Multidimensional treatment foster care for adolescents: Processes and outcomes. In J. R. Weisz & A. E. Kazdin (Eds.), *Evidence-based psychotherapies for children and adolescents* (pp. 243–259). New York: Guilford Press.

Smith, J. A. (2015). You can count on goodness. *Shambhala Sun, 24*(4), 58–63.

Soll, J. B., Milkman, K. L., & Payne, J. W. (2015, Winter). Outsmart your own biases. In *Leadership: The art of decision-making. Harvard Business Review OnPoint*, pp. 2–48.

Spetzler, C., Winter, H., & Meyer, J. (2016). *Decision quality: Value creation from better business decision.* Hoboken, NJ: Wiley.

Sprenkle, D. H., Davis, S. D., & Lebow, J. L. (2009). *Common factors in couple and family therapy: The overlooked foundation for effective practice.* New York: Guilford Press.

Stanton, M. D. (1984). Fusion, compression, diversion, and the workings of paradox: A therapeutic systemic change. *Family Process, 23*(2), 15–167.

Stanton, M. D., & Todd, T. C. (1982). *The family therapy of drug abuse and addiction.* New York: Guilford Press.

Stark, K. D., Streusand, W., Krumholz, L. S., & Patel, P. (2010). Cognitive-behavioral therapy for depression: The ACTION treatment program for girls. In J. R. Weisz & A. E. Kazdin (Eds.), *Evidence-based psychotherapies for children and adolescents* (pp. 93–110). New York: Guilford Press.

Steinberg, L. (2014). *Age of opportunity: Lessons from the new science of adolescence.* Boston: Houghton-Mifflin.

Steiner, T. (2014). *Encourage adolescents to optimize their risk and support care-takers to cope with it.* Workshop presented at the Just Suppose . . . International Solution-Focused Brief Therapy Conference, Amsterdam, The Netherlands.

Sternberg, R. (1981). Intelligence and non-entrenchment. *Journal of Educational Psychology, 73,* 1–16.

Stinnett, N., & O'Donnell, M. (1996). *Good kids: How you and your kids can successfully navigate the teen years.* New York: Doubleday.

Stokes, P. (2008). *Philosophy: 100 essential thinkers.* New York: Enchanted Lion.

Sukel, K. (2016). *The art of risk: The new science of courage, caution, and chance.* Washington, DC: National Geographic Society.

Sunstein, C. R., & Hastie, R. (2015). *Wiser: Getting beyond groupthink to make groups smarter.* Boston: Harvard Business Review.

Swift, J. K., & Callahan, J. L. (2008). A delay discounting measure of great expectations and the effectiveness of psychotherapy. *Professional Psychology: Research and Practice, 39,* 581–588.

Swift, J. K., & Greenberg, R. P. (2015). *Premature termination in psychotherapy: Strategies for engaging clients and improving outcomes.* Washington, DC: American Psychological Association.

Szapocznik, J., Hervis, O., & Schwartz, S. (2003). *Brief strategic family therapy for adolescent drug abuse* (Therapy manuals for drug abuse, manual 5). Bethesda, MD: U.S. Department of Health and Human Services, National Institutes of Health, and National Institute on Drug Abuse.

Szapocznik, J., & Kurtines, W. M. (1989). *Breakthroughs in family therapy with drug-abusing and problem youth.* New York: Springer.

Szapocznik, J., Schwartz, S. J., Muir, J. A., & Brown, C. H. (2012). Brief strategic family therapy: An intervention to reduce adolescent risk behavior. *Couple and Family Psychology, 1*(2), 134–145.

Taffel, R., & Blau, M. (2001). *The second family: How adolescent power is challenging the American family.* New York: St. Martin's.

Talgam, I. (2015). *The ignorant maestro.* New York: Penguin.

Tatarsky, A. (2007). *Harm reduction psychotherapy: A new treatment for drug and alcohol problems.* Lanham, MD: Rowman & Littlefield.

Tetlock, P., & Gardner, D. (2015). *Superforecasting: The art and science of prediction.* New York: Crown.

Tomm, K. (1987). Interventive interviewing: Part II. Reflexive questioning as a means to enable self-healing. *Family Process, 26*(1), 167–183.

Tomm, K., St. George, S., Wulff, D., & Strong, T. (Eds.). (2014). *Patterns in interpersonal interactions: Inviting relational understandings for therapeutic change.* New York: Routledge.

Tormala, Z. L., Jia, J. S., & Norton, M. I. (2012). The preference for potential. *Journal of Personality and Social Psychology, 103*(4), 567–53.

Tryon, G. S., & Winograd, G. (2011). Goal consensus and collaboration. In J. C. Norcross (Ed.), *Psychotherapy relationships that work: Evidence-based responsiveness* (2nd ed., pp. 153–168). New York: Oxford University Press.

Tugade, M. M., Shiota, M. N., & Keirby, L. D. (Eds.). (2014). *Handbook of positive psychology.* New York: Guilford Press.

Turkle, S. (2011). *Alone together: Why we expect more from technology and less from each other.* New York: Basic Books.

Turkle, S. (2015). *Reclaiming conversation: The power of talk in a digital age.* New York: Penguin.

Tyler, R. (2015). *Jolt: Shake up your thinking and upgrade your impact for extraordinary success.* Chichester, UK: Capstone.

van der Kolk, B. A. (2014). *The body keeps the score: Brain, mind, and body in the healing of trauma.* New York: Viking.

van der Kolk, B. A., McFarlane, A. C., & Weisaeth, L. (Eds.). (2007). *Traumatic stress: The effects of overwhelming experience on mind, body, and society.* New York: Guilford Press.

Velasquez, M. M., Crouch, C., Stephens, N. S., & DiClemente, C. C. (2016). *Group treatment for substance abuse: A stages-of-change therapy manual* (2nd ed.). New York: Guilford Press.

Waldron, H. B., & Brody, J. L. (2010). Functional family therapy for adolescent substance use disorders. In J. R. Weisz & A. E. Kazdin (Eds.), *Evidence-based psychotherapies for children and adolescents* (pp. 401–416). New York: Guilford Press.

Wallerstein, J. S., Lewis, J. M., & Blakeslee, S. (2001). *The unexpected legacy of divorce: The 25 year landmark study.* New York: Hachette.

Watzlawick, P., Weakland, W. H., & Fisch, R. (1974). *Change: Principles of problem formation and problem resolution.* New York: Norton.

Weeks, G. (Ed.). (1991). *Promoting change through paradoxical therapy* (rev. ed.). New York: Brunner/Mazel.

Weeks, G., & L'Abate, L. (1982). *Paradoxical psychotherapy: Theory and practice with individuals, couples, and families.* New York: Brunner/Mazel.

Weersing, V. R., & Brent, D. A. (2010). Treating depression in adolescents using individual cognitive-behavioral therapy. In J. R. Weisz & A. E. Kazdin (Eds.), *Evidence-based psychotherapies for children and adolescents* (pp. 126–140). New York: Guilford Press.

Weiner-Davis, M., de Shazer, S., & Gingerich, W. (1987). Building on pretreatment change to construct the therapeutic solution: An exploratory study. *Journal of Marital and Family Therapy, 13*(4), 359–363.

Weintraub, P. (2015). The voice of reason. *Psychology Today, 48*(3), 50–59, 88.

Weisbord, M., & Janoff, S. (2007). *Don't just do something stand there!: Ten principles for leading meetings that matter.* San Francisco: Berrett-Koehler.

Weisinger, H., & Pawliw-Fry, J. P. (2015). *Performing under pressure: The science of doing your best when it matters most.* New York: Crown Business.

Weiss, B., Han, S., Harris, V., Catron, T., Ngo, V. K., Caron, A., et al. (2013). An independent randomized trial of multisystemic therapy with non-court-ordered adolescents with serious conduct problems. *Journal of Consulting and Clinical Psychology, 81,* 1027–1039.

Welch, S. (2009). *10/10/10.* New York: Scribner.

Whitaker, C. (1989). *Midnight musings of a family therapist.* New York: Norton.

Whitaker, C., & Keith, D. V. (1981). Symbolic experiential family therapy. In A. Gurman & D. Kniskern (Eds.), *Handbook of family therapy* (pp. 187–225). New York: Brunner/Mazel.

White, M. (2007). *Maps of narrative practice.* New York: Norton.

White, M. (2011). *Narrative practice: Continuing the conversations.* New York: Norton.

White, M., & Epston, D. (1990). *Narrative means to therapeutic ends.* New York: Norton.

Willard, C., & Saltzman, A. (Eds.). (2015). *Teaching mindfulness skills to kids and teens.* New York: Guilford Press.

Williams, L., Patterson, J. E., & Edwards, T. (2014). Attitudes, skills, and knowledge: The ingredients to becoming a research-informed clinician. *Family Therapy Magazine, 13*(5), 24–28.

Wilson, K., & DuFrene, T. (2012). *The wisdom to know the difference: An acceptance and commitment therapy workbook for overcoming substance abuse.* Oakland, CA: New Harbinger.

Wittgenstein, L. (1953). *Philosophical investigations.* New York: Macmillan.

Zeig, J. K. (1980). *A teaching seminar with Milton H. Erickson.* New York: Brunner/Mazel.

Zhu, R., & Argo, J. J. (2013). Exploring the impact of various seating arrangements on persuasion. *Journal of Consumer Research, 40*(2), 336–349.

Index

Parents. *See also* Parenting strategies
  collaborative team meetings and, 101–102
  engaging powerful reluctant adolescents and,
    36
  engaging reluctant fathers and, 45–49
  intervention development and, 112–118
  lack of consensus among regarding treatment
    goals, 91–95
  parental unity and teamwork and, 151–152
  problem-determined systems and, 8
  resolving long-standing conflicts and, 60–64
  treatment goals and, 83–95
Passions, 112–113, 130–131
Pathway thinking, 139
Pattern intervention strategies, 159–160. *See also*
  Systemic approaches
Pattern recognition, 13
Peer relationships, 4, 39–40, 172–173, 264–265
Percentage questions, 100–101. *See also*
  Questioning
Perceptual ability, 270–271
Perspective changing, 116
Perspective-taking skill, 129. *See also* Social skills
  training
Persuadability, 68–69
Pessimism, 87–91
Pessimistic questions, 89. *See also* Questioning
Photography therapeutic experiments. *See* Art
  and photography therapeutic experiments
Playfulness, 44–45, 51, 115–116, 276–278
Popcorn meditation, 120–121. *See also*
  Mindfulness meditation
Positive consequences, 144. *See also* Parenting
  strategies
Positive moods photography album activity,
  137–138. *See also* Art and photography
  therapeutic experiments
Positive regard, 26, 28
Positivity, 67–68
Possibility scenario planning, 72–73, 75
Post hoc, ergo propter hoc, 246
Postmodern systemic therapy models, 16, 23
Power, 58–59
Precontemplative stage of change, 31–32, 250,
  260–261, 262. *See also* Stages-of-change
  model
Predictive bias, 245–246. *See also* Biases
Premature termination, 53–54. *See also* Dropping
  out of treatment; Termination
Preparation stage of change, 33, 262. *See also*
  Stages-of-change model
Presenting ideas, 70–71
Presenting problems, 21–22
Presuppositional questions, 80–81. *See also*
  Questioning
Pretend the miracle happened experiment,
  148–149. *See also* Parenting strategies
Pretreatment change, 20–22, 112–113
Problem comebacks, 170–171
Problem focus, 249
Problem-determined systems, 7–8
Problem-solving strategies, 96, 112–113, 119–120.
  See also Self-generated solution strategies;
  Solution strategies
Propelling questions, 102. *See also* Questioning

Psychological reactance levels, 34
Purpose in life, 49, 129–131. *See also* Intervention
  development and selection

Question storming, 116, 117–118. *See also*
  Questioning
Questioning
  collaboration and, 21–22, 24, 69–70
  engaging powerful reluctant adolescents and,
    44
  relapse prevention and, 164–166
  solution strategies development and, 116–118
  team meetings and, 100–101, 102
  therapeutic artistry and, 272, 286, 290–292
  treatment goals and, 78–83, 87, 89–91, 92,
    164–166
  treatment mistakes and failures and, 253, 256

Reactivity, 34
Readiness for change, 30–33, 262–263. *See also*
  Change; Stages-of-change model
Reasonable man or woman bias, 246. *See also*
  Biases
Referral process, 184–185, 208–209
Referring persons, 94–95
Reflecting team consultation method, 176–177
Reflection-in-action, 14–15, 253–254
Reflection-on-action, 14–15, 253–254
Reframing, 49, 51–52
Relapse prevention
  action steps planning, 168
  case illustration of a high-risk suicidal
    adolescent, 228–230, 231–233
  case illustration of a violent adolescent, 201,
    202, 203–204
  collaborative strengths-based family therapy
    (CSBFT) model and, 24
  consolidating gains and amplifying changes
    and, 164–166
  family–social network and, 163–164
  high slip rates and prolonged relapsing
    periods and, 175–181
  mindfulness regarding impending slips and,
    174–175
  positive slip prevention management skills and
    strategies, 168
  solution-oriented behavioral rehearsing and,
    168
  tools and strategies for, 169–174
  treatment mistakes and failures and, 265–266
  triggers and, 166–167
  worst-case scenarios and, 168
Relationships, 39–40. *See also* Peer relationships;
  Therapeutic relationship
Reluctance, 34–45
Representative bias, 240–241. *See also* Biases
Residental treatment, 7, 221–225
Resiliency, 143–144
Resourcefulness, 112–113
Resources, 67–68
Respectful curiosity. *See* Curiosity
Retention strategies
  engaging powerful reluctant adolescents and,
    43–45
  engaging reluctant fathers and, 48–49